THE Y PLAN
COUNTDOWN

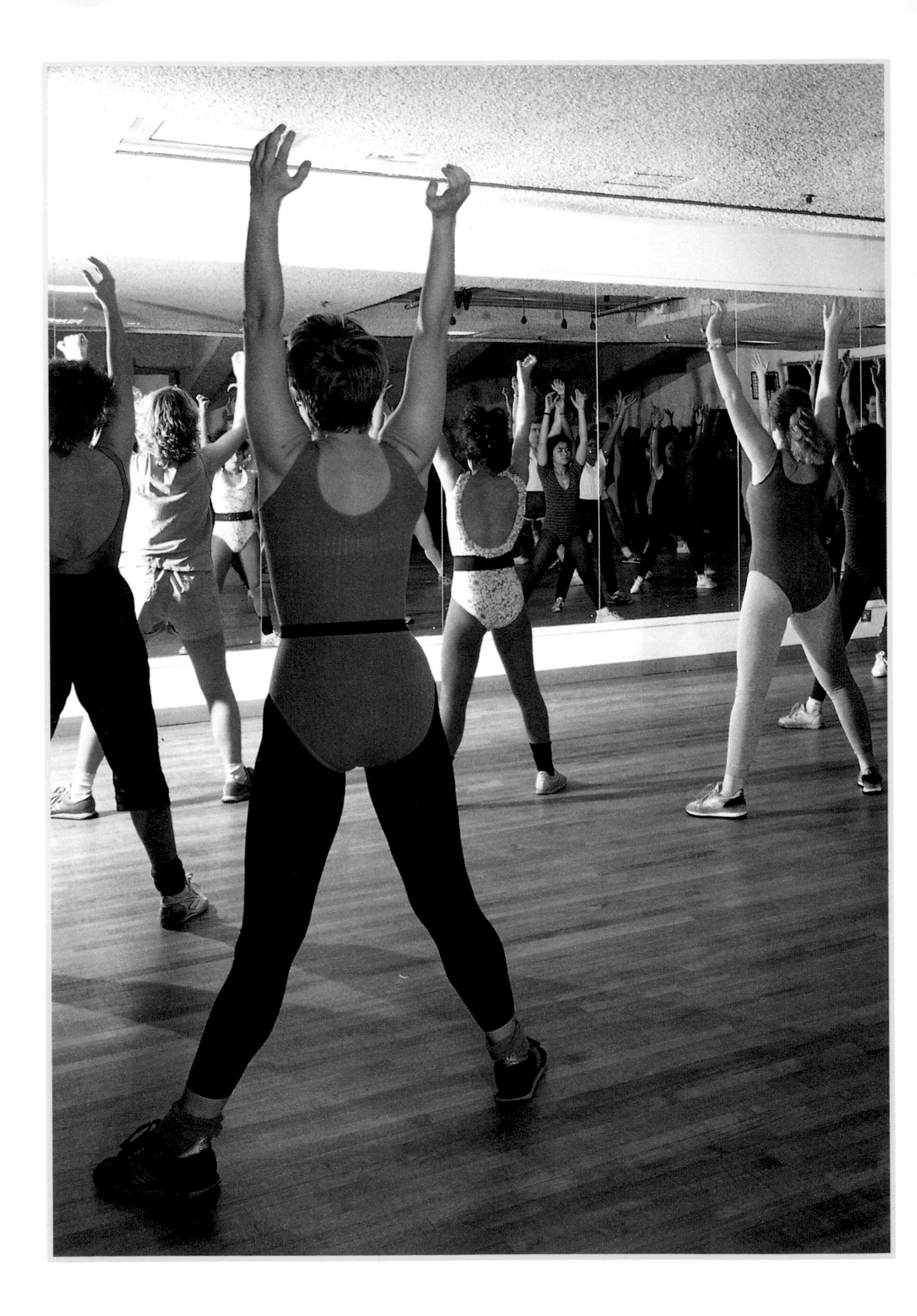

THE Y PLAN COUNTDOWN

A GREAT NEW SHAPE IN 36 DAYS

LESLEY MOWBRAY
AND
JILL GASKELL

HAMLYN

LESLEY MOWBRAY, Director of Training and Development, London Central YMCA, is the leading figure in Britain in health related fitness teacher training. Having graduated in Art and Science of Movement from Dartford College in Kent in 1973, she pioneered the training of exercise to music teachers and was co-author of the English YMCA Guide to Exercise to Music. She has been instrumental in setting up a nationally independent validation scheme for the qualifying of Exercise To Music teachers.

Following on from this she lead her department into a whole range of Health Related Fitness Training Courses, fitness, 501, Ante and PostNatal etc. She is the co-author and co-founder of the Y Plan home exercise series which has produced to date two books and three videos.

JILL GASKELL, Development Director Training and Development, London Central YMCA, graduated in Sports Science and Physical Education from Loughborough University. She has a special interest and expertise in the teaching of Ante and Post-Natal exercise, particularly in the development of exercise opportunities for pregnant mothers. She is co-author and co-founder of the Y Plan home exercise series, and presenter of all the Y Plan exercise videos.

She has made numerous appearances on television and radio and gives lectures, workshops and seminars on health related fitness to exercise teachers as well as to other health professionals throughout Britain.

ACKNOWLEDGEMENTS

We would like to extend a big thank you to all our colleagues in Training and Development Department at London Central YMCA, especially Maria and Ruth, for their support and help during the intensive weeks of writing this book and to Dr Craig Sharp, former director of the British Olympic Medical Centre for his continuing support and encouragement throughout the Y Plan series.

We would also like to make acknowledgements to Rodney Cullum, Operations Director London Central YMCA and William Campbell, Managing Director Lifetime Vision, for making this book possible; and to Anthea Turner, Chris Smith and Sue Atu for their help with the photographs for this book.

Finally we would like to say a big thank you to our husbands, for putting up with us during the writing and for their support, assistance and encouragement throughout.

Available from MCEG Virgin Vision

THE Y PLAN COUNTDOWN VIDEO

from all good high street video stockists.

Published in 1992
by Octopus Illustrated Publishing
part of Reed International Books Limited
Michelin House, 81 Fulham Road, London SW3 6RB

Hamlyn is an imprint of Octopus Illustrated Publishing

ISBN 0 600 57509 8

A catalogue record for this book is available from the British Library

Printed in Great Britain by The Bath Press, Avon

Contents

Foreword

Many people and institutions have, over the past decade, claimed to be expert in the field of physical activity, exercise and health. Few have produced programmes in which the individual can help themselves, at their own pace and level, to achieve and maintain a healthy way of life. Only the YMCA Training and Development Department have trained individuals and also 'the trainers' of individuals in safe and effective exercise to such a high and respected level.

They are held in the highest regard both nationally and internationally for the expertise and experience that they have accumulated and passed on, so successfully, to others.

All of this experience has been put together into the 'Y Plan' series. It deals with fitness facts, not fads that quickly lose their appeal and effectiveness. They have tried to get away from exercise being seen as a fad, fashion or a chore. All too often, people find that other exercise programmes are not all that they claim to be or that they are too difficult and far too time consuming. Rather than motivating you to be more active, they in actual fact put many people off continuing and stop others from starting.

The 'Y Plan' does not promise miracle results in days. What it does offer is a ***safe***, ***effective*** and ***progressive*** programme, that encourages participants, at whatever level, to monitor their progress and learn and understand more about their fitness and condition.

This philosophy of catering for the individual and ensuring that an activities are both safe and effective are the keys to success of any exercise programme. Long may the YMCA continue to follow and communicate this formula.

Peter Gardonyi,
Activity and Health Officer,
Health Education Authority.

Introduction

What is the YMCA?

The London Central YMCA is an international and charitable organization whose purpose is the development of mind, body and spirit for individuals of all ages and backgrounds. It has been at the forefront of keeping people fit and healthy since 1844.

This philosophy, combined with a clearly identified need in the community for well-trained teachers of health-related exercise, led to the development of the London Central YMCA's nationally recognized training courses in the teaching of exercise and exercise to music. The Training and Development Department is the premier health and fitness teacher-training organization in the country and has taught over 5,000 exercise teachers.

Y trained teachers are running classes all over the country and establishing high standards in teaching safe and effective exercise. However, the percentage of the population who actively attend fitness classes is very low. The national fitness survey published in the spring of 1992 has highlighted the nation's tremendous lack of fitness and absence of participation in any type of 'active' physical exercise. Therefore, we feel it is important to make the principles of the YMCA fitness programmes more readily available to people who perhaps do not have the time or confidence to go out and attend exercise classes.

With the support and guidance of Dr Craig Sharp we launched the Y Plan series. Dr Sharp, former Senior Lecturer at Birmingham University for 20 years and former Director of the British Olympic Medical Centre for five years, continues to be our consultant and a leading figure in the field of fitness and fitness testing.

What is the Y Plan?

The Y Plan series of exercise books and videos was launched in March 1990. It was devised by the London Central YMCA's most experienced fitness teachers and widely based on the most up-to-date Sports Science research. The YMCA's aim was to produce a series of well-researched exercise programmes for anyone to perform in the comfort of his or her own home.

The Y Plan programmes are proving to be overwhelmingly successful, with the original Y Plan continuing to be one of the top-selling exercise programmes.

Y PLAN

The first in the series called, 'The Y Plan', is a joint book and exercise video which has formed a base for further exercise books and videos. With clear guidelines for the participants on which level to start, the Y Plan progresses through four colour-coded levels of difficulty and at each level there is a toning programme and an aerobic programme. These programmes are only 12 minutes long. The programmes are each performed twice a week, the toning programme firming and shaping the body's muscles, the aerobic programme keeping the heart and lungs fit and strong. The Y Plan is safe, effective and fun, and because it requires only 12 minutes of exercise every other day it can easily be incorporated into a daily routine.

Y Plan Countdown

The Y Plan 36 Day Countdown was developed from the feedback from the original Y Plan. The video of the Countdown has been in the Top 10 since its release in March 1991. The same scientifically approved principles have been followed and similar professional advice sought, with the aim of providing a programme to tone up and shape the body of both the avid Y Plan follower and the 'couch potato'. The Countdown is a progressive programme with three colour-coded levels. At each level there are two workouts, one targeting the muscles of the hips and thighs and the other the bums, tums and arms. These workouts are performed alternately for six days of the week.

This Countdown book is an adapted version of the Countdown video with additional in-depth information about the body and safe exercise. It allows the participant to do a workout at any time and in any place, with the added advantage of moving at his or her own pace rather than at the pace dictated by the music as in the video.

Y Plan Before and After Pregnancy

The Y Plan Before and After Pregnancy is the third exercise video in the Y Plan range. The YMCA has devised and runs the only nationally recognized training programme for the specialist teaching of ante- and post-natal exercise in the country. The course has the approval of The Association of Chartered Physiotherapists specialising in Obstetrics and Gynaecology (ACPOG) and The Royal College of Midwives (RCM).

This unique YMCA exercise to music programme on video, which was devised in close consultation with health professionals, allows pregnant women who have not necessarily exercised before to exercise safely throughout all stages of pregnancy and the post-natal period.

Sue, Chris, Anthea and Jill - The Y Plan team.

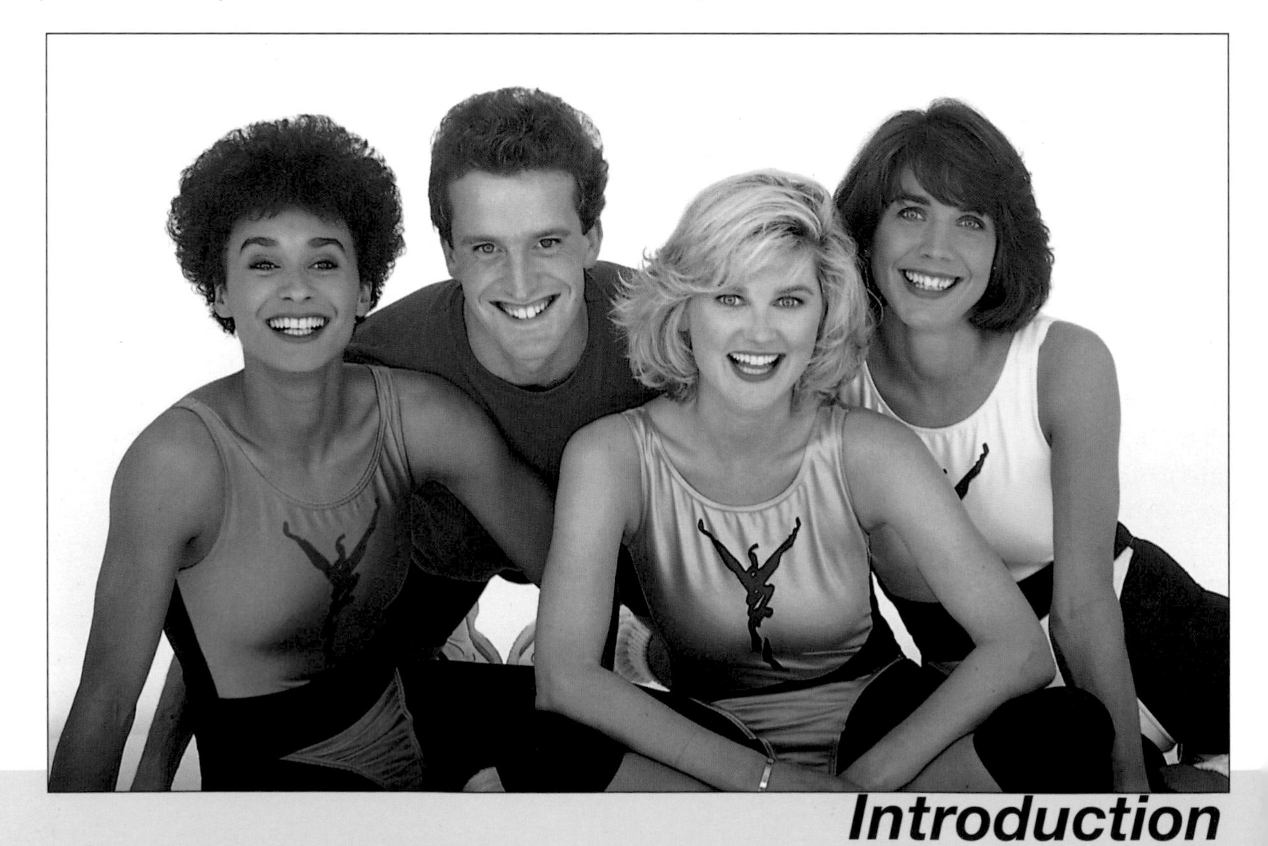

Why Countdown?

In Search of Something

What affects everyone? What are most people concerned about? Is it how their body functions? Is it how they look? Some people will tell you the body is not as important as the mind – the body just needs to be in good working order to get them from A to B. On the other hand, others place more importance on how they look even to the detriment of how the body functions. Let's face it, if we are looking good we often feel good. All members of the 'Y' team involved with developing the Y Plan aim to provide a range of exercise programmes that will keep the 'whole body' active, healthy and fit from birth to grave and we do realize that inextricably linked with this aim is the necessity to help people look trim, slim and make them feel good about themselves, so that they can take charge of their whole lifestyle.

Why the Countdown?

There are many different ways of exercising and different benefits to be gained from it. The Y Plan Countdown was developed because we identified a particular need. A large proportion of people we came in contact with were so concerned about changing their body shape that they would spend endless amounts of time and money on the latest exercise fads and diets. Unfortunately, too often the outcome was failure because they either set themselves unrealistic targets or followed programmes or advice that was technically unsound.

The Countdown, therefore, is an exercise programme that concentrates predominantly on improving body shape and tone. We have carefully selected toning exercises that blitz the major muscles of the whole body. We have paid particular attention to common areas of the body that people usually need to slim and trim; hips and thighs; tums, bums and arms.

Because we are particularly experienced in teaching exercise and are familiar with the current scientific knowledge and exercise principles, the Countdown programme provides the best results in the shortest possible time while ensuring complete safety to the body structure.

The 36 Day Countdown consists of an optimum 12-minute daily toning programme, with one day a week rest, consisting of three levels. This makes Countdown accessible to both men and women of all ages and stages of fitness who have a limited amount of time available for achieving a firmer, shapelier body for a special event such as skiing or a summer holiday, or a wedding day.

The Countdown toning programme will succeed, provided that care is taken to do the exercises properly and consistently.

Once you have completed the 36 Day Countdown programme, working gradually through the levels, you will wish to maintain your newly toned and shaped body. This can be achieved by moving on to our specially designed 14-minute Supertone maintenance programme.

Countdown Video Feedback

One of the problems of home exercise is deciding between the many programmes on offer on the shelf. How can you judge which programme is going to suit your needs, be safe and do the job it claims it will do?

To help you with this dilemma and substantiate the Countdown we thought we would draw on some feedback from the people who have been successfully following the Countdown video. We hope that their opinions and comments may help you to get the best from our programme.

The following comments are taken from the Countdown questionnaire and are just a few of the many responses we have had. They come from a wide range of people including a 14-year-old schoolgirl, a 55-year-old PA, students, housewives, secretaries, physiotherapists, shopkeepers, part-time models and even prison officers – but very, very few of them are men. We hope that this will change, as most male bodies are in need of toning too!

These are some of the comments:

Brilliant
Well presented, clear instructions
Easy to do – no extras
Exercise I did before put too much pressure on my back
I enjoyed it and it assisted me in losing 2½ stone
It's short but effective
Others have noticed a difference
Booklet invaluable
I like Jill Gaskell and the way she explains everything so plainly and makes this tape extremely easy to follow, even for a beginner
I like the way it took you in stages so you could build up slowly
Easy to follow, just long enough for home exercise
Jill is fun and explains everything very well
I feel my body shape has improved
I like the fact that it is suitable for all levels of fitness and not too easy
Doing the 12/14 minutes didn't bite into my already busy timetable
For the first time I am still doing the exercises 12 weeks later - a miracle I assure you

Countdown and Body Shape

BODY TYPE

Before you embark on any programme that you hope is going to give you a new body shape and tone, you must first be in possession of the full facts. It is no good expecting to acquire a certain body shape if it is is going to contradict your basic body type (known as somatotype). There are three main body types and we all fall roughly into one or other of them.

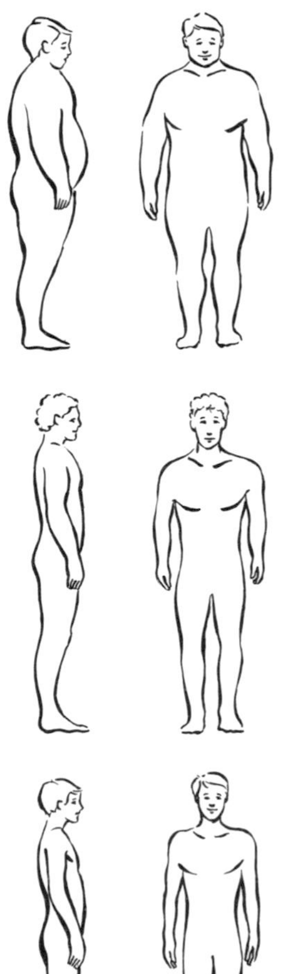

ENDOMORPHS *are pear-shaped, short and wide hipped, they tend to be rounded and gain weight*

MESOMORPHS *are triangular-shaped and quite muscley, with broad shoulders and narrow waist and hips.*

ECTOMORPHS *are long and lean, with little fat or muscle bulk.*

If you are born an 'endomorph', no amount of exercise or diets will turn you into an 'ectomorph'. However, all body types and shapes can be improved.

We all have fat stores, but the size of them and where they are proportioned are directly related to our body type. Obviously, ectomorphs, by eating large amounts and being inactive, may become fat. However, if they wish to reduce the amount of food they eat and take up exercise they always have the potential of returning to their natural body shape.

Endomorphs, however, should not lose heart, thinking they are a hopeless case, because although their body type means their shape is naturally more rounded, exercise combined with a sensible diet will develop muscle tone and a slimmer, trimmer, more pleasing figure.

BODY SHAPE AND DIET

If you do not control your eating, it is very easy to eat more calories than you use up and gradually there will be an increase in the fatty tissue deposited beneath your skin. The body has certain places where it stores most of its fat. In the case of women it is usually waist, hips and thighs and the backs of the arms, whereas with men, fat is stored predominantly around the abdomen. Everyone has his or her own problem area, where more fat gets stored in one particular place, creating unsightly bulges.

If you have developed excessive amounts of surplus body fat it is necessary to follow a strict, calorie-controlled diet in order to become slim again. However, if you only diet you may not be left with an attractive body. It is muscle which gives the body its natural form and muscle tissue wastes if the body is inactive. Therefore, you could be left with a slim body but saggy skin and flabby muscles. Diet plus exercise is the answer.

When you do diet, you should take care in your choice of regime. Weight should be lost gradually. Strict, unbalanced diets can have unnatural effects on the body. The body compensates for excessive eating habits by altering its metabolism; in excessive dieting it will soon learn to function on fewer calories. Therefore, each time you diet your body needs an even lower intake of calories before you will begin to see weight reduction. It gets more and more difficult to lose weight through diet alone. Consequently, exercise has a valuable role to play.

BODY SHAPE AND EXERCISE

To get rid of fatty tissue you must expend more calories than you ingest. By increasing activity you will speed up the weight loss still further. Programmed exercise also affects the body's muscle mass, which in turn affects the body's daily energy expenditure as fitter muscles tend to burn more calories than unfit muscles. It has also been discovered that if you diet continuously without exercising, the diet adds to the wasting of lean muscle tissue; when dieting stops the body compensates and takes up more fatty tissue. This reinforces the fact that any diet should always be accompanied by a safe, effective exercise programme such as the Y Plan series.

Most of us have modest amounts of surplus fat but have areas of the body where, with sensible eating and a bit of exercise, the muscles would tone up and immediately improve the look of the body. Some people are unhappy with their tummy and other areas such as thighs and the bum. Body shape is peculiar to each individual.

Those of you who have felt that dieting is easier than exercise, think again! Exercise can be fun and there are more chances of succeeding. Some diet programmes are successful when those following them have the required will-power and motivation to persevere.

Countdown consists of specially designed exercises to improve body shape by toning the muscles and developing their firmness. The exercises increase the circulation and blood supply to the working muscle and encourage growth of the muscle fibres. The greater blood supply and the development of the muscle fibres fill out the muscle, giving it better shape and tone. This can only be achieved and then maintained through regular exercise – 'use it or lose it' is the reality of good muscle tone.

If you do not exercise your muscles, whatever your age, they waste away. You may have had a limb put in plaster for several weeks and observed that, once the plaster was removed, the immobilized muscle was very much thinner than it had been before. Muscle, then, is vital for good body shape.

It is our belief that by prescribing an effective toning programme,such as Countdown, and by giving you some simple principles, we provide the opportunity to greatly improve your shape.

Exercise and Daily Living

Most people feel that their appearance is important, but just as vital is the effect that inactive muscle has on how the body functions. Weak muscles mean a lack of strength or stamina to perform daily tasks such as carrying shopping, walking up stairs and leisure activities.

Muscles are vital to keep the body upright as well as for movement. Poor tone in muscle means that the muscles do not have the ability to hold the bones in their proper place. Poor joint and bone alignment leads to aches and pains and, in many people, disabling back pain. All of this contributes to poor posture which is unattractive, makes the figure look overweight and accentuates the bulges.

Muscles are the powerhouse of the body. Weak muscles lead to inactivity and more inactivity leads to weaker muscles. It can become a vicious circle and the body is likely to become prone to injury and illness which, in turn, can not only affect what you look like but how you live and what you feel like. A body that is inactive and overweight will be a softer body to touch and a saggy body to look at. Physical ageing begins at 21, and an ageing body with poor muscle tone is not attractive to look at.

Exercise and Ageing

Those of you who think that exercise is only for the young, think again! Research shows that regular exercise can reduce and is some cases prevent the normal problems associated with ageing.

As we get older, we allow ourselves (and indeed society encourages us), to adopt a more sedentary lifestyle. We tend to accept a gradual increase in weight, a lack of flexibility, a reduction in strength and speed, and we may become prone to illness, aches and pains. In fact, these symptoms often have very little to do with the ageing process of the body but are actually attributable to inactivity. The Y Plan Countdown is a safe and progressive programme and if you work gradually through it there is no reason why it cannot take you successfully into your fifties!

Countdown and Fitness

By being conscientious and successfully completing the Countdown you will reap the rewards, both in how you feel and how you look. Your friends and family will see the difference too, and you will probably receive comments such as 'You've lost weight', 'You look good', and 'You look happy!'

Health and Fitness

You may look fit and healthy with Countdown, but is that enough? If you are going to get the most out of our exercise programme you need to put it into the context of the whole picture of fitness and health. Being fit is not the same as being healthy – the two are quite separate. Very fit athletes can be medically unhealthy and, on the other side of the coin, medically healthy non-athletes can be very unfit. However, the effect of fitness on health is becoming increasingly apparent. Increased physical activity cannot cure such illnesses as diabetes, emphysema and hypertension, and it cannot always prevent disease. However, studies on the general public have shown that people who are more active have a lower risk of heart attacks and have significant health benefits in a number of areas.

Benefits of Exercise

1 *It improves heart and lung health.*
2 *It assists appetite control.*
3 *It helps to reduce body fat.*
4 *It reduces blood fat and excessive cholesterol.*
5 *It helps lower blood pressure.*
6 *It maintains and increases bone density.*
7 *It can improve mood.*
8 *It reduces the impact of ageing.*

If you are going to capitalize on these benefits you must understand more about exercise and fitness. Total fitness includes many facets of our lifestyle, as shown in the chart below.

All of these aspects are important individually and collectively, as each will influence the other. Our experience and research tell us that physical fitness, with good nutrition and good health, can also improve our emotional and social well-being. In fact, it is a powerful medication to prolong an active and healthy life.

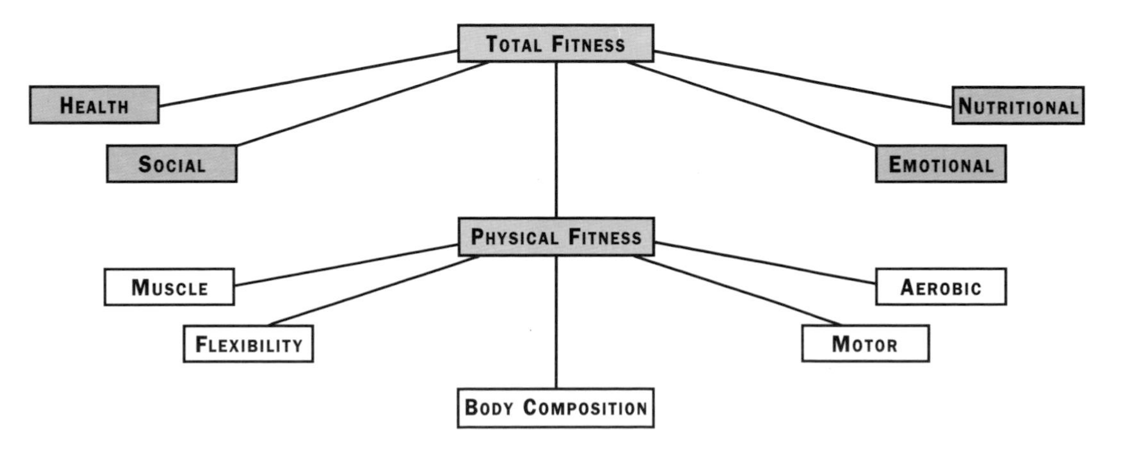

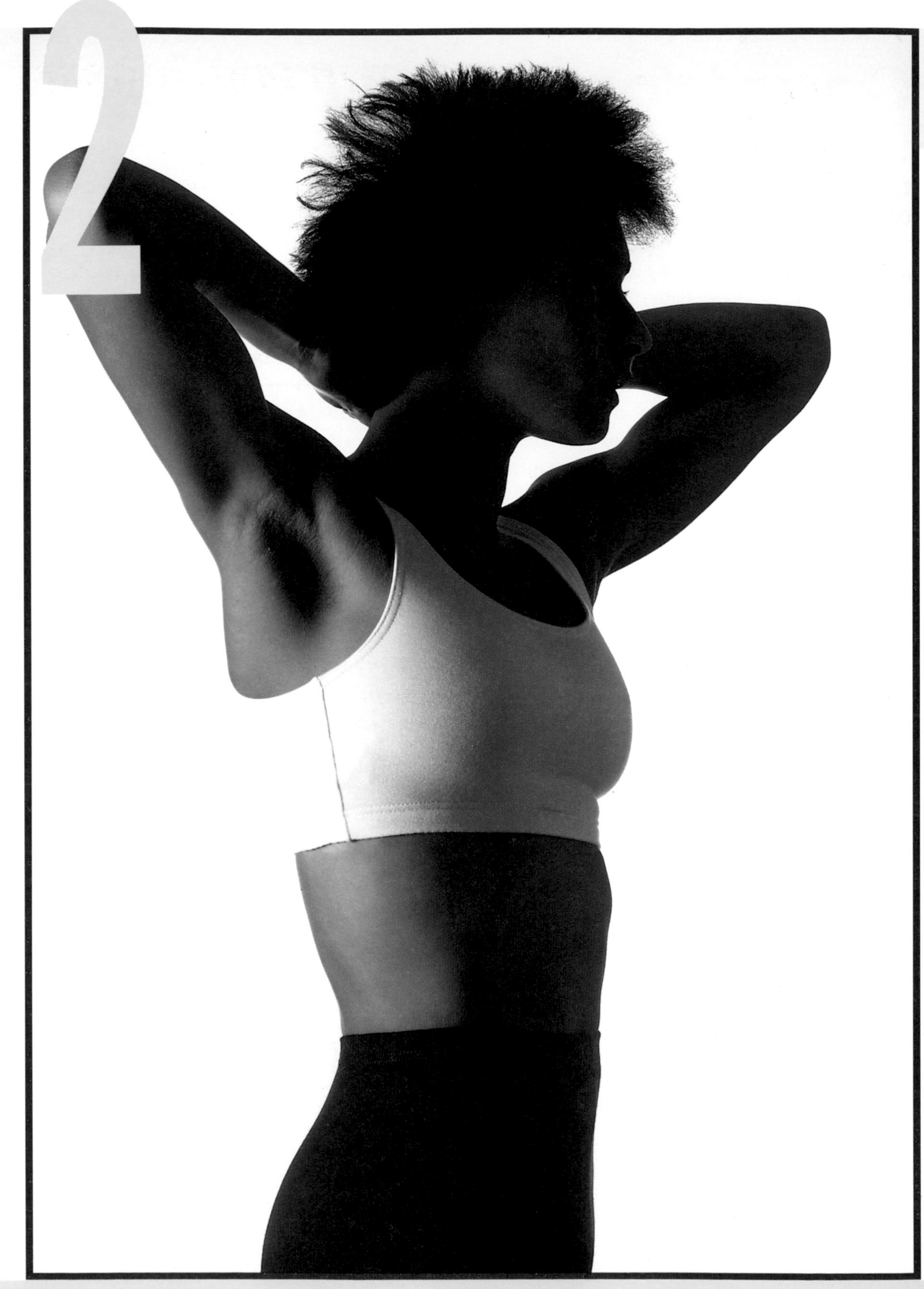
2

Countdown and Components of Physical Fitness

MUSCLE FITNESS

Y Plan Countdown as a toning programme is predominantly designed to develop this component of fitness. Muscle fitness can be broken down into two types, both vitally important.

Muscle strength refers to the ability to lift a heavy object or perform strenuous exercises. The heavier the object or the harder the exercise the stronger the muscle needs to be. A weight-trainer will become stronger by increasing the weight lifted. The Countdown exerciser will get stronger because the related exercises get progressively harder (see pictures below left).

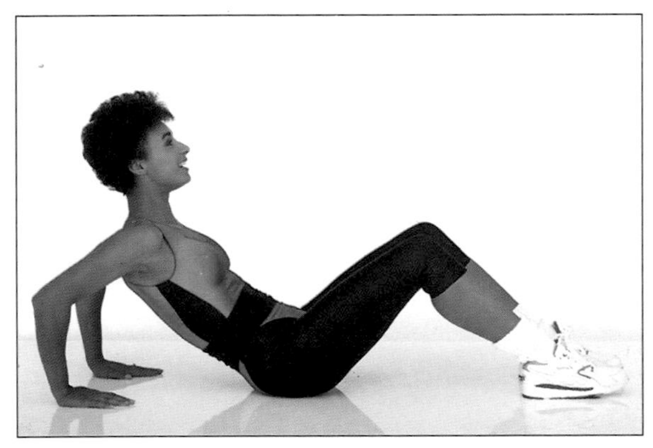

Above: *Seated Dips from Level 2.*
Below: *Dips from Level 3.*

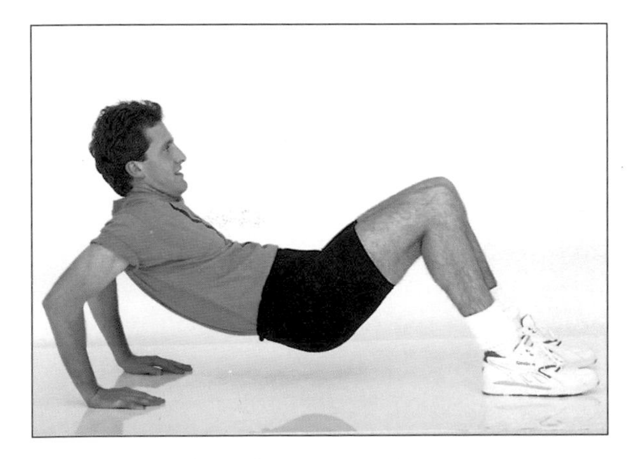

Muscle endurance refers to your ability to work for an extended period of time. The capacity of a muscle to continue carrying the object, or to repeat continuously an exercise, is developed in the Countdown exercise blocks by performing a high number of repetitions of a comparatively easy exercise (see pictures above).

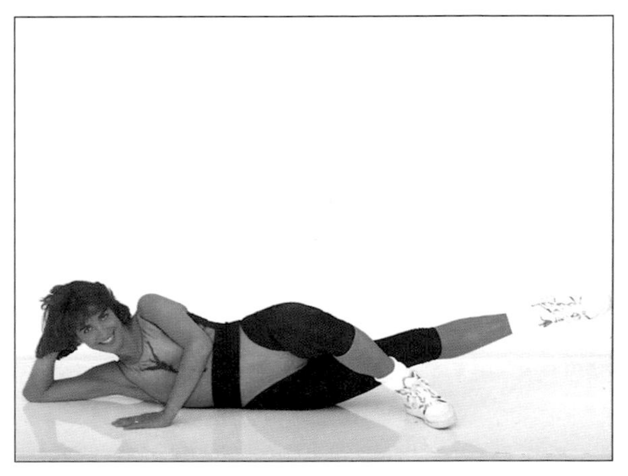

Above: *Lying Inner Thigh Raises Level 2 (2 x 12).*
Below: *Lying Inner Thigh Raises Level 3 (32 + 16).*

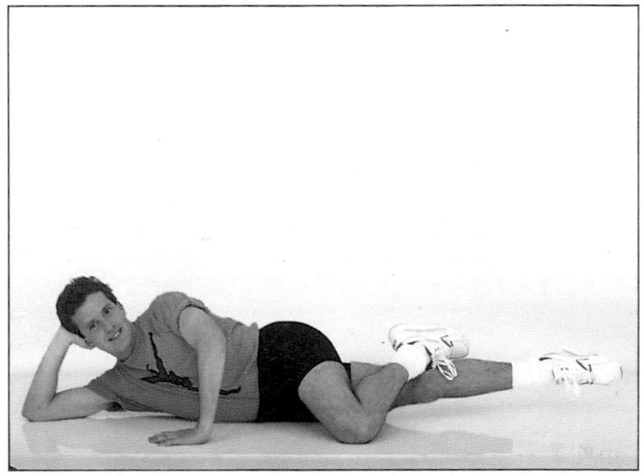

The development of strength and endurance in the muscles is usually related

– once you have gained the strength to perform an exercise correctly Countdown develops your endurance by increasing the number of times you do it.

FLEXIBILITY

This refers to the ability of your muscles and joints to move through a full range of movement. Flexibility or suppleness is developed by the stretching exercises in the warm-up and cool-down sections of the Countdown. It is very important, as a more supple body moves more freely and makes many daily tasks easier to perform. Physiotherapists use careful stretching exercises when trying to repair a muscle injury.

MOTOR FITNESS

Motor fitness is skill related fitness and it tends to be very specific to the type of exercise. It refers to body management (mind over muscle control), agility, balance, co-ordination. All Y Plan programmes, including the Countdown, are careful to include all of these skills in their exercise routines. We introduce motor skills gradually, making the exercises more taxing as you progress through the levels. Our opinion is that these trained skills are transferable to everyday life so they keep the body active and alert, willing and able to meet all kinds of challenges. An unfit, sluggish body will be lazy, unco-ordinated and inefficient, and in the long term will advance the negative aspects of ageing – for example, difficulty getting out of a chair, falling asleep regularly and so on.

BODY COMPOSITION

Body composition does not relate to a specific type of exercise as in the case of the other components of fitness but it may be significantly affected by all forms of activity. Body composition is the term used to describe the proportions of muscle, fat, bone and organs. Lean body weight refers to the weight of the muscle, bones, tissues and organs. Fat weight refers to the amount of total fat stored. Regular exercise increases lean body weight and decreases fat weight. The ratio between these two is associated with optimal fitness and health.

AEROBIC FITNESS

Aerobic fitness is sometimes referred to as stamina or endurance. It actually refers to the efficiency of the heart and lungs, which is fundamental to a well-functioning body; aerobic fitness forms the basis of overall fitness and brings about most of the health benefits. Aerobic fitness is achieved by sustained, moderate exercise that makes you breathe deeply, for example a brisk walk. The Countdown does not train aerobic fitness but the original Y Plan book and video do, so if you have the time mix and match your 'Y' Plan programmes. Otherwise, try to include a brisk walk, a cycle or a swim two or three times a week. All of these activities are good forms of aerobic exercise.

Muscle fitness, flexibility, motor fitness, body composition and aerobic fitness all have an impact on physical fitness and health. By understanding the difference between them you can now be more selective about the type of exercise you choose in order to achieve your aims. You can review your daily activities and try to get a balance by including something from all of the components of fitness in your weekly activity.

3 Countdown and Toning

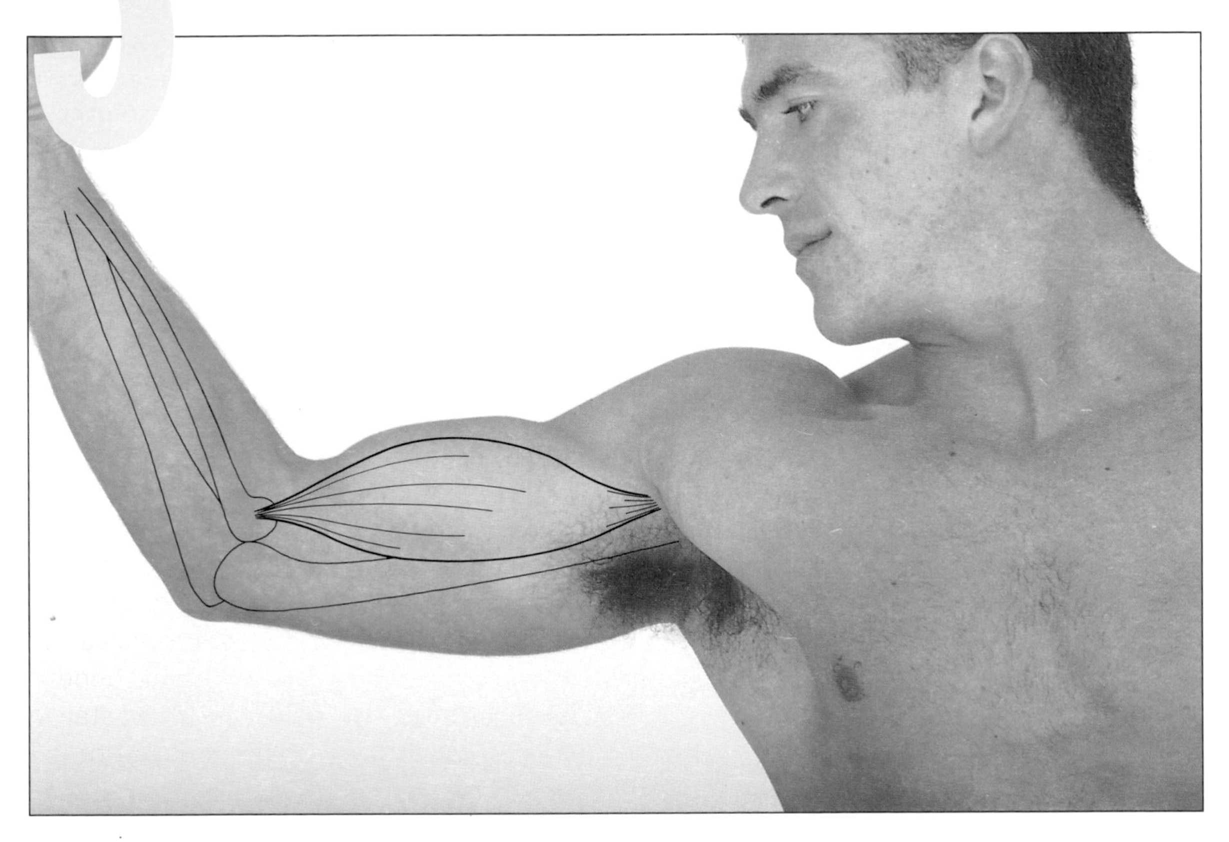

What is muscle tone?

All muscle, provided it is not injured or diseased, has a natural tone. Young muscle has a firm, elastic look and feel to it whereas older muscle, due to lack of use and training, tends to deteriorate and appear more flabby. The toned appearance is due to the condition of the muscles, the development of the actual muscle fibres and the circulation within the muscle itself.

All of these factors are improved by developing the strength and endurance of the muscles through exercise. The degree of natural muscle tone and the potential to develop it is very individual, being affected by factors within our genetic make-up (including levels of hormones) and social and cultural influences.

Toning Exercise

Muscles consist of bundles of long, narrow fibres held together by connective tissue. The ends of the muscle fibres form tendons which attach the muscle to the bone. Messages are sent from the brain to the muscle via nerves which signal the muscle fibres to shorten. Many muscle fibres receive these messages so the whole muscle shortens. Muscles cross joints and joints are the points at which two bones meet. To allow movement the joints can bend, straighten and even rotate, although the types of movement possible depends on the structure of the joint. The elbow for example is a single hinge joint (see above). When the arm muscle shortens it pulls on the two bones and produces movement.

3

Obviously the co-ordination of many different muscle actions together with varying amounts of contraction (shortening) and relaxing (lengthening) to bring about movement is very complicated. By understanding and applying this information we have been able to choose the most appropriate exercises for your Countdown programme making it totally safe and very effective.

Types of Toning Exercises

In order to improve your tone or muscle strength and endurance, what types of exercise do you need? Let us have to look again at how the muscle works. It can either work statically (known as an isometric contraction) or can shorten and lengthen as it works (isotonic contraction).

ISOMETRIC EXERCISES

Isometric exercises were introduced to the public in the 1950s by Charles Atlas and have regained popularity in the 1980s with Callanetics. This form of exercise does improve muscle tone but not to the extent often claimed and with some risk of injury.

An example of an isometric exercise with static muscle contraction would simply be to squeeze your elbows together while standing upright with your arms in front of you at shoulder height and your elbows bent so that your fists point up towards the ceiling (a static pec squeeze) .

To be effective the muscle contraction should be held for at least six seconds and then repeated several times if the tone of the specific muscles is to be improved. There are several limitations to this type of exercise, however. The first is the fact that the strength of the muscles is mainly improved in this position (the point at which the contraction is held) and in order to gain strength throughout the full range of movement the exercise would have to be repeated at various stages throughout the muscles' whole range of movement. The second, and even more significant, limitation of isometric exercise is the fact that a strong isometric contraction accelerates the pumping of blood from the heart while restricting blood flow back to the heart. After 10 seconds of holding an isometric contraction there begins a marked rise in blood pressure which is potentially very dangerous in certain people.

Isometric muscle contractions are, however, common in certain exercises and activities of everyday life. Muscles often have to work statically to support the body, for example when standing still, when sitting upright and when holding your tummy in for good posture. The difference between situations where isometric contractions are acceptable and where they are not, is to do with the effort or strength required to perform the exercise or task, together with the total amount of isometric exercise performed. In any exercise programme, some isometric contractions are inevitable. This holds true for the Countdown exercise programme, which even includes static contractions for the tummy muscles and the inner thighs. These are relevant and safe toning exercises because they are minimal, light and easy.

Exercise programmes, however, that are based totally on isometric contractions are not recommended because of the accumulative effect of the work involved. Some exercise programmes that are based on this type of muscle contraction adapt it slightly. Instead of holding the muscle completely still for a short time the exercise requires that the movement hovers around the fixed point

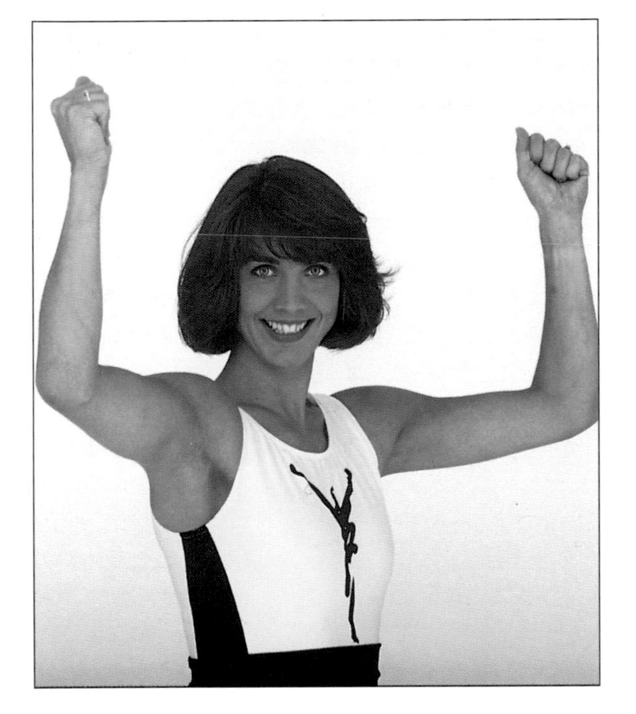

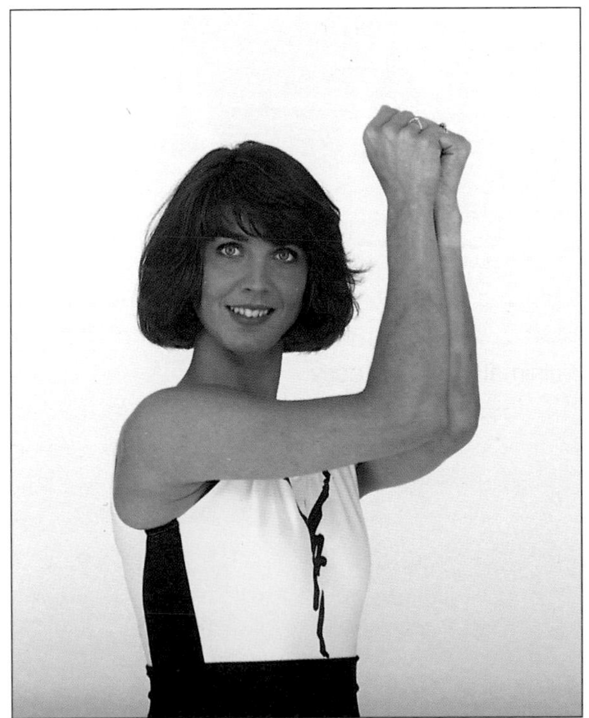

(moving about an inch either way) for an excessive number of times. Such a programme is obviously very repetitious and tedious. Moreover, by asking the body to perform 50 or 100 or more repetitions, the joints and muscles are put under unnecessary stress and over many months of exercising in this way, soft tissue injuries may be caused. These injuries can occur at any time, not necessarily during the exercise session and, therefore, they are not always seen as exercise-related injuries. Strong caution should be taken when offering such exercise programmes to the elderly, overweight or unfit.

ISOTONIC EXERCISES

We feel this form of exercise is more appropriate for general exercise programmes and therefore Countdown consists predominantly of isotonic exercises.

In isotonic exercise the muscle is strengthened throughout its natural range of movement as it lengthens and shortens during the contraction. If we return to the example of the pec squeeze, two movements are involved: first, the arms are opened to the side (see picture at top) and then they are closed again with a little squeeze of the elbows when they come together (see picture left).

Over the past few years there has been much research into strength training, leading to the development of sophisticated weight-training machines that alter the amount of weight according to the strength of your muscles. However, we do not need to concern ourselves with this detail of training. The Countdown programme is more than enough exercise for everyday living and to achieve good body shape and tone.

Countdown's Target Muscles

As we have previously explained, exercise is specific and therefore, to achieve a shapelier and toned body, it is necessary to exercise the particular muscles that affect the relevant areas. The following section explains these muscles in a little more detail.

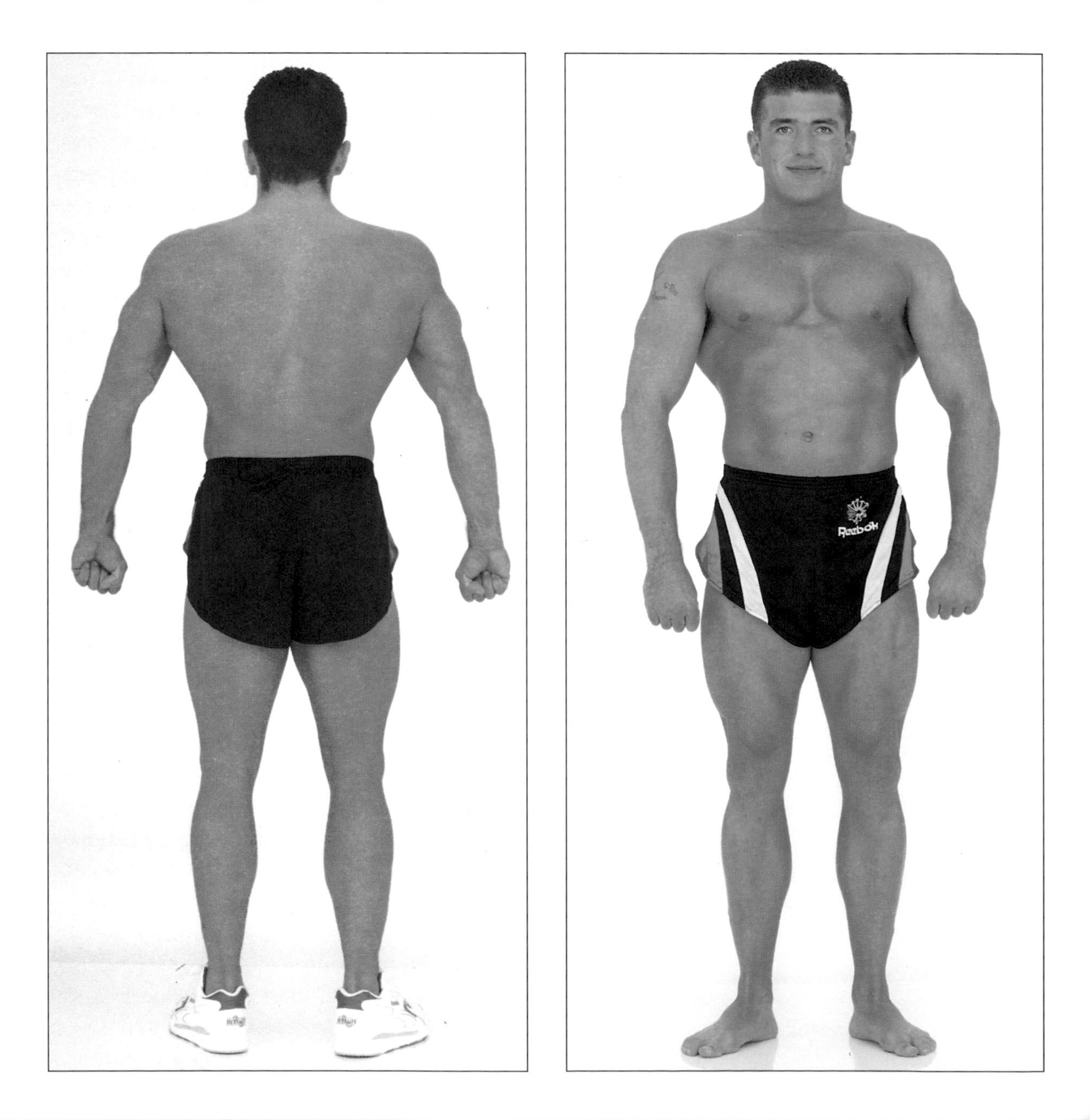

ABDUCTORS (HIPS AND OUTER THIGHS)

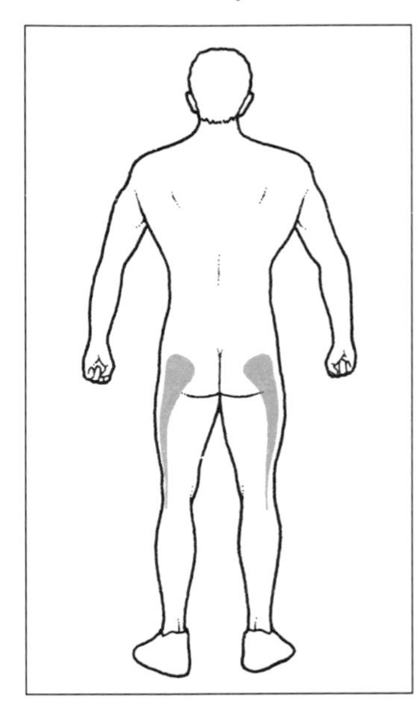

The abductors run down the side of the hip and thigh and are part of the group of muscles that form the buttocks. Keeping them toned helps to keep the hips trim and shapely. They play an important role in stabilizing the hips and protecting them from stresses and strains.

ADDUCTORS (INNER THIGHS)

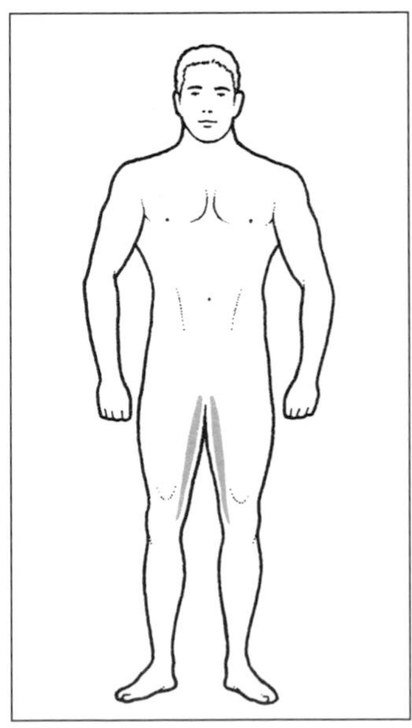

The adductors are attached to the pelvis and inside of the thigh. They are a difficult group of muscle to tone as the choice of suitable exercises is limited. Many women seem to suffer flabby inner thighs. Squeezing your legs together for a count of two (then relaxing) when standing still or squeezing your knees (for short periods) when sitting will provide extra toning for these muscles.

QUADRICEPS (FRONT OF THE THIGHS)

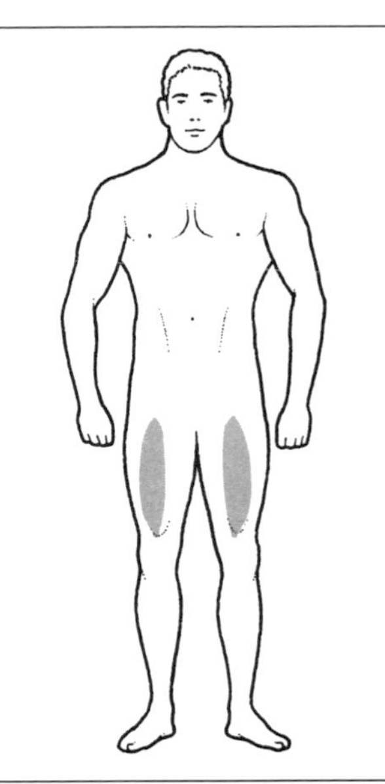

The quadriceps are attached to the front of the pelvis and the front of the leg just below the kneecap. These are large and powerful muscles. They are easily exercised in most day-to-day activity such as walking, climbing the stairs and so on. Strong quads are important for lowering and squatting and, along with correct technique, can protect the back from unnecessary injury during exercise. The thighs are not such a common fat store as the hips and tummy but they do need to be kept toned to maintain a good look and shape.

HAMSTRINGS (BACKS OF THE THIGHS)

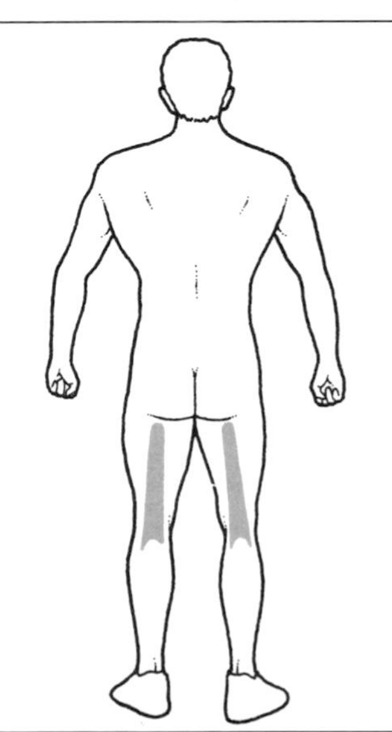

The hamstrings are attached to the back of the pelvis and the back of the leg just below the knee. These work in conjunction with the big, powerful quadriceps (front of thigh). When the quads contract the hamstrings relax and vice versa.

These muscles are often neglected in conditioning programmes, creating an imbalance between the two groups so the hamstrings are prone to injury. A particular problem with hamstrings is that they need to be frequently stretched to work efficiently and reduce the risk of injury. Tight hamstrings can lead to muscle tears, as is frequently the case for many athletes, although pulled hamstrings can just as easily happen in recreational activities with the family. The hamstrings are important postural muscles; lack of flexiblity here also pulls the vertebral column out of line, resulting in lower back pain and discomfort.

GLUTEALS (BUTTOCKS)

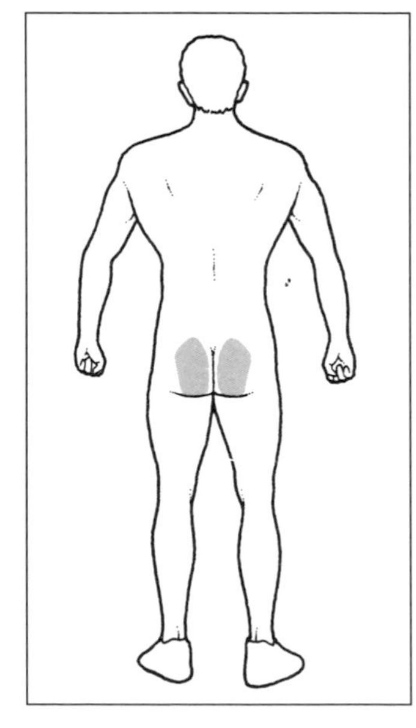

These muscles are large and rounded, although the male buttocks tend to be more angular and muscular. They are attached to the pelvis and to the outside of the top of the thigh bone. Toned, strong buttocks, apart from looking more attractive, help with posture and are powerful muscles that help us run and squat. They too protect the back in lowering and lifting activities. Unexercised buttocks tend to sag and flatten. Women tend to store fat particularly around the hips, forming a 'saddle' effect.

TRICEPS (BACK OF THE ARMS)

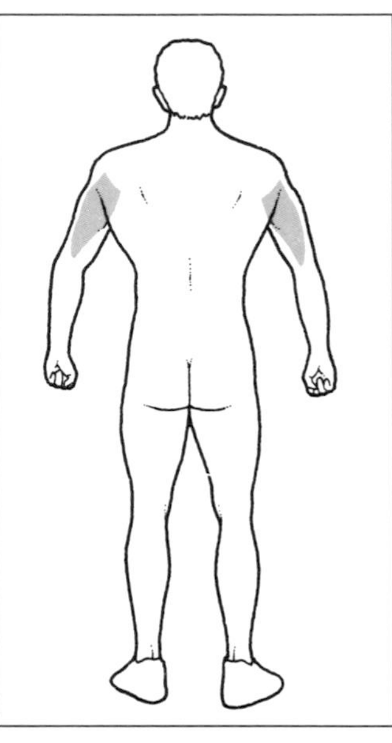

The triceps are attached to the shoulder and the arm, below the elbow. Women are traditionally weaker in their arms and upper body; they often find toning these areas hard work, and do not always recognize the same need to exercise them as they do the hips and thighs. However, the backs of the arms is another of the major fat stores for the female body. They should be kept exercised and toned to prevent the unsightly, flabby arms that are familiar in aging women. The press-up, a popular arm exercise, also works the chest muscles – an area of interest to many women!

PECTORALS (CHEST)

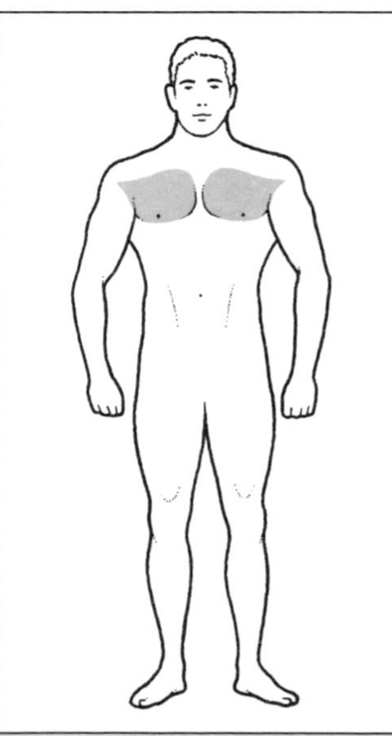

The chest muscles are broad, thick triangles attached to the bone down the middle of the chest (sternum) and the upper arm. Highly developed chest muscles, (pecs) are pursued by male body builders.

The breasts are attached to these muscles so well-toned pectorals will be of benefit to this area and help to prevent the breasts sagging. The size and shape of the breasts are very individual; diet and exercise can only improve them, not drastically alter them.

Today, more and more women resort to plastic surgery in pursuit of the perfect breast, but there is growing concern that some kinds of implants are causing cancer.

ABDOMINALS (TUMMY)

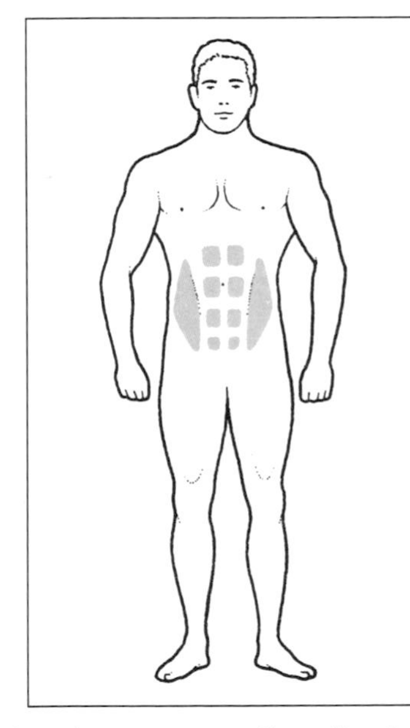

The abdominals are more often referred to as the tummy muscles. They consist of four muscles that run down and across the front of the abdomen and together form a sort of corset for the middle of the trunk. They play an important role in keeping all the vital inner organs in place, supporting the back and preventing back problems, and maintaining good posture. This corset of muscles is attached to the bottom front of the rib cage and the front of the pelvis Well-toned abdominals hold the tummy flat, which gives a more flattering outline. By constantly holding your tummy in during the day, whatever you may be doing, you will provide extra toning for these muscles.

This area of the body is susceptible to large fat stores especially in the male, forming the paunch but also bulbus layers of fat in women. Surplus fat in this area will put greater stress on the back and scientists have found a direct correlation between large waist measurements and heart attacks in men.

Toning and Progression

To strengthen a muscle we must apply sufficient force to create a resistance as the muscle contracts. In general, to progress with any exercise programme the level of exercise must create an extra demand on the body's systems usually known as overload. If the body's systems are overloaded its physiological make-up adapts to accommodate this extra exertion These adaptations are known as the training effect

Once the body adapts to the existing level of exercise, the latter should be increased to provide the overload necessary to continue the progression. This gradient of difficulty is very important because, if the exercise programme does not take into account different types of individuals and their varying levels of fitness, the level of overload could be too high for some and not high enough for others. This could result, at the worst, in injury and, at the least, in demotivating the exerciser.

Effective progressive improvement in training is related to the frequency, the intensity, the duration or time and the type of exercise. This is referred to as the principles of training and is often abbreviated to FITT.

***FREQUENCY* – HOW OFTEN TO EXERCISE**

In the case of the Y Plan Countdown, because we have chosen to get results as quickly as is feasibly possible, the programme was specifically designed to operate for six consecutive days for six weeks, with one day's rest each week. The design of the programme means that you exercise different muscle groups on alternate days – the hips and thighs on Mondays, Wednesdays and Fridays, and the tums, bums and arms on Tuesdays, Thursdays and Saturdays. This allows each muscle group that vital day for rest, recovery and adaptation between workouts

Allowing the muscles time to recover between workouts is very important; even serious weight trainers follow this principle of alternating muscle groups in successive workouts. It must be noted that in our opinion it is not possible to achieve the desired results from the Countdown in less than six weeks.

INTENSITY – HOW HARD TO EXERCISE

The Countdown toning programmes employ a commonly used technique of training known as 'sets' and 'reps'. This entails repeating a particular exercise a certain number of times until the muscle aches a little and needs a rest. This is known as a set of repetitions. After a short rest, the set of exercises for that particular muscle group is repeated. This process of working the muscle until it tires, resting and then working it again provides overload and induces the desired training effects

Determining how hard to exercise in order to achieve optimum results is a vital balancing act. When starting each set you should be able comfortably to perform the exercise prescribed and be able to maintain good technique throughout. As the muscles tire it becomes more difficult to maintain technique and as soon as this occurs you must rest. Countdown progresses the intensity through the levels in some cases by making the exercise harder and in other cases by increasing the number of repetitions (see below).

TIME – HOW LONG TO EXERCISE

The distinctive trademark of the 'Y' Plan is its 12-minute workout, which allows just enough time to get results without taking too much out of a busy schedule or getting bored.

TYPE – CHOICE OF EXERCISE

We have chosen exercise that concentrates on isolating the muscle group to be worked. We have worked the muscles predominantly isotonically, so they are being toned throughout their full range of movement.

In the different levels there is often a combination of exercises that work a specific

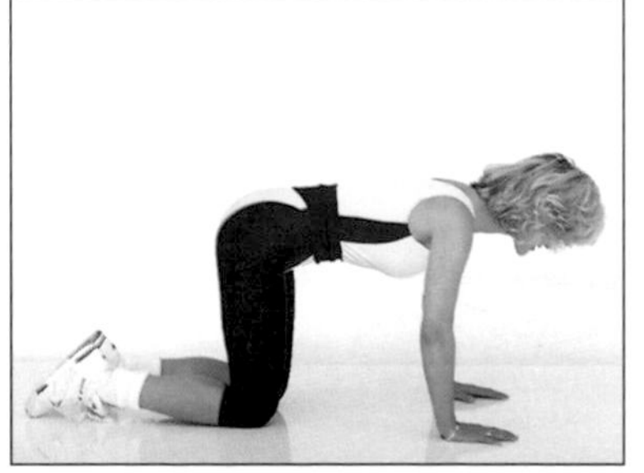

Box Press Up Level 1
Repetitions 2 x 8

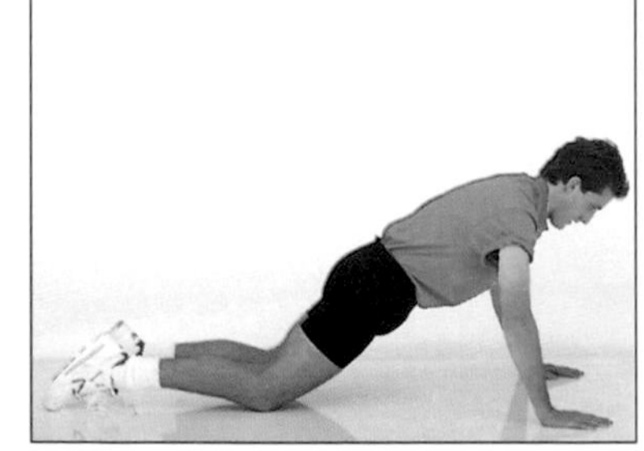

Three-Quarter Press Up Level 2
Repetitions 4 x 4

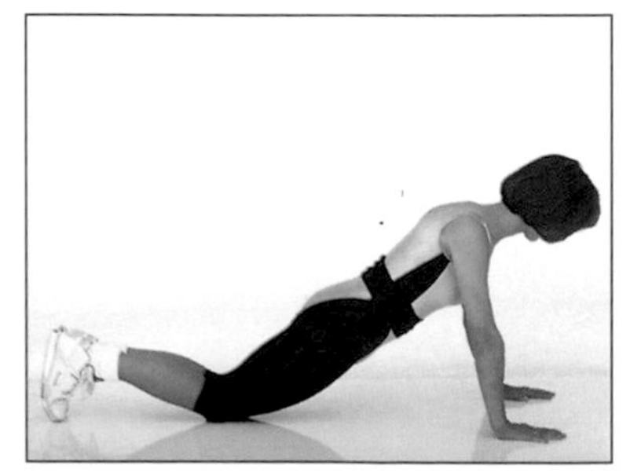

Three-Quarter Press Up Level 3
Repetitions 2 x 12

muscle group. This not only provides variety and maintains interest in the programme, it also develops the motor skill component of physical fitness (see below).

Every exercise programme should be governed by FITT. Through the levels of Countdown, the exercises become harder and build on the technique mastered in the previous level. The repetitions (and number of sets) may increase and speed may alter.

It is, therefore, vital to be clear about the technique of every exercise and the changes when moving on to a new level and new exercises. Any experienced exercise teacher will have the ability to use the formula FITT to plan a safe and effective exercise programme and provide alternatives should an exercise be uncomfortable.

Specificity

Any exercise programme is designed according to its particular requirements. Exercise is specific – for instance, if you want to develop specific muscle tone around your tum or chest there is little point in doing aerobic exercise such as walking. If you want to be good at running, there is little point in doing a lot of swimming.

Reversibility

It is worth noting here that toning effects are reversible. If you stop the exercise or the exercises are not frequent enough or hard enough, your gains will be lost. However, if you develop a high level of toning as in the 36 Day Countdown you can reduce your training levels to those given in the Supertone programme and still maintain what you have achieved.

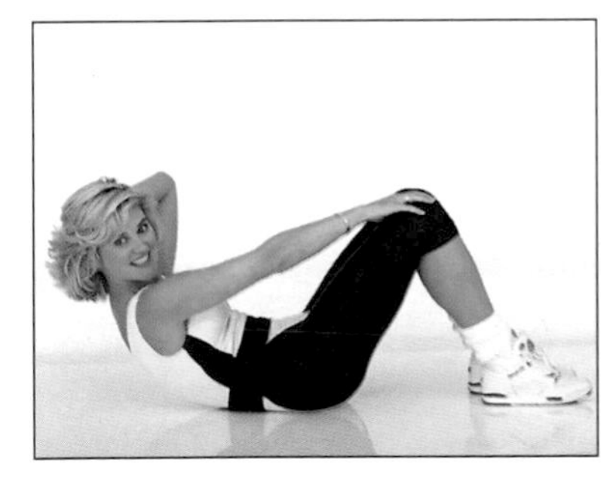

Above and below: *Level 1*

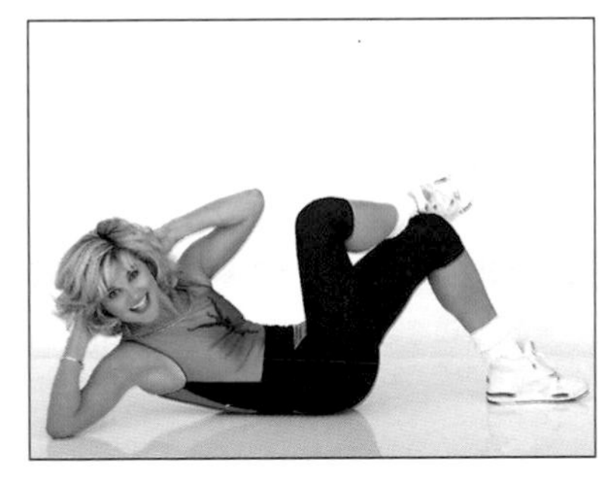

Above and below: *Level 2*

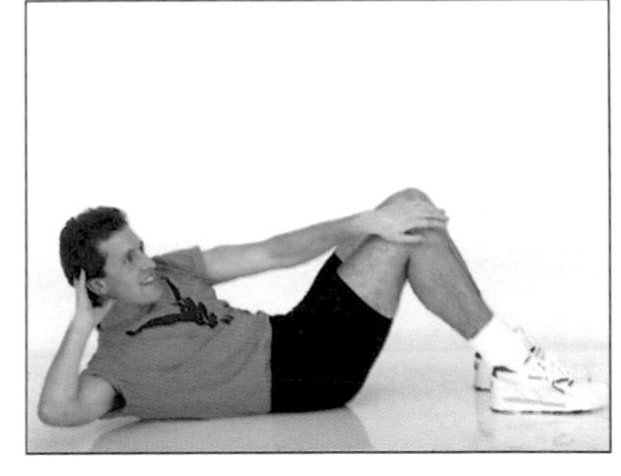

Above and below: *Level 3*

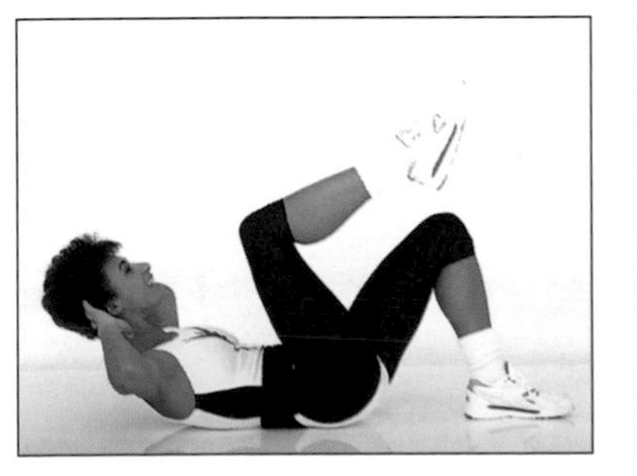

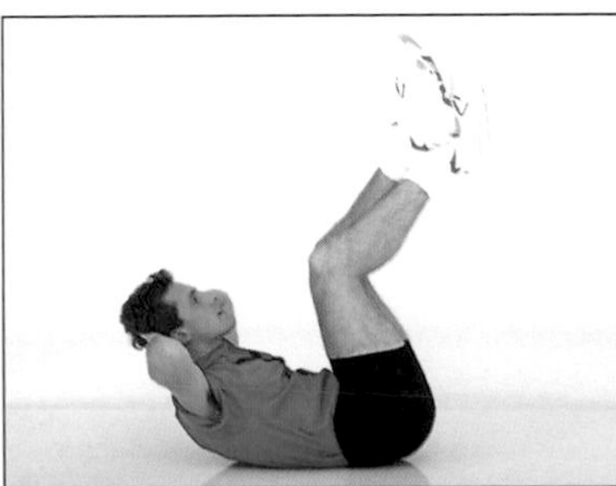

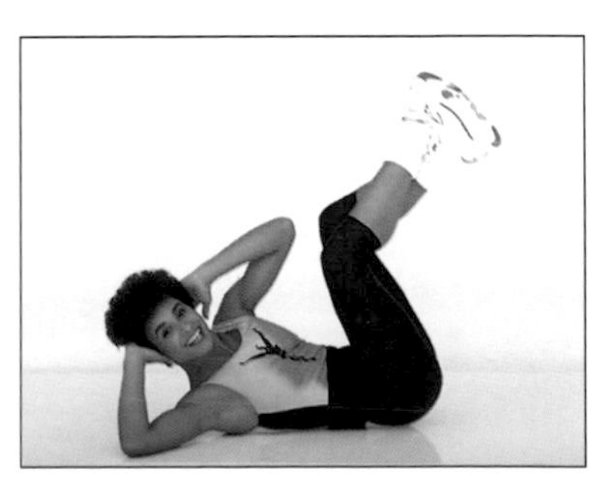

4 How Countdown Works

Diagram A

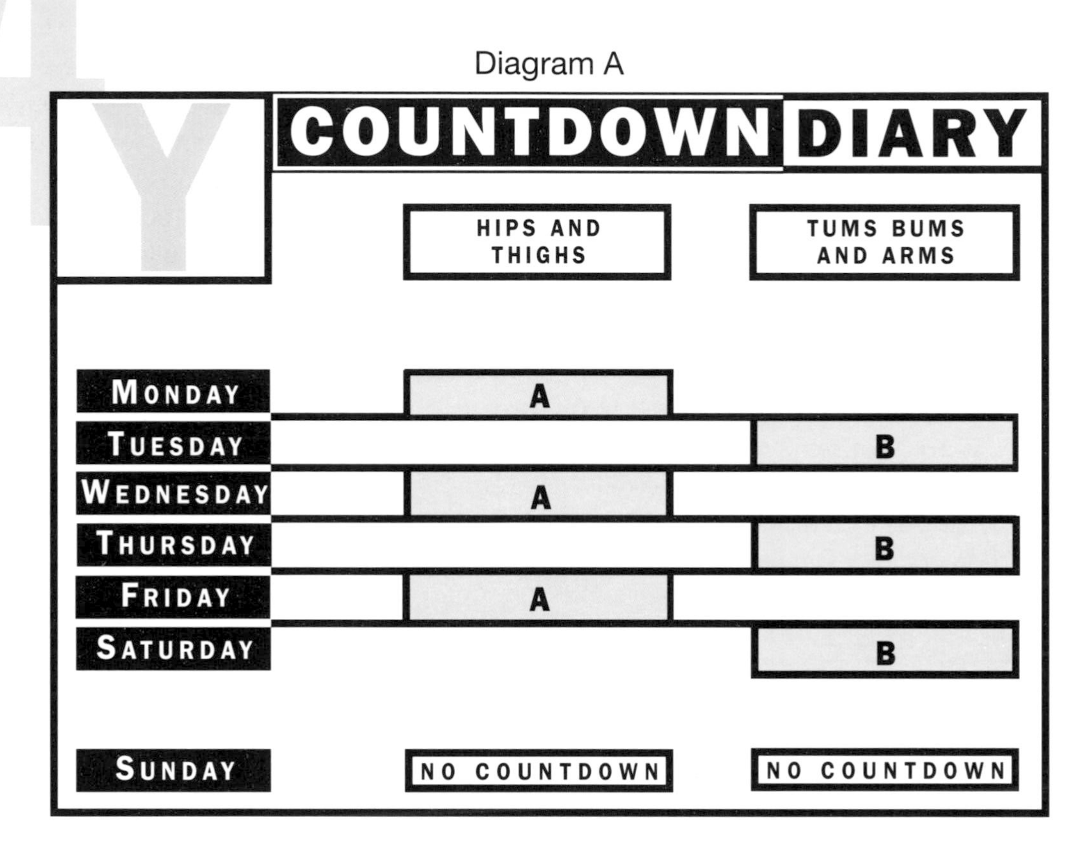

Diagram B

THE Y PLAN COUNTDOWN

	12 MINUTES	12 MINUTES
LEVEL 1	A	B
LEVEL 2	A	B
LEVEL 3	A	B
	HIPS AND THIGHS	TUMS BUMS AND ARMS

Structure of Countdown

Countdown consists of six 12 minute blocks of toning exercises. There are two types of exercise blocks which are performed on alternate days. Mondays, Wednesdays and Fridays are for Toning Block A, exercises for the hips and thighs, and Tuesdays, Thursdays and Saturdays are for Toning Block B, exercises for tums, bums and arms. Sunday is a rest day (see diagram A opposite).

The Countdown exercise blocks come in three colour-coded levels: yellow for Level 1, blue for Level 2, and pink for Level 3. Begin at Level 1, which is appropriate for everyone, and progress to the other levels (see diagram B opposite).

Each level is performed for six days followed by a rest day and then a further six days before moving on to the next level. Once you have completed the 36 Day Countdown programme, progressing gradually through the three levels, you should have worked your body hard enough to bring about the desired effect of a toned, shaped body.

The diagram below sets out the 36 day Countdown diary. By following the programme you will perform each level before moving on. To adapt this programme to your individual needs, refer to the section on monitoring your progress (see page 30).

Diagram C

LEVEL		1		2		3	
WEEK		1	2	3	4	5	6
MON	A HIPS & THIGHS	1	7	13	19	25	31
TUES	B TUMS BUMS & ARMS	2	8	14	20	26	32
WED	A HIPS & THIGHS	3	9	15	21	27	33
THURS	B TUMS BUMS & ARMS	4	10	16	22	28	34
FRI	A HIPS & THIGHS	5	11	17	23	29	35
SAT	B TUMS BUMS & ARMS	6	12	18	24	30	36
SUN	R	E	S	T	D	A	Y

Supertone programme

Once you have worked hard and achieved a newly toned body shape, you need only do the unique 14 minute Supertone programme three times a week (colour code purple). This programme consists of one exercise block which is the same degree of difficulty as Level 3 of the 36 Day Countdown. It incorporates all of the muscle groups at one time.

SUPERTONE DIARY

Monday	*Supertone*
Tuesday	*Rest*
Wednesday	*Supertone*
Thursday	*Rest*
Friday	*Supertone*
Saturday	*Rest*
Sunday	*Rest*

Countdown exercise blocks

The Countdown toning blocks are each 12 minutes long. Each block consists of a 3 minute warm-up section, a 7 minute toning section and a 2 minute cool-down section.

Block A: Hips & Thighs

1 2 3	4 5 6 7 8 9 10	11 12
Warm Up	Toning Exercises For Hips And Thighs	Cool Down

Block B: Tums, Bums & Arms

1 2 3	4 5 6 7 8 9 10	11 12
Warm Up	Toning Exercises For Tums, Bums And Arms	Cool Down

Every kind of exercise programme, no matter how simple, should incorporate a warm-up and a cool-down for safety and effectiveness.

The warm-up section

The warm-up exercises protect the muscle, joints and heart from doing too much too soon and so prevent the risk of injury. These exercises have two elements which combine to ensure that you are physically and mentally prepared for your Countdown workout throughout the 36 days.

MOBILITY AND PULSE-RAISING ELEMENT

These exercises make up the first part of each warm-up section. The mobility exercises are designed to loosen up the joints used in the workout. The aim is to move each joint slowly and thoroughly throughout the full range of movement. This increases the joint lubrication and promotes easier movement and shock absorption.

Pulse-raising exercises consist of large, rhythmic movements. Their scale and frequency put greater demands on the muscles which therefore require more oxygen, and as the muscles (including the heart) work harder, heat is generated and released, literally warming the muscle up and eventually the body.

STRETCHING ELEMENT

These exercises make up the second element of the warm-up and further prepare the muscles and joints for the workout. Stretching exercises are slow and controlled movements. They relax the muscles and lengthen them by taking the muscles and joints right to the end of their range of movement. Holding the stretch for up to 8 seconds in the warm-up is necessary for it to be effective.

The stretching exercises in the warm-ups of the Countdown concentrate on the muscle groups specific to the target areas of the body for that workout. Block A stretches the muscles of the hips and thighs and Block B stretches the muscles of the tum, bum and arms.

CHECKPOINTS FOR SAFE AND EFFECTIVE STRETCHING

Muscles are able to stretch and lengthen better after the warming process. Without it, not only will the results of the exercises be less effective but actual damage could occur. All stretches should be static – never bounce or jerk as this could damage the muscles or joints. Always ensure that you feel the stretch in the correct place and that the position is not uncomfortable or painful. Breathe naturally when stretching – never hold your breath. You will require something to hold on to for balance for some of the stretches in the hip and thigh blocks.

The toning section

The toning sections incorporate a variety of exercises that target the relevant part of the body. The muscles are worked using the training principle of reps and sets incorporated into standing or floorwork routines. The routines are designed so that the exercises flow easily from one to the next.

For the standing routines you require a support for balance. Find something that is conveniently on hand for you, such as the wall or the edge of a table. Anything that is about waist height will do as long as it is stable and will not impede movement. For the floorwork routines make sure you have a soft, comfortable and secure surface to work on, such as a thick carpet or an exercise mat.

The cool-down section

Once you reach this part of the block, all the hard work is done. The cool-down aims to reduce any tension in the muscles as a result of the workout and it is also an excellent time to relax and improve your flexibility. Take your time to get comfortable in each exercise and then relax into the stretch. Remember never to bounce or jerk as injury could occur.

The cool-down stretches are held for longer than the warm-up stretches because the muscles are much warmer after the workout and are therefore more responsive to stretching. In many of the cool-down stretches, you are encouraged to 'develop the stretch', through a technique known as developmental stretching.

DEVELOPMENTAL STRETCHING TECHNIQUE

To do this, check that you are comfortable in the stretch then concentrate on trying to relax the muscles being stretched. If, after about 10 seconds, you feel they have become accustomed to the initial stretch position, try to lengthen the muscles by stretching just a little bit further. For example, try a developmental stretch for the inner thigh (see page 64).

Sit up comfortably with your knees bent and the soles of your feet together, as close to your crutch as possible. Let your knees drop out towards the floor until you feel the stretch in the inner thigh muscles. When these are first stretched, they tend to contract to resist the movement and guard against overstretching. This reaction can be minimized by moving slowly and carefully into the stretch. After holding the stretch for about 10 seconds the muscles should begin to relax as they become acclimatized to the stretch position. To develop the stretch, try very gently to ease your knees down a little further towards the floor until you feel the stretch in the inner thighs again and hold this for another 10-15 seconds. This process can be continued, holding the stretch for as long as you like – a technique used in yoga.

This technique of developmental stretching is not suitable for all stretches in the cool-down – some stretches by their nature do not facilitate sufficiently relaxed positions. Do not expect to get this technique right first time around, but persevere and you will find that you can ease further into the stretches and improve your suppleness. It will benefit you to extend the length of the cool-down whenever possible – the longer you hold the stretches the more improvement you will see.

Progression through the levels

THE WARM-UPS AND COOL-DOWNS

Level 1 introduces a core of warm-up and cool-down exercises that form the basis of the warm-ups and cool-downs in subsequent levels. Detailed explanations of the exercises are given the first time they appear; the exercises are then represented pictorially as we progress through the levels. Two new warm-up and cool-down exercises are introduced for variety and effectiveness in both Level 2 and 3.

Familiarity with the warm-up exercises will enable you to work more fluently, making the warm-up more effective. Familiarity with the cool-down exercises allows the stretches to be held for longer, reducing muscle tension and increasing flexibility.

TONING

The toning exercises progress through the levels, in line with the principles of training (FITT). The exercises themselves become harder, either by demanding more strength for correct performance as in the three-quarter press-ups (Level 2), or by requiring more body awareness and movement control as in the curl-up combination (Level 3). The number of repetitions and/or sets increase, which in turn continues to develop muscular endurance.

The total number of repetitions in each block also increases without significantly increasing your total exercise time, as familiarity with the exercises should mean that the whole session progresses smoothly.

As you progress to the next level, allow time to learn the new exercises thoroughly and do not expect to be able to perform the block completely the first time. Give yourself at least a couple of sessions to adapt to the increased level of exercise. If any of the new exercises do not suit you, choose an alternative with the same purpose from another level.

Monitoring your progress

If you are not familiar with exercise you may be uncertain as to whether or not you are exercising at the right level. The three categories opposite will help.

As you work through your 36 Day Countdown the following should apply: at the beginning of each level the exercises should be hard to challenging; by the end of the 12 days of exercise at that level, the exercises should be easily managed. If they remain a challenge it is worth continuing at that level until you feel the exercises are more easily managed, then move on to a higher level. Exercise has to be demanding if it is to be effective but it must not be painful.

1) STRUGGLING, UNCOMFORTABLE, HARD WORK

Are you unable to do the exercises properly? Do you have a burning sensation in your muscles? Do your muscles feel like jelly? Do you feel that you need to stop, before completing the routine? Do you experience extreme aches and pains in your joints and muscles which make them very uncomfortable to move a day or more later? If yes drop a level.

2) HARD TO CHALLENGING

Are you able to perform the exercises well even though they take a lot of effort? Do your muscles get warm, then tire? Are you just able to finish the routines? Do you experience slight stiffness in your joints and muscles 24-48 hours after your exercise? If yes stay on this level.

3) EASILY MANAGED

Are you able to perform the exercises with ease and without concentration? Do your muscles feel as though they do not have to work against any resistance? Do you feel you are ready for more at the end of your exercise routine? If yes move on a level.

Remember, if the exercises are too easy the muscle will not improve in tone because it has not been overloaded. Similarly, if the exercises are too difficult the muscles will become fatigued and injury could result.

Ideally, the programme is designed to take 36 days but listen to your body – there is nothing wrong with exercising at Levels 1 and 2 for 36 days and moving on to Level 3 and Supertone in your own time. Similarly, if you find Level 1 too easy, move on to the next level and work for longer at a level you find challenging. The aim, however, is not only to find the right level but to sustain regular, challenging exercise for a minimum of 36 days for the Countdown to work effectively. Do not be in a hurry to move on until you have perfected the technique of the exercise at that level. Once you have reached Supertone the aim changes to become one of maintenance.

Supertone maintenance level

This exercise block should only be performed once you have worked through all 3 levels for 36 days. It is 14 minutes long, consisting of a 3 minute warm-up, 9 minutes of toning and a 2 minute cool-down.

Because the muscles have achieved good shape and tone, you need only do this block three times per week.

The Supertone block is one block of exercise that incorporates much of what has been established in the A and B blocks over the first three levels. The exercises continue to be taxing and one or two new exercise combinations are even more intricate, so be prepared to take time to learn the programme so that you get the most out of the exercises. You will need a weighted object, such as a bag of sugar, to hold during the standing toning section. Supertone is an all-over body programme so that you get the most out of the exercises. You will need a weighted object, such as a bag of sugar or can of beans, to hold during the standing toning section. Supertone is an all-over body programme packed into 14 minutes of exercise.

1 2 3	4 5 6 7 8 9 10 11 12	13 14
Warm Up	Toning Exercises For Hips, Thighs, Tums Bums And Arms	Cool Down

Performance criteria for maintaining supertone level

You should feel your muscles tire by the end of each set of repetitions.

You should be able to complete all exercises with the Supertone programme.

You should feel warm and worked after the session.

You should be able to perform each exercise well, with purpose and control. If you want variety you can return to Level 3 and mix and match it with Supertone.

If Supertone becomes easily manageable you will need to lengthen your exercise session. You could double up on the toning section, combine it with the toning block of Y Plan 1 Level 3 or attend an exercise class.

It is worth noting if you do not concentrate on doing the exercises properly, they may seem easier than they actually are.

TIPS FOR SUCCEEDING WITH COUNTDOWN

PLANNING AND PREPARATION

The Countdown programme relies on a commitment for 36 days, so do not start it just before going on holiday or moving house! Plan the right time for this programme to work.

1 *Find a time in the day that becomes your exercise time and stick with it.*

2 *Make sure the time you choose doesn't compete with anyone else's needs.*

3 *Make sure that family or flatmates know you are not available at your exercise time. Shut yourself away in a quiet and private area.*

4 *Make room to do your exercises safely. Make sure there is no furniture to obstruct your movements.*

5 *Plan ahead. If an important engagement clashes with your exercise time, find another time that day or do two Countdown blocks the following day.*

6 *If you miss an odd day of exercise, do not worry. Try to double up the next day or pick up where you left off and persevere to the end.*

7 *It is not essential to wear shoes for this programme but if you do, wear shoes with a good grip, all round support and cushioning.*

8 *If you don't feel well, do not exercise. Pick it up another day. This applies even if you only have a cold.*

9 *If, due to illness or unforeseen problems, you have a break of more than a week in the Countdown programme, be prepared to start again at the beginning to achieve the best results.*

10 *Don't exercise too soon after eating a heavy meal – wait about two hours before you begin your workout.*

11 *Drink a little water while exercising if you need to.*

12 *Don't rush – be prepared to learn the exercises correctly.*

13 *Don't expect your first attempts at exercise to be effortless. If you feel that some of what you are doing is too hard, don't give up hope. Starting is the hardest part and you have already done that. Try to remember what you are doing for your body and why.*

14 *You may find it helps you at first to have someone read the instructions to you. He or she can check your position and it may allow you to put the moves together more swiftly.*

Preparing to Exercise

Safe exercising

The Y Plan series has set extremely high standards for safe exercise by not only ensuring that the choice of exercise is graduated according to the ability of the participants, but also that the purpose of each exercise and the correct way to perform it is understood while there are many exercises that are contraindicated, that is, exercises that should be avoided (see page 37), any exercise can be controversial. It is its performance that makes a specific exercise safe or potentially dangerous. Incorrect exercise technique causes unnecessary stresses and strains to joints and muscles from which injury, temporary or more permanent, can result.

Getting the most out of your exercise

In the Countdown blocks the exercise descriptions are accompanied by a few checkpoints so you can ensure that your performance is correct and you are getting the most out of your programme. Always take time to check these thoroughly and use a mirror or a helper to make sure you have interpreted the instructions correctly. If you find you do not 'feel' the exercise in the way described, check your position carefully; if you are sure it is correct, put more effort into the performance of it. Some common faults in the technique of certain popular exercises are explained on page 35; familiarize yourself with these to enhance your own exercise performance.

To make the most of your exercise programme you need to perform each exercise with purpose as well as correct technique. This aspect is both subtle and more difficult to achieve as it requires concerted effort and more body awareness. Simply getting to the end of the session is not what matters; what does matter is how you get there and the energy you expend on the way. The well-known adage 'the more you put in the more you'll get out' certainly applies here.

As you get fitter you will feel the exercises getting easier, by putting more effort into the exercises as they become familiar, you will get more out of them. Always remember that it is quite normal for the exercise to feel easier some days than others. You should always listen to your body and exercise at your own level.

Aim to find a rhythm for each exercise that suits you and ensure that you complete each exercise every time with control and precision. You may find it helps you to exercise to music, or to the regular beat of a ticking clock or metronome – but be careful that the beat is not too fast. A good way of checking this is to ensure that you can stop during any part of the exercise.

Increasing the speed of the exercises is often interpreted as the way to make them harder. However, fast movements of an arm or a leg often require less muscle work because the limb is carried along by the momentum of the movement rather than by the actions of the muscles themselves.

Muscles as stabilizers

Good body alignment is important in order to maintain correct technique throughout the exercise. To do this, many muscles have to work statically to hold the body in place. For example, in the standing side leg raises (page 56) the muscles of the supporting leg, in particular those at the side of the hip, have to work hard to maintain the balance on one leg.

Muscles working in this way, acting as stabilisers, are referred to as fixators. They will also be toned by the exercise.

You may find that the fixators tire before you have completed a particular set of exercises. If so, give the muscles a short rest and then you will be able to resume safely. The abdominal or tummy muscles should work as fixators in most exercises in order to stabilize the spine and protect the back. Using them well in this way (as well as using them to maintain good posture throughout the day) will result in additional toning for these muscles.

Exercise adaptations

Many people have particular characteristics over and above their level of fitness, body type and experience of exercise that affect their ability to perform certain exercises. These may be the result of hereditary make-up (for example, length of legs related to length of arms, muscle bulk or level of natural flexibility), variation in the components of physical fitness (for example muscular strength, much stronger muscles in the lower body compared to those in the upper body) or past or recent injuries .

The Countdown exercise blocks provide adaptations offering minor variations to some exercises that we know often cause a problem. These are nearly always illustrated by a small picture accompanying that exercise. Exercise should never be painful or uncomfortable; it is very individual and what is suitable for one person is not necessarily suitable for another. Listen to your body and always respond to discomfort (which is sometimes not felt until afterwards or even the next day). If you do suffer from delayed discomfort, try to find out which exercise is causing it and avoid that in future workouts – use an alternative exercise from another block that has the same purpose.

Specific exercise technique

The following section looks more closely at specific exercises that appear frequently in Countdown and highlights some of the common problems that occur through incorrect exercise technique. Many of these exercises are fundamental to any exercise programme.

THE CURL-UP

The Countdown exercise blocks incorporate many variations of the basic curl-up to provide variety and maintain interest in the programme. You will find that the variations become more difficult in intensity and co-ordination as you progress through the levels. Some of the exercises work the oblique muscles – these are actually the part of the tummy muscles that form the waist.

All the variations on the basic curl-up produce similar results – the toning of the tummy muscles – and the same principles of good technique apply to them all.

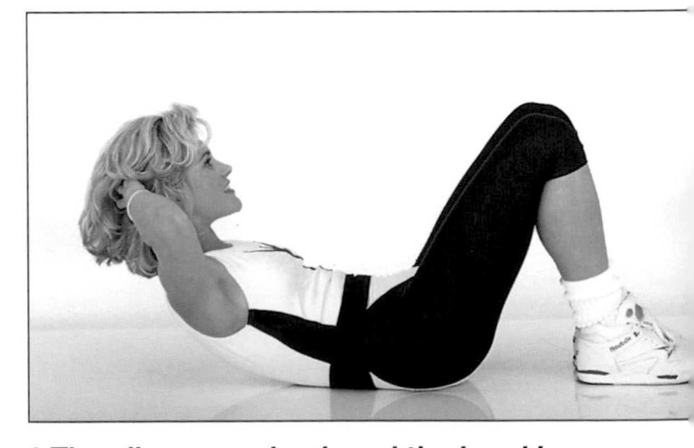

1 The elbows are back and the head is resting in the fingertips
2 The tummy is held in flat during the curl-up
3 Breath is exhaled on the way up and inhaled on the way down

Some common faults in the technique of the curl-up

PULLING ON THE HEAD

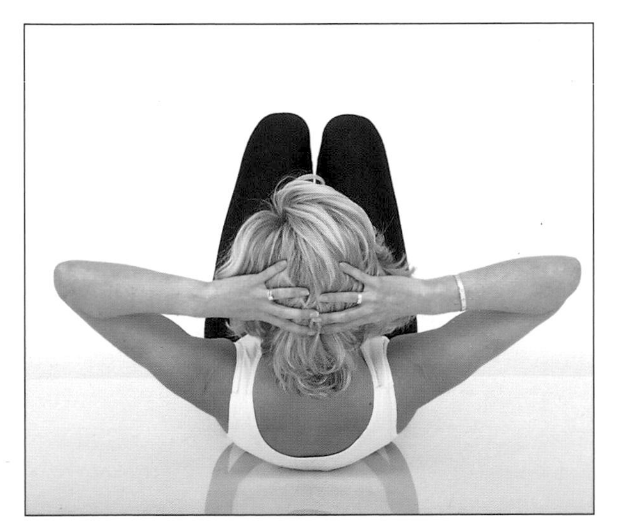

CORRECT – *FINGER TIPS ONLY*
The head is resting lightly in finger tips to prevent neck ache

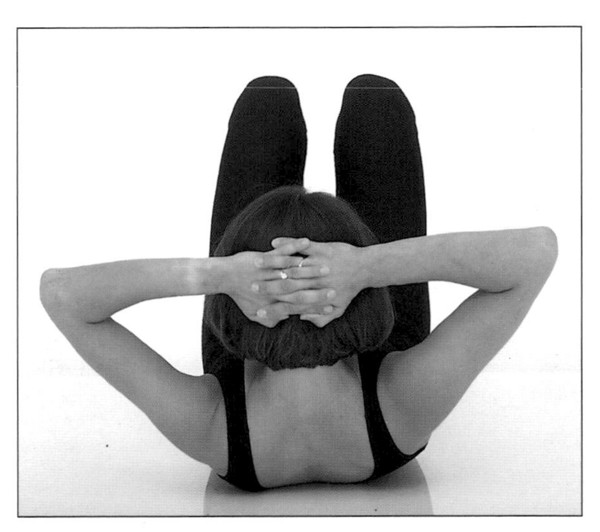

INCORRECT- *HANDS BEHIND HEAD*
The hands are clasped behind the head and pulling it forwards, straining the neck

DOMING

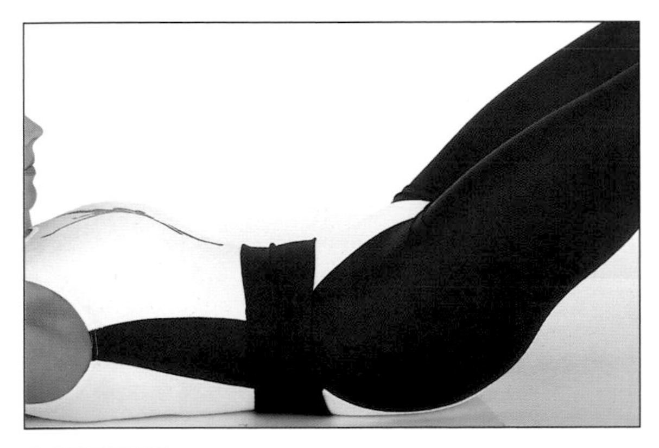

CORRECT
The tummy is pulled in and held flat during the curl-up

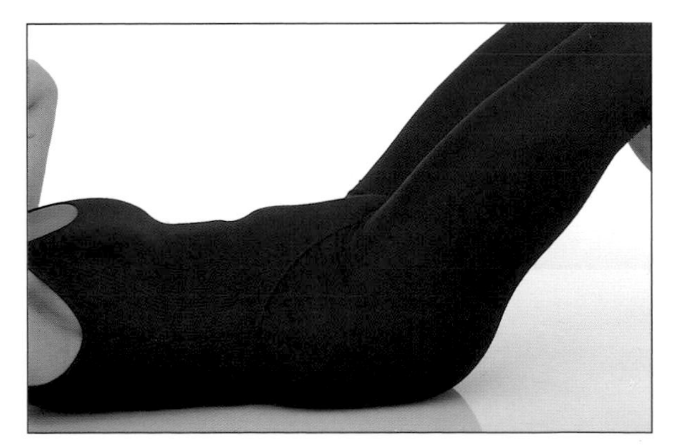

INCORRECT
The tummy is domed during the curl-up

THE REVERSE CURL

Back problems associated with the tummy exercises are also a common problem. The reverse curl can sometimes be a useful alternative. Use this exercise instead of any of the tummy exercises in any level of the Countdown where the curl-up or the variations on the curl-up are unsuitable.

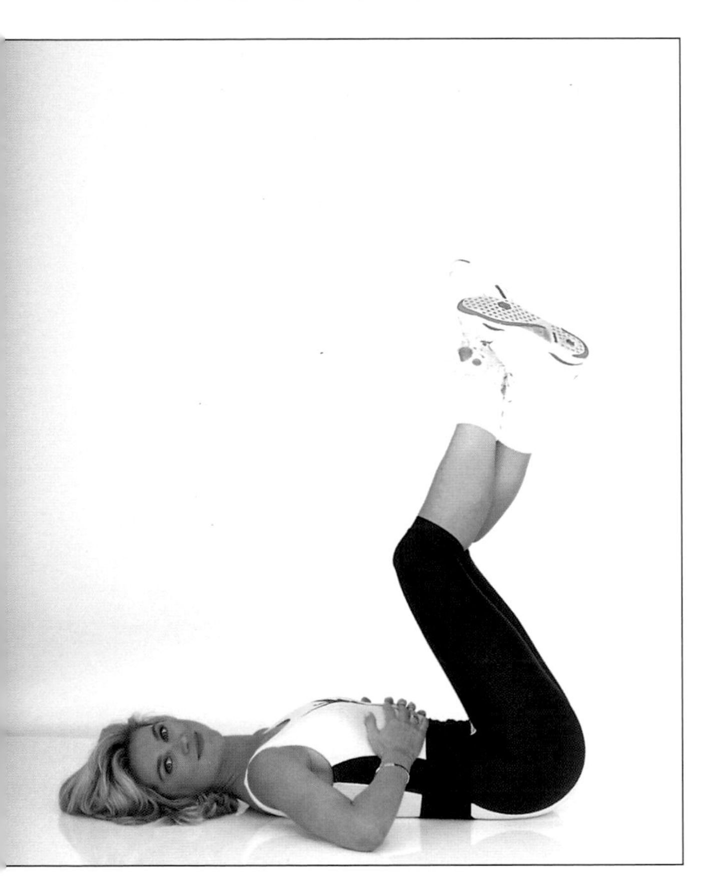

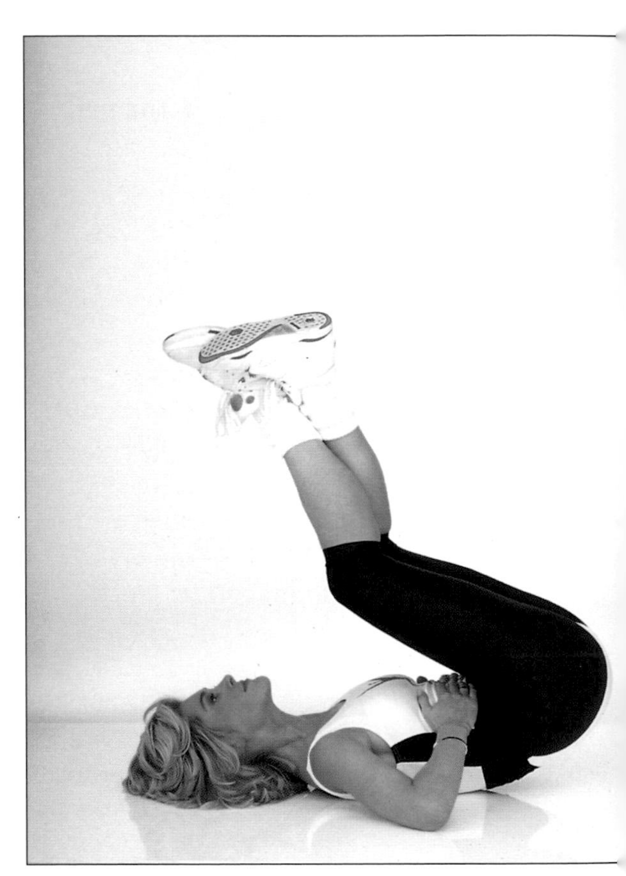

- Lie on your back with your legs bent and your knees over your chest.

- Keeping your head and shoulders relaxed back on the floor, and without swinging your legs, pull in your tummy muscles and very gently curl your buttocks and lower back off the floor. Relax.

You may find it easier at first to place your hands on the floor beside you and push down on them to assist the movement.

Feel your tummy muscles working

Think of squeezing your knees in towards your chest.

Rest your hands on your ribs

KNEE BENDS

Establishing the correct technique in the knee bend is crucial to a safe exercise programme because the movement is a fundamental part of many exercises.

CORRECT

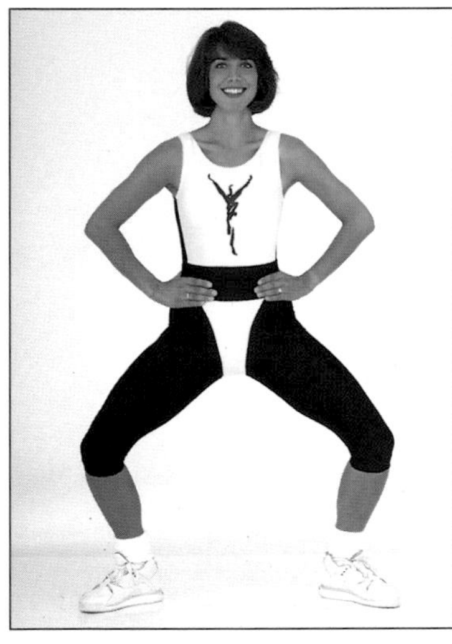

1 The feet are hip- or shoulder-width apart, flat on the floor and pointing forwards or slightly out.
2 The knees are bent, pointing in the same direction as the feet (in the exercise descriptions this is referred to as 'knees over the feet').

INCORRECT

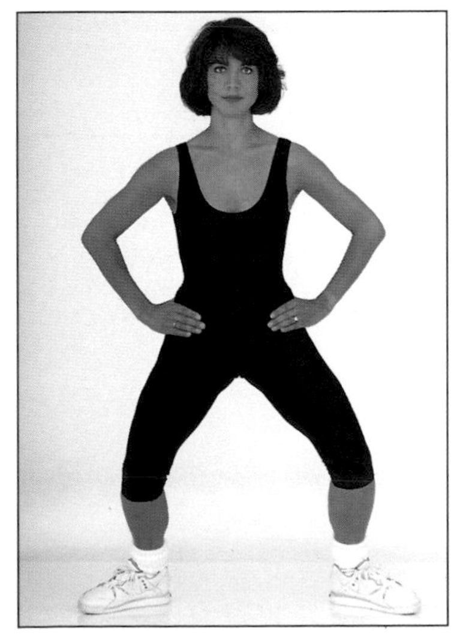

1 The feet are turned too far out.
2 The knees are rolling in, straining them.

LOCKING OUT THE ELBOWS AND KNEES

A common fault in exercise is to lock out the elbows or knees. This means that the joint is completely straight when it is supporting the body and so it, the joint, rather than the muscles which are designed for the purpose, takes the strain.

In any exercise involving bending and straightening the legs or arms, always ensure that you straighten them with control and approach the end of the range of movement with a great deal of care.

Exercises Which Should Be Avoided

The safety and effectiveness of exercise programmes have developed considerably over the past 15 years. The desire to exercise for fitness is not new, and many of the exercises incorporated into programmes today were practiced many years ago.

However, since the start of the exercise boom which happened in the late 1970s, the significant developments made in the understanding of how the body works – together, unfortunately, with surveys of the injuries that result from exercise classes – have made us realize that some of the exercises from these old PT programmes are not as suitable for general exercise programmes as was once thought. The old adage or saying 'no gain without pain' has been proven to be untrue and the message that must be learnt now is, 'if it hurts don't do it'.

The exercises on the following pages (38 to 39) should be avoided as the risks of injury outweigh the benefits. The results they provide can be just as easily achieved, without the risk of injury, through much safer alternatives.

5

INTENDED PURPOSE:
TO STRENGTHEN THE ABDOMINALS
Problem: strains the back
Alternative: the curl-up with bent knees

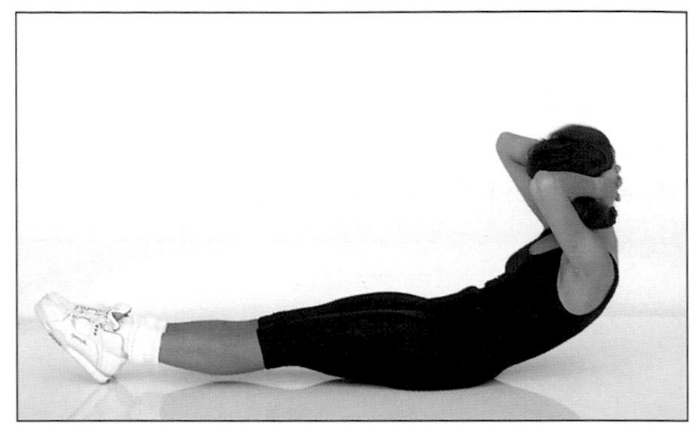

STRAIGHT LEG SIT-UPS

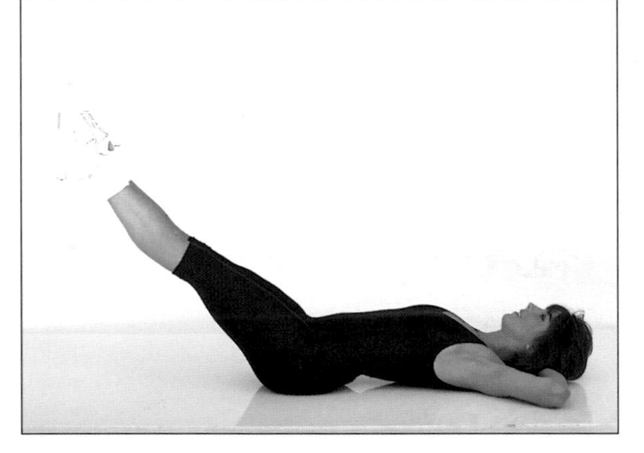

STRAIGHT LEG RAISES

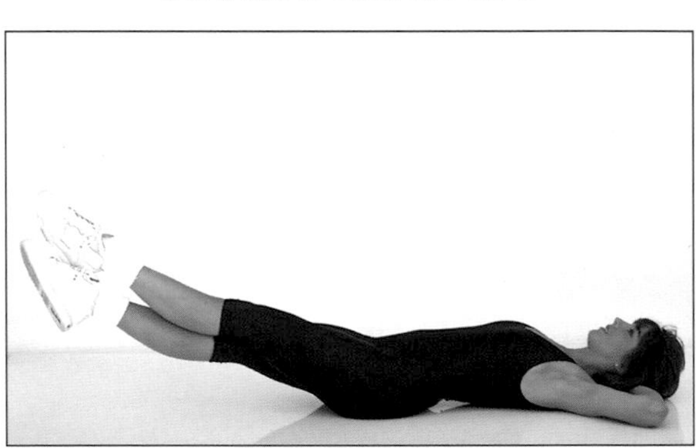

CRISS CROSSES

INTENDED PURPOSE:
TO STRETCH THE HAMSTRINGS
Problem: strains the back
Alternative: seated hamstring stretch

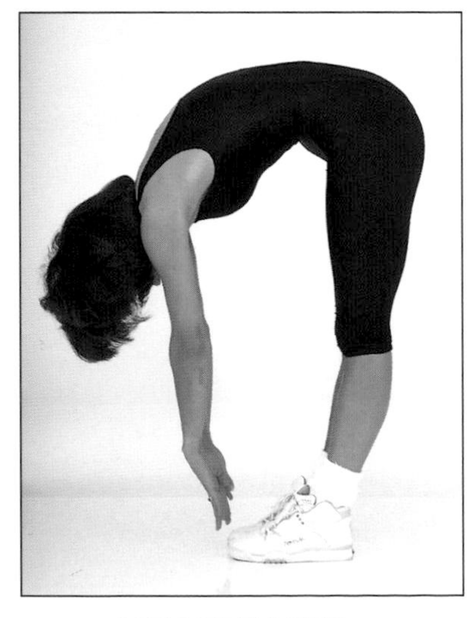

TOE TOUCHES

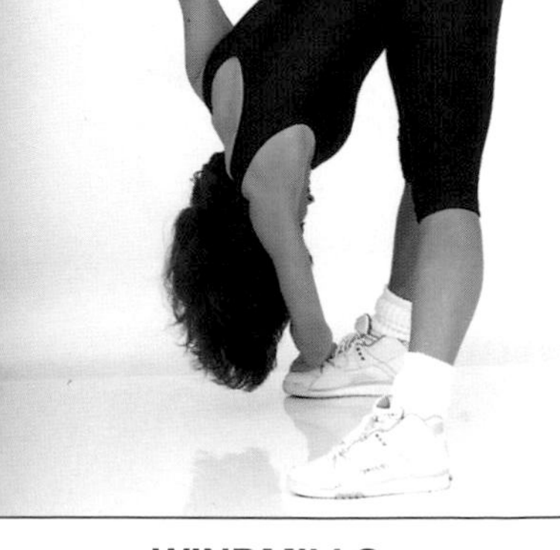

WINDMILLS

INTENDED PURPOSE:
TO STRETCH THE HAMSTRINGS AND LOOSEN THE BACK
Problem: stresses the neck and back
Alternative: forward hamstring stretch

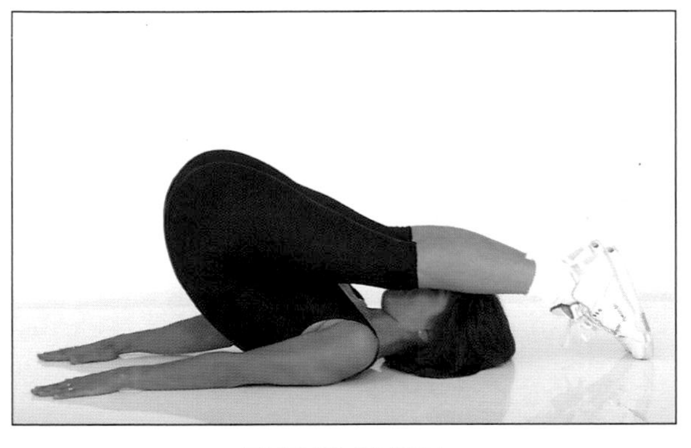

THE PLOUGH

INTENDED PURPOSE:
TO STRENGTHEN THE QUADS
Problem: stresses the knees
Alternative: knee bends

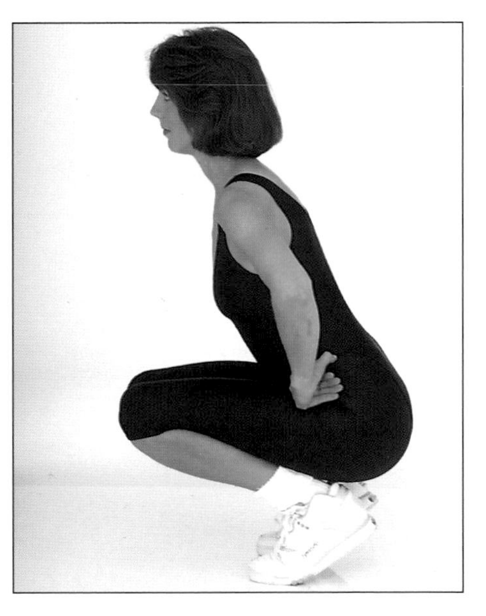

DEEP KNEE BENDS

INTENDED PURPOSE:
TO STRETCH THE SHOULDERS AND ABDOMINAL MUSCLES
Problem: stresses the back
Alternative: shoulder stretch and tum stretch

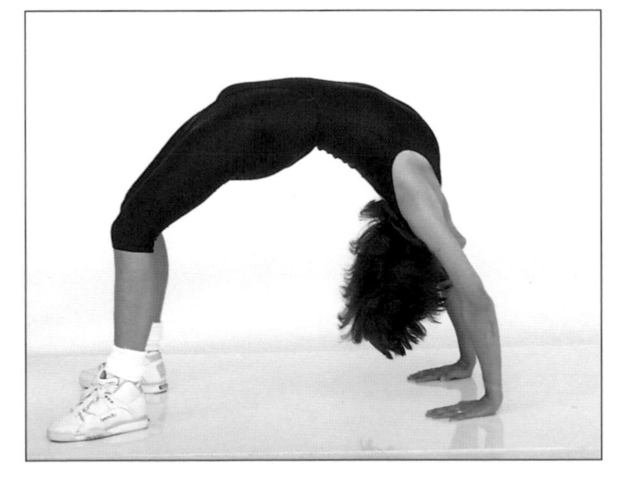

THE BRIDGE

INTENDED PURPOSE:
TO STRETCH THE QUADS
Problem: stresses the knees
Alternative: side lying quad stretch

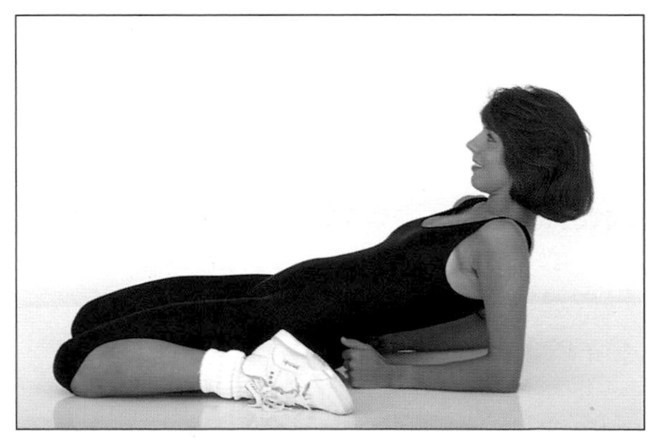

SEATED QUAD STRETCH

6 The Countdown Exercise

Posture

Correct posture is a must, not only when exercising, but also throughout our daily activities. Good posture (meaning good body alignment from the head to the heels) is automatic for some people, whereas for others it has to be learnt.

Some of the benefits of good posture are:

1 *Improved self confidence.*
2 *Improved self image.*
3 *Improved body shape.*
4 *Excellent training for all muscle tone.*
5 *Protection of structure and joints of the body.*
6 *Stresses and strains of the body, in particular the back, are alleviated.*

Backcare and the Spine

The spine is a very complicated and delicate part of the body and correct posture is a particular area of concern in respect of back care. Throughout the book, exercise technique and muscle toning and stretching have been highlighted as essential for protecting the back, as it is nearly always directly or indirectly involved in exercise. If any part of the back feels distressed or painful during exercise, the exercise should be stopped and medical advice sought.

The spine consists of a complex structure of small bones (vertebrae) and discs (cushioning pads of cartilage), muscles and ligaments. Bad posture causes muscle fatigue resulting in backache. Perpetual backache can cause more long-term damage to the ligaments of the back as they bear the strain of the fatigued muscles. The discs between the vertebrae can also be affected. This in turn can affect nerves, producing pain in not only the back but in other areas as well.

There is a natural arch in the lower back that equips it to support a considerable weight – that of the upper body. In many people this natural arch is exaggerated, which can be due simply to poor posture, or to added weight at the front – as in pregnant women and men with a paunch! An exaggerated curve in the lower back is often compensated for by an exaggerated forward curve in the upper back and neck, leading to the common bad posture of an arched lower back and round shoulders.

Good v Bad Posture – Your Self-Help List

Stand side-on to a mirror (see pictures opposite) and try to improve your posture from the following pointers. Your tummy should be pulled in (you shouldn't, however, be holding your breath), and the curve in your lower back should only be slight. Think of pulling up tall from the top of the back of your head right throughout the body and lengthening your spine; you should feel (and be) a couple of inches taller. We are often shorter at the end of the day than we were in the morning. This is because the muscles and structures that support the spine tire and sag and we tend unconsciously to let ourselves droop as the day goes on; also, the discs become thinner during the day. As we get older we reduce in height which is also due to shrinking of the discs between the vertebrae, and to loss of tone and elasticity in the muscles.

A little effort to 'train' your posture every day will soon start to show positive effects on how you look and feel.

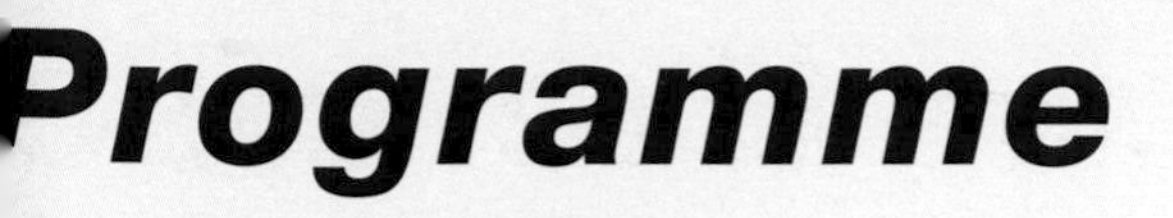
Programme

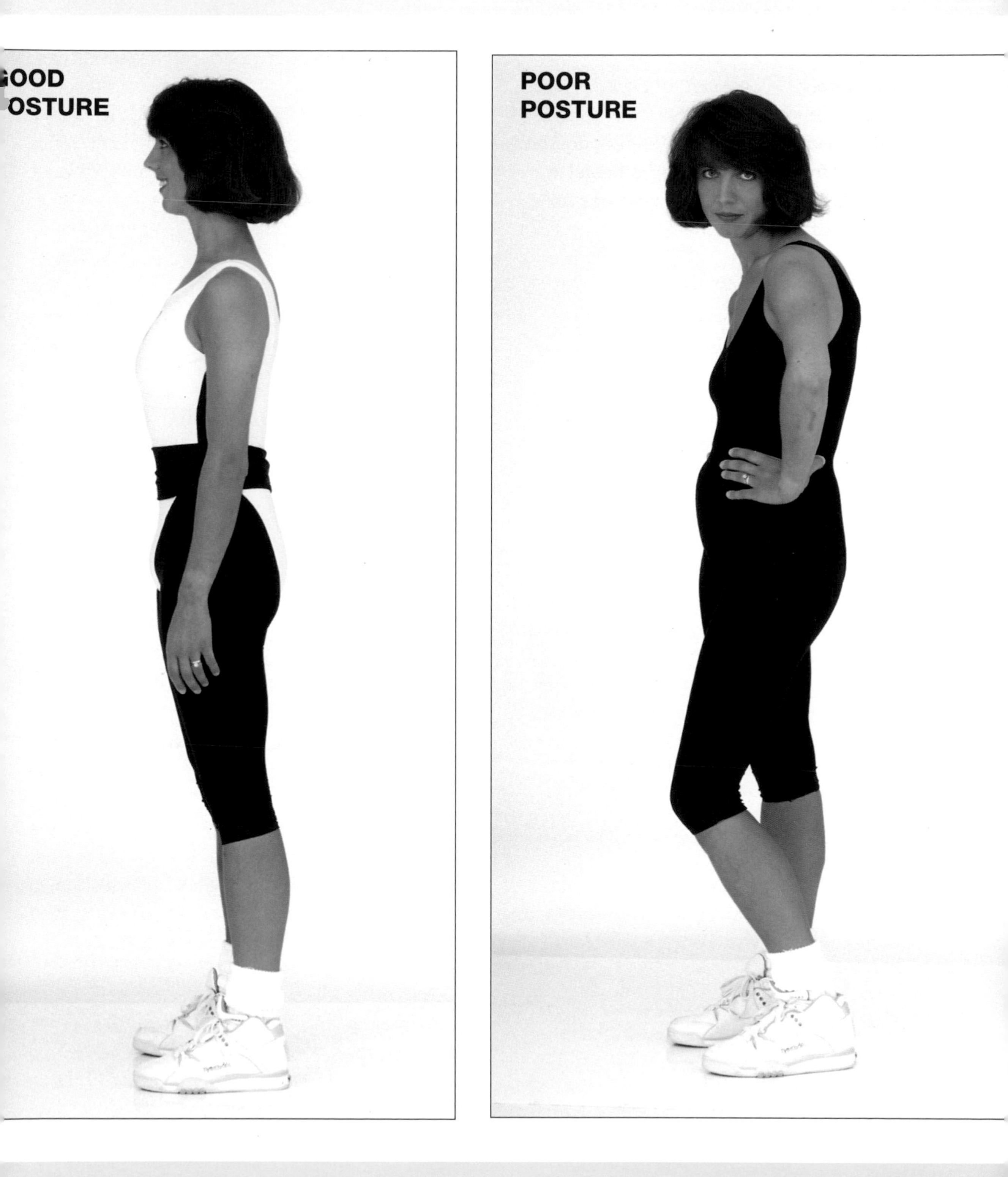
OOD
OSTURE
POOR
POSTURE

The Pelvic Tilt

The pelvis is the bony basin that connects the legs to the trunk. The pelvic tilt is a fundamental part of good posture and safe exercise technique, as it affects the position of the lower back. The correct pelvic tilt is constantly referred to throughout the Countdown.

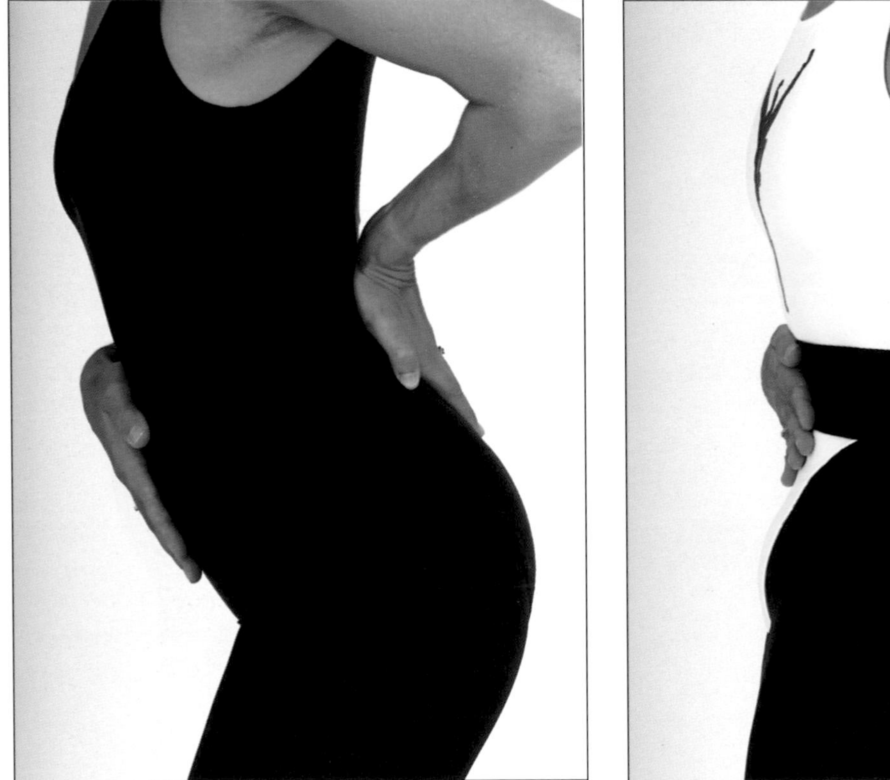

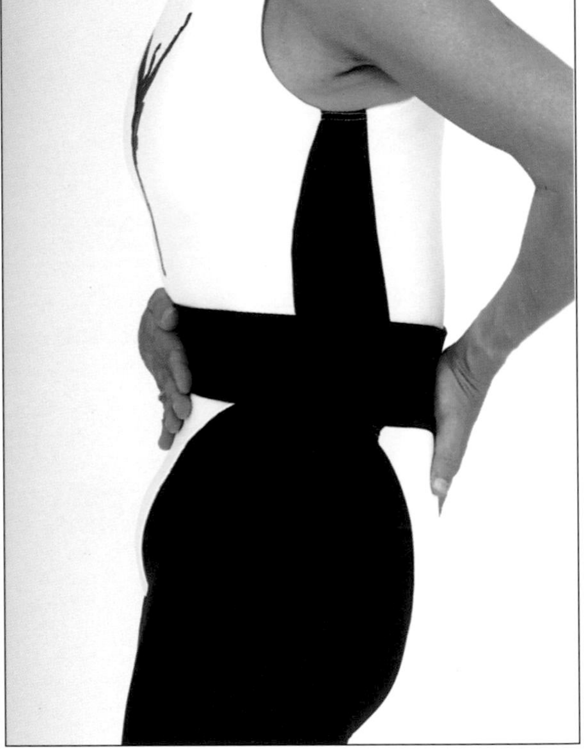

THE PELVIC TILT

- Stand with your feet hip-width apart.
- Bend your knees slightly to make it easier and place one hand on your tummy and the other on your lower back.
- Start from the position of an incorrect pelvic tilt (above left) with your back hollowed, tummy and bottom stuck out.
- To correct the pelvic tilt, pull in your tummy muscles and tilt your pelvis (above right). Imagine that with your hands you are pushing down at the back, smoothing out the curve in your lower back, and pulling up at the front, pushing your tummy in.
- Without holding your breath, try to maintain this correct pelvic tilt with your bottom tucked under as you straighten your legs.

Feel your tummy muscles working to maintain the end position – the correct pelvic tilt.

The Pelvic Tilt and Tummy Toning

Because of its excellent toning effect for the tummy muscles, a pelvic tilting exercise is actually incorporated into Level 1B of the Countdown. By maintaining a correct pelvic tilt throughout the day you will be toning your tummy muscles and gaining a flatter stomach at the same time as you are improving your posture and looking after your back.

Centre Control

Centre control is a term that refers to the correct pelvic tilt and the stability of your hips and lower back. The tummy muscles, as well as maintaining the correct pelvic tilt, support the base of the spine. This role is made even harder during exercise because of the movement of the arms and legs that encourage the back to move out of postural alignment. For good centre control, tighten your tummy muscles to support your back and maintain the correct pelvic tilt and contract your buttocks, squeezing them tightly to stabilize the hips.

The Pelvic Floor

The pelvic floor is a criss-cross layer of muscles at the base of the pelvis that supports the organs in the abdominal cavity. It is a very important group of muscles as it controls the bladder, vagina and bowel. Many women, especially following childbirth, can suffer from an embarrassing condition known as stress incontinence. This is leakage of urine on sudden exertion as in sneezing, laughing or exercising. A toned pelvic floor muscle can dramatically reduce and often eliminate the problem altogether.

Toning exercise for the pelvic floor consists of specific isolated contractions for that muscle while the rest of the body is relaxed. When performing this exercise a common fault is to hold the breath or squeeze the knees and buttocks. Regular practice will enable you to isolate the muscle effectively. To do the exercise correctly follow these instructions carefully and aim to do it as often as possible – at least half a dozen times a day. As well as reducing or eliminating any problems of stress incontinence, a well-toned pelvic floor can lead to a more enjoyable sex life!

THE PELVIC FLOOR CONTRACTION

1 *It is a good idea to learn the pelvic floor contraction sitting down at first. Just make sure that your knees are bent and slightly apart, with your feet flat on the floor.*

2 *Think of drawing the pelvic floor muscles up inside, squeezing around the back, middle and front passages. Make sure that you concentrate on taking the contraction right the way to the front, tensing the muscles as if to hold back from urinating.*

3 *Hold this for a count of four then let go.*

4 *Repeat this again, this time checking that you are not holding your breath or squeezing any other muscles at the same time.*

Once you have mastered the above technique, remind yourself to practise it by associating the exercise with some of your daily activities, from talking on the telephone to doing the washing up! You should then vary the timing of the contractions, performing one long one held for a count of 10 followed by four quick ones held for about one second each.

Men also have a pelvic floor that needs to be exercised in the same way. However, they are lucky in that they are not as likely to suffer from stress incontinence to the same degree as women.

6

Starting Positions

When exercising with Countdown you must be sure that you get the starting position correct for each exercise. These vary throughout the programme and sometimes the differences are quite subtle. The two most common standing positions entail the feet being hip-width or shoulder-width apart. In either position you must be careful that your feet are pointing only slightly out and not to the sides, which can strain your knees. 'Knees slightly bent' is also important to the correct starting positions because this makes it easier to achieve the correct pelvic tilt and maintain good centre control. Having your knees any more than very slightly bent makes the position a static contraction for the quads, which becomes very tiring.

Starting position, feet hip-width apart

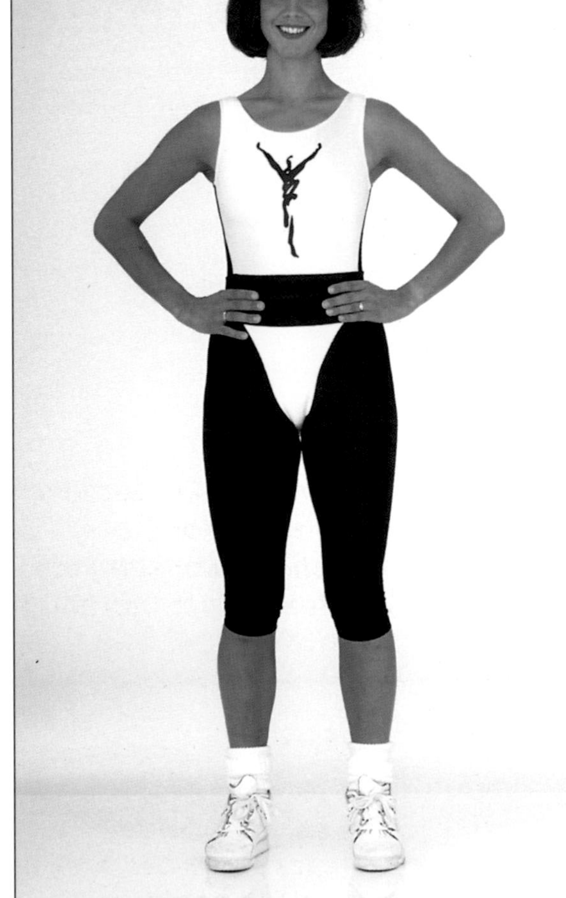

Starting position, feet shoulder-width apart

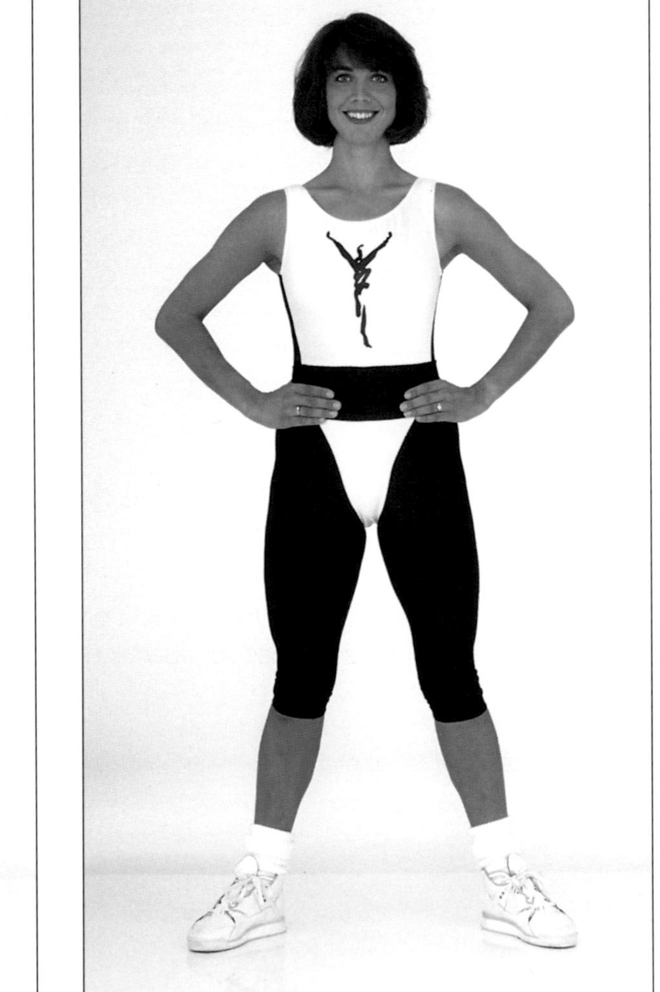

London Central YMCA Training and Development

PRE-EXERCISE QUESTIONNAIRE

BEFORE STARTING ANY EXERCISE PROGRAMME IT IS IMPORTANT TO COMPLETE THE QUESTIONNAIRE THAT FOLLOWS.
Read the questions carefully and answer as accurately as you can.

	YES	NO
1 Has your doctor ever said you have heart disease, high blood pressure or any other cardiovascular problem?		
2 Is there a history of heart disease in your family?		
3 Do you ever have pains in your heart and chest especially associated with minimal effort?		
4 Do you often get headaches or feel faint or dizzy?		
5 Do you suffer from either pain or limited movement in any joints which has been caused by exercise or might be aggravated with exercise?		
6 Are you taking medication at the moment or recuperating from a recent illness or operation?		
7 Are you pregnant?		
8 Are you unaccustomed to exercise and aged over 50?		
9 Do you have any other medical condition which you think may affect your ability to participate in exercise?		

If you have answered 'Yes' to one or more questions, consult your doctor prior to starting a graduated exercise programme.

If you have answered 'No' to all questions, this is reasonable assurance that it is safe for you to begin.

Level 1a Hips and Thighs

EXERCISE 1

KNEE BENDS

REPETITIONS *4*
PURPOSE:
To warm the muscles

- Stand with your feet just over shoulder width apart, toes pointing very slightly out.
- Keeping your heels pressed into the ground, your pelvis correctly tilted and your back upright, slowly bend and straighten your legs.
- Do this 4 times.

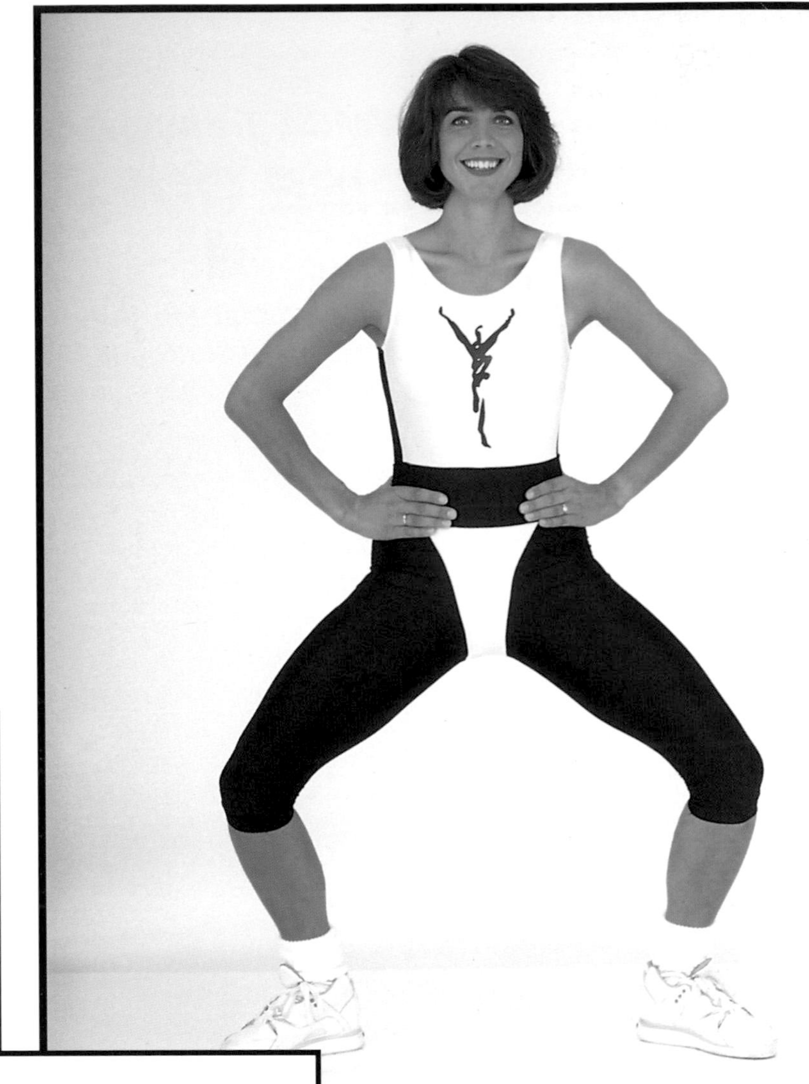

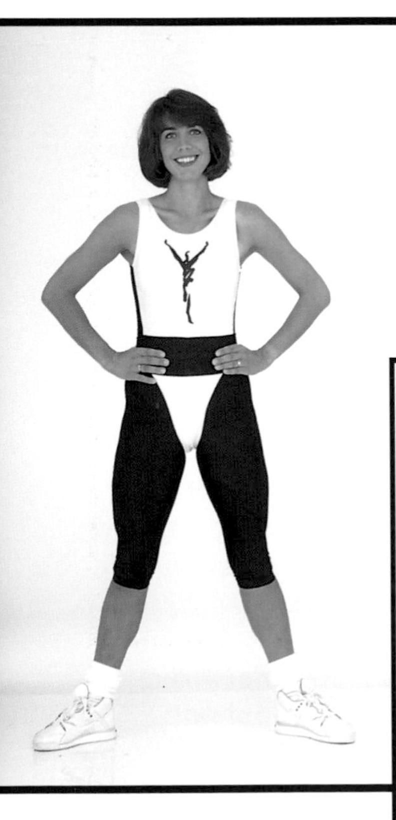

Check that your knees point in the same direction as your feet and that your feet are not too turned out

Straighten legs with care to avoid snapping the knees straight

To make the exercise a little more effective, try to bend slightly lower, but do not let your hips drop below the level of your knees

During these initial warm-up exercises think carefully about warming and loosening your muscles and joints. Move with effort and control, concentrating on what you are trying to achieve. The stretching exercises are aimed specifically at preparing the muscles and joints for the hip- and thigh-toning exercises. When stretching, remember to move into each stretch position gently and with control. Feel the stretch and hold the position – don't bounce.

EXERCISE 2

SIDE BENDS

REPETITIONS *4*
PURPOSE:
To mobilize the spine

- Stand with your feet shoulder-width apart, knees slightly bent and with a correct pelvic tilt.
- Bend to your right side, sliding your right arm down the side of your right leg to about the level of your knee.
- Slide your left arm up the left side of your body.
- Repeat this to the other side then repeat the whole exercise.

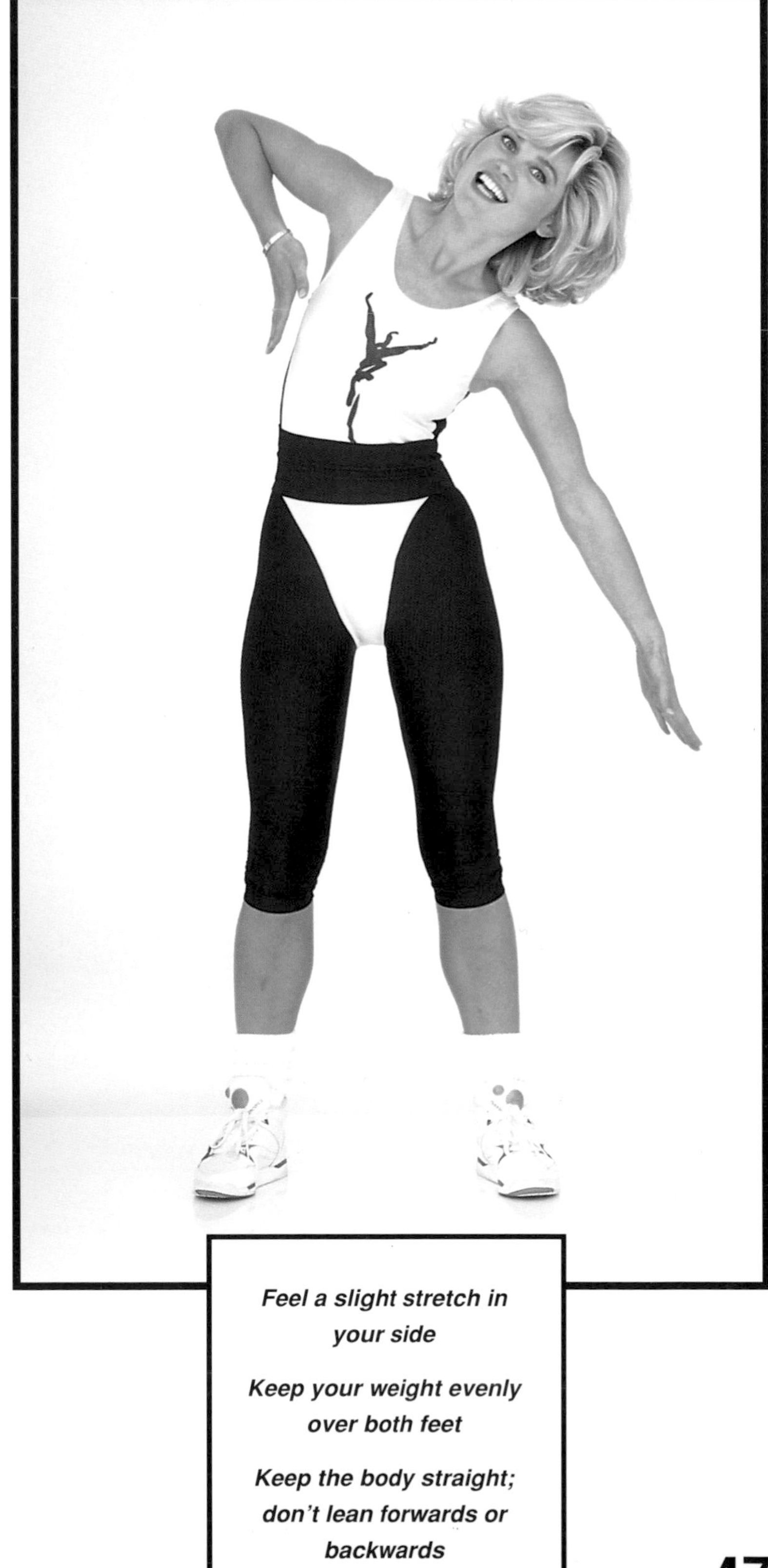

Feel a slight stretch in your side

Keep your weight evenly over both feet

Keep the body straight; don't lean forwards or backwards

EXERCISE 3

SWAYS

REPETITIONS *8*
PURPOSE:
To warm the muscles

- With your hands on your hips and your tummy held in tight, stand with your weight over your right leg and your left leg extended to the side.
- Transfer your weight over both feet and slowly bend your knees.
- Gently straighten your legs moving your weight over your left leg and extending your right leg to the side.
- Repeat this until you have done 8 sways in total.

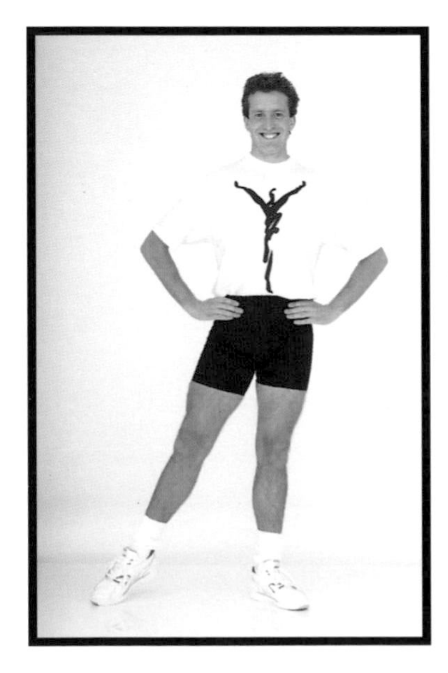

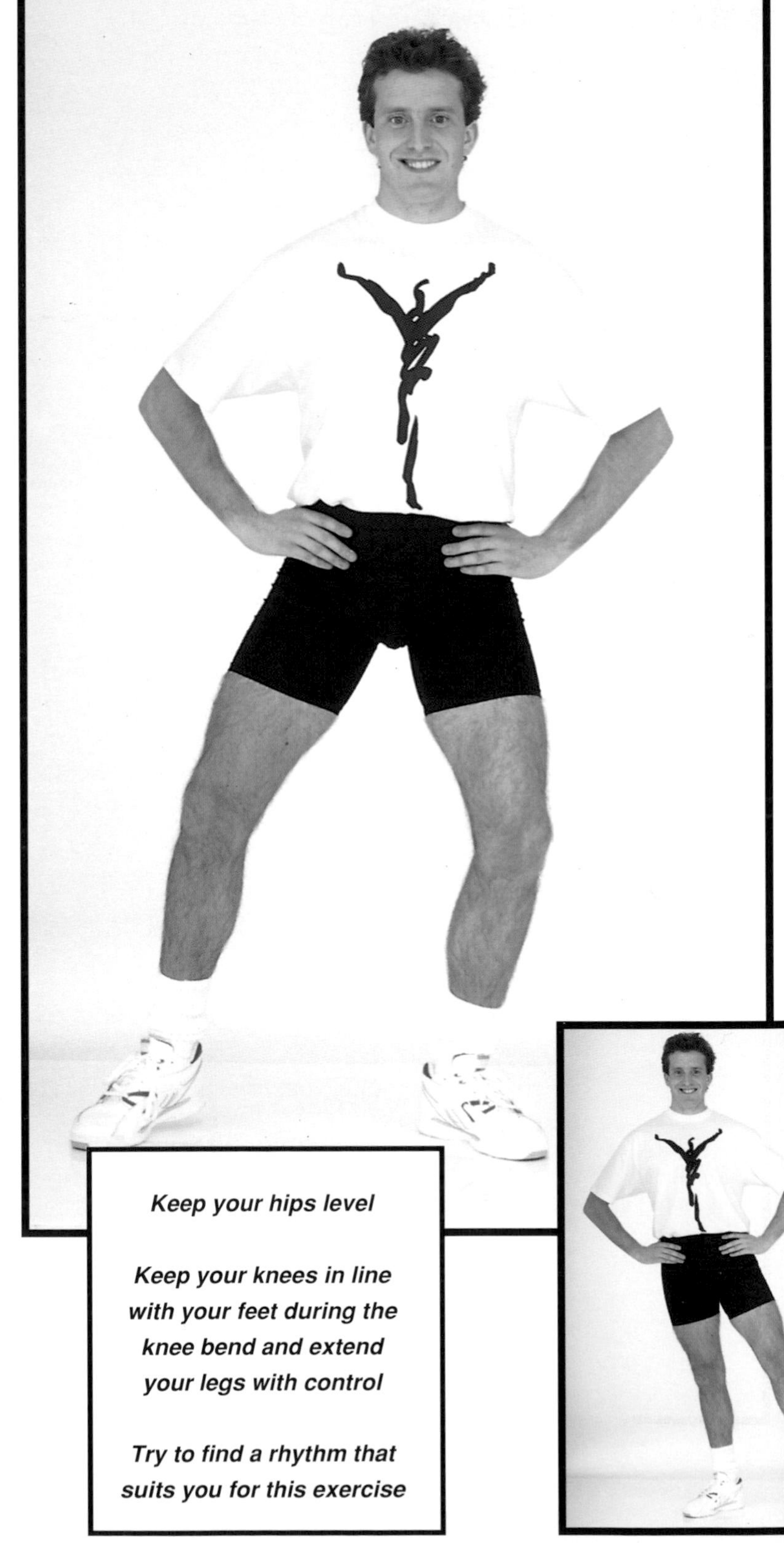

Keep your hips level

Keep your knees in line with your feet during the knee bend and extend your legs with control

Try to find a rhythm that suits you for this exercise

EXERCISE 4

SHOULDER SQUEEZES

REPETITIONS *4*
PURPOSE:
To loosen the shoulders and upper back

- Stand with your feet shoulder width apart and your arms hanging loosely by your sides.

- Letting your head and arms move slightly forwards, pull your shoulders forwards and slightly round the top of your back while breathing out.

- Then open your chest by looking up and pulling your shoulders and arms back and down, squeezing your shoulder blades together and taking a deep breath in.

- Do this four times.

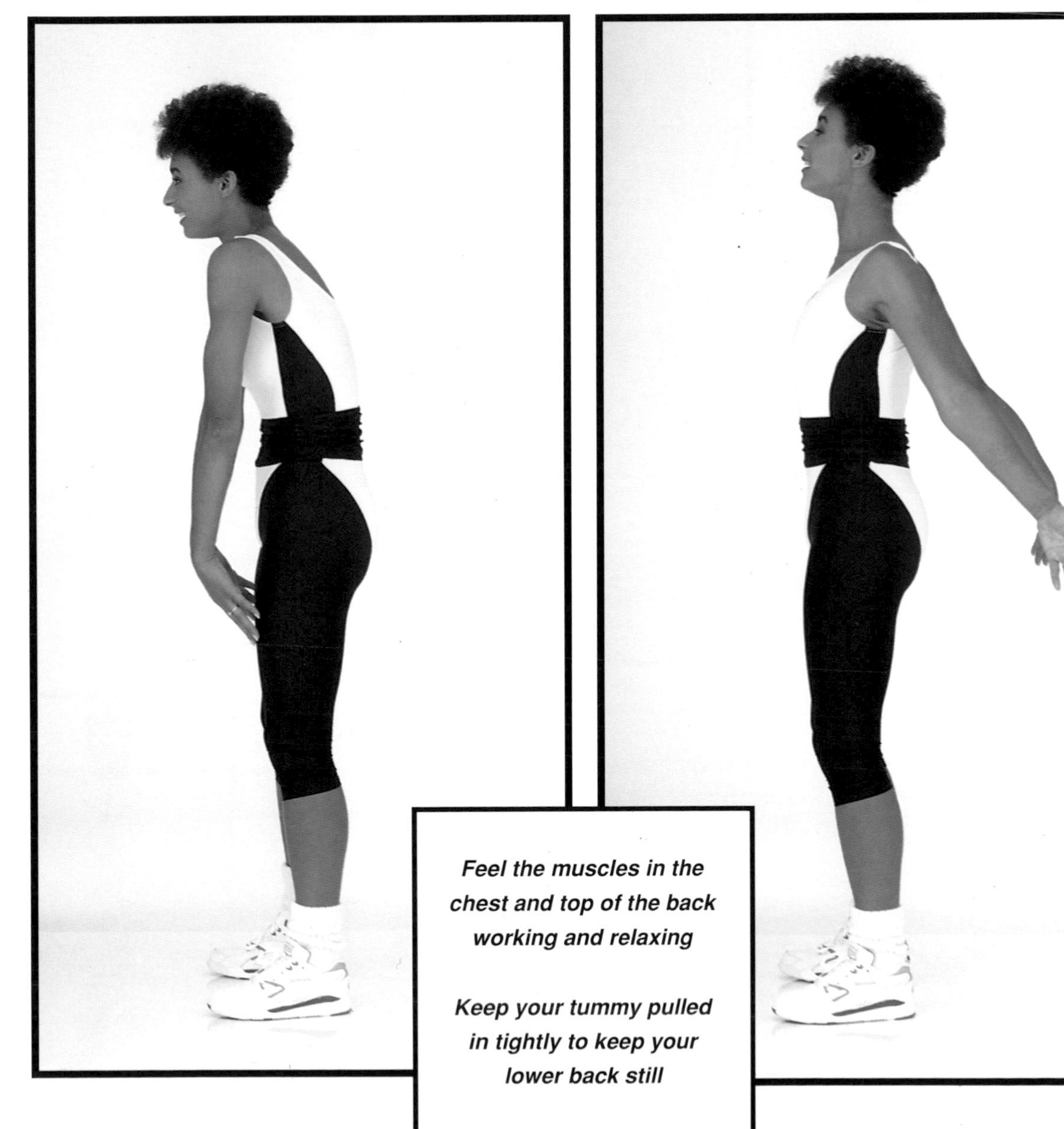

Feel the muscles in the chest and top of the back working and relaxing

Keep your tummy pulled in tightly to keep your lower back still

Make sure you only move around the top of your back

EXERCISE 5

HIP CIRCLES

REPETITIONS
2 Right 2 Left
PURPOSE:
To mobilize the lower back

- Stand with your feet shoulder-width apart, your knees slightly bent and your hands on your hips.

- Circle your hips by taking them to the right, backwards, to the left, then forwards.

- Do this once more then repeat twice going the other way.

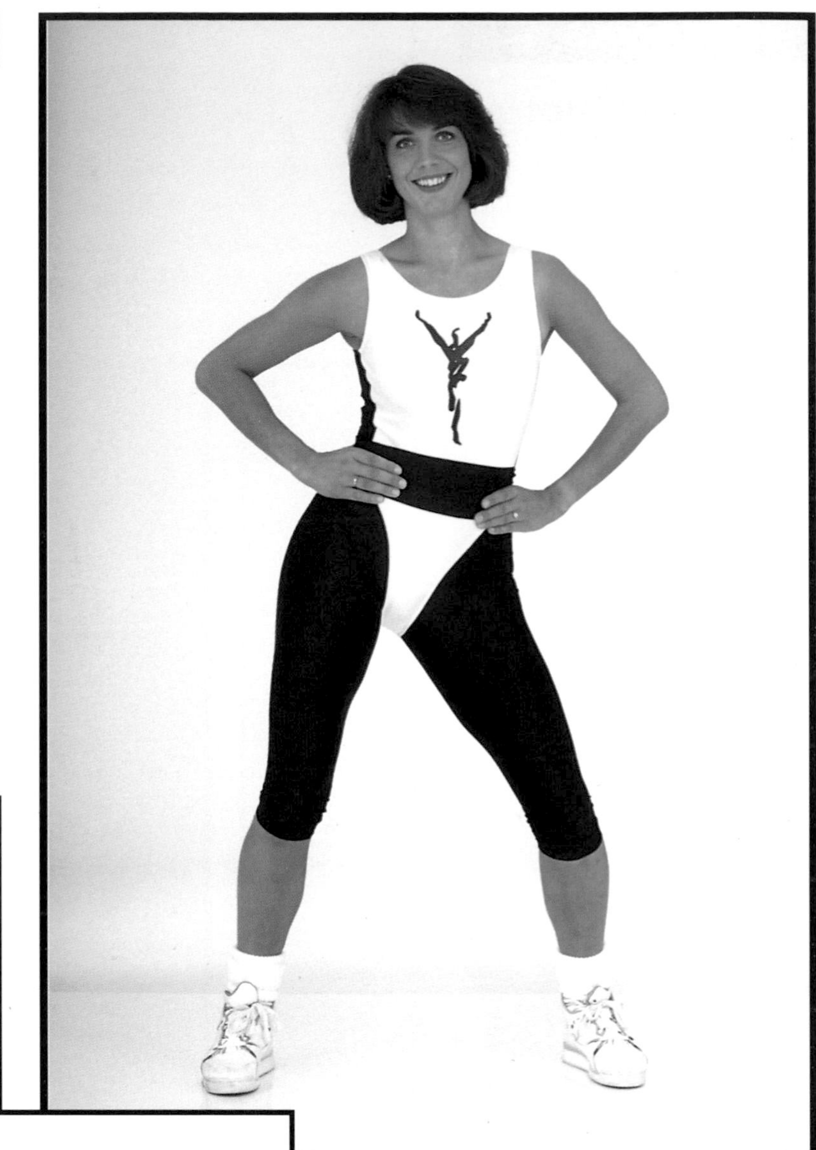

Feel the exercise relax the muscles in the lower back

Use your tummy muscles to bring about the movement

Isolate the movement to the lower back by keeping your shoulders and knees still

EXERCISE 6

FORWARD ARM CIRCLES

REPETITIONS
2 Right 2 Left
PURPOSE:
To mobilize the shoulders

- Stand with your feet shoulder-width apart and your toes pointing forwards.

- Keeping your hips facing forwards all the time, circle your right arm by taking it forwards and up, brushing your ear with it as it goes round and down, drawing as large an imaginary circle as possible with your middle finger.

- Do this once more then repeat it twice using the other arm.

Feel the movement loosening any stiffness in your shoulder joint

Try to keep your arm straight throughout the exercise

To get the most out of this exercise, as your arm circles down, keep it behind you as much as possible and keep your palm facing out

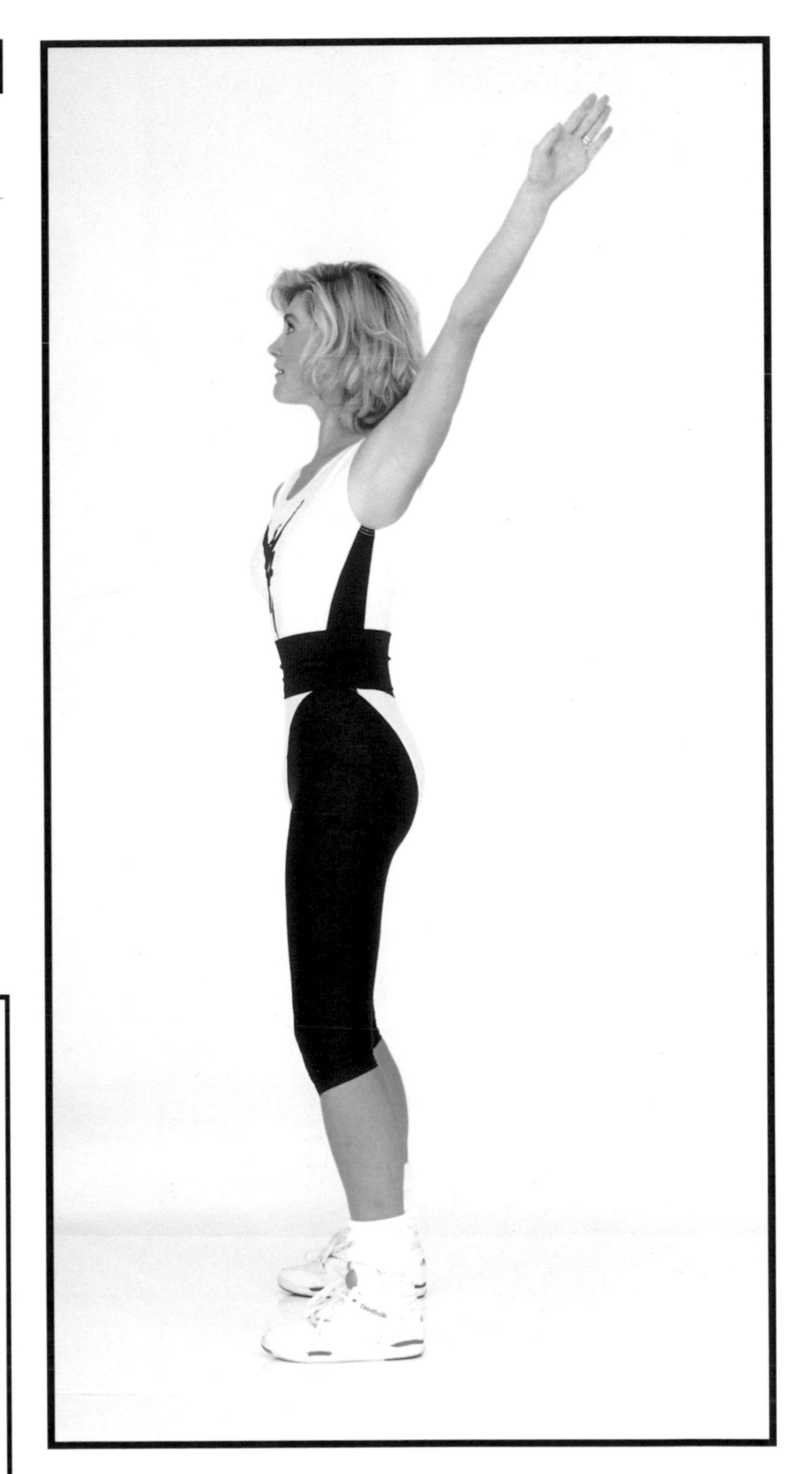

Level 1a Hips and Thighs

EXERCISE 7

SQUAT AND REACH WITH HEEL RAISE

REPETITIONS *4*
PURPOSE:
To warm the muscles

- Stand with your feet just wider than shoulder-width apart and your arms hanging loosely by your sides.

- Bend your knees and tap them with your hands, then gently straighten your legs touching your shoulders with your hands, rise up on to your toes (keeping the weight over your big toe) and stretch both arms up towards the ceiling as much as possible.

- Do this 4 times.

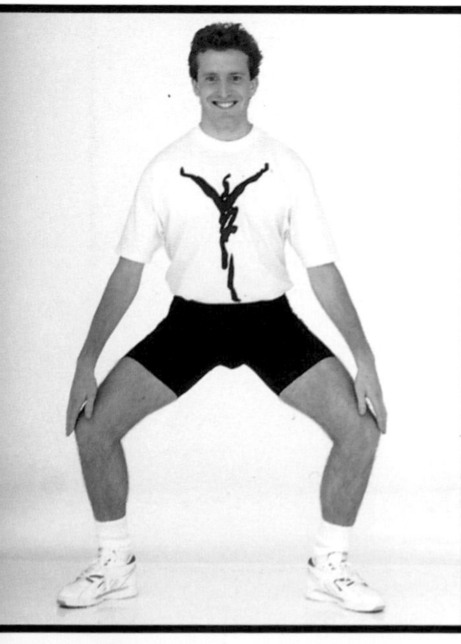

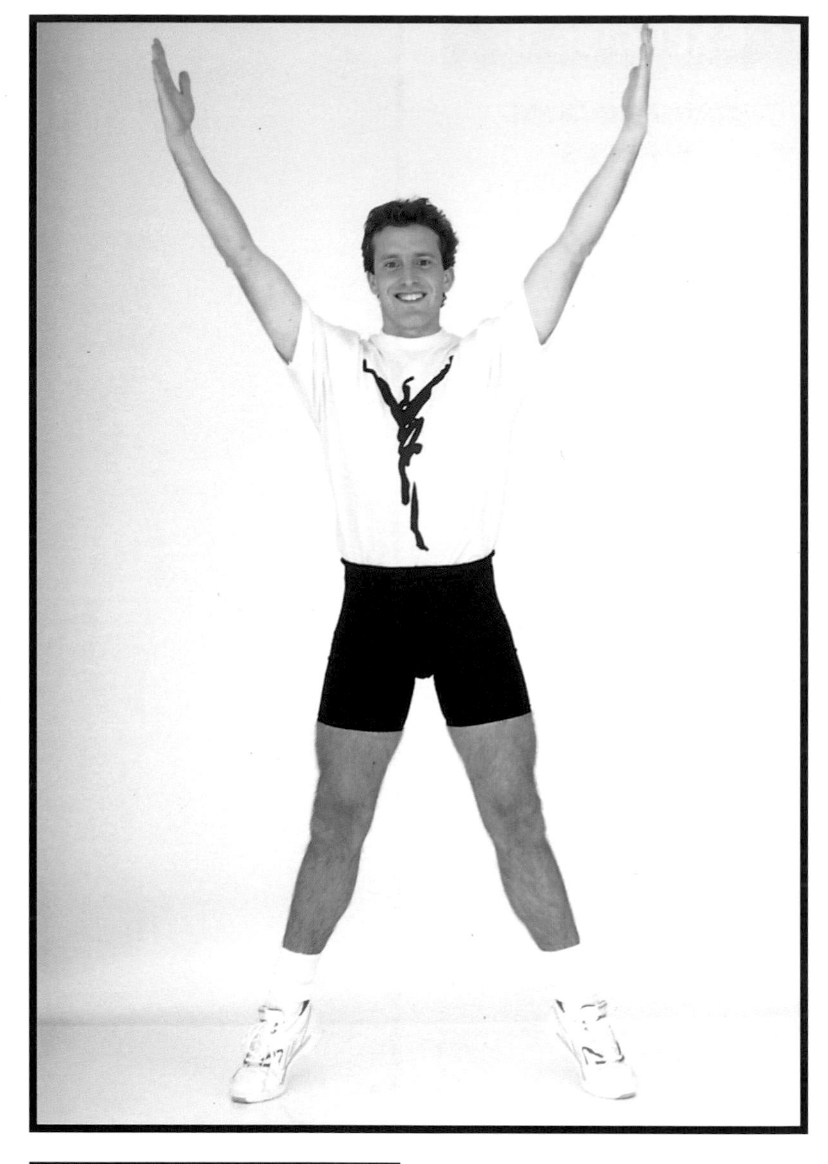

Keep your tummy pulled in tight to maintain the correct pelvic tilt

Now go back to the beginning (Exercise 1) and repeat each exercise again (the specified number of times) before moving on to the warm-up stretches that follow.

EXERCISE 8

STANDING QUAD STRETCH

PURPOSE:
To stretch the quadriceps (front of the thigh)

- Face a wall or chair for support. Transfer your weight to your left leg, bend your knee slightly and tuck your bottom under as for the pelvic tilt.

- Bring your right heel back and up towards your buttocks, and using your right hand on your ankle to assist, lift your heel towards your buttocks until you feel the stretch down the front of your thigh.

- Hold for a count of 8, then repeat, using the other leg.

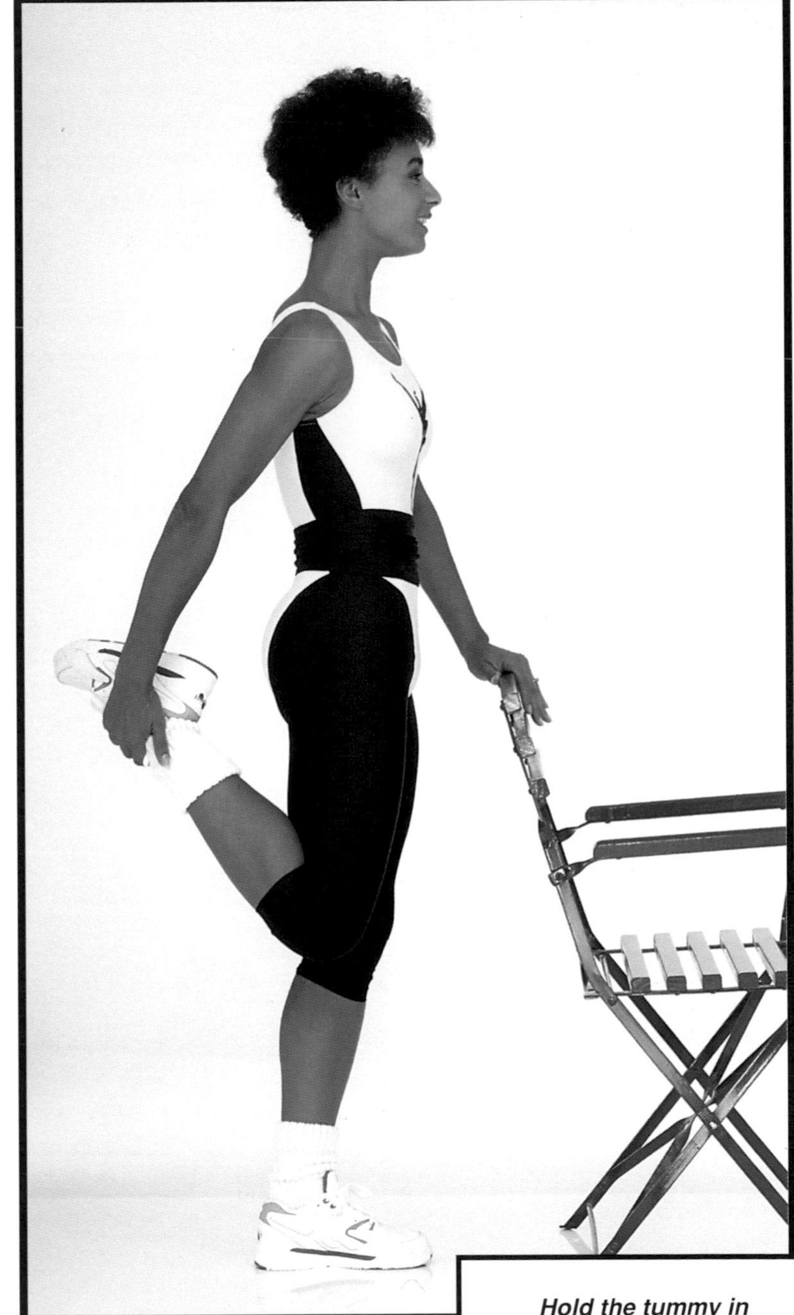

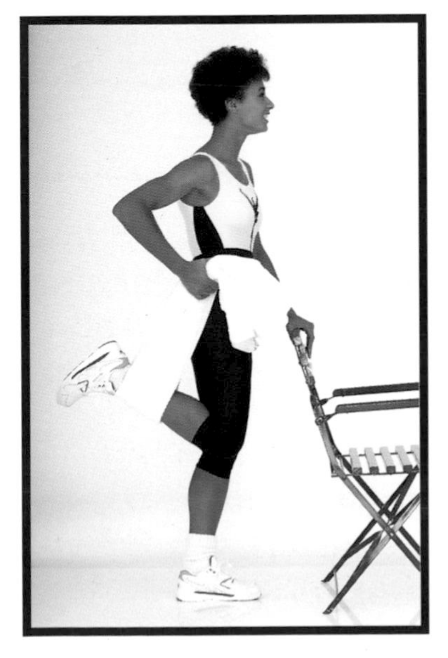

If you have difficulty reaching your ankle, try looping a towel round it and pulling on this to lift your foot up towards your buttocks.

Hold the tummy in tightly to stop the lower back arching

Keep the thighs parallel

Exercise 9

STANDING INNER THIGH STRETCH

PURPOSE:
To stretch the adductors (inner thigh)

- Stand with your feet wide apart and your toes pointing slightly out.

- Bend your left knee in line with your left foot, then slide your right leg away sideways until you feel a stretch in your inner thigh.

- Hold for a count of 8, then repeat for the other side.

If you don't feel a stretch, check that your feet are wide enough apart and your weight is evenly distributed between them.

Keep both hips facing forwards and both feet flat on the floor

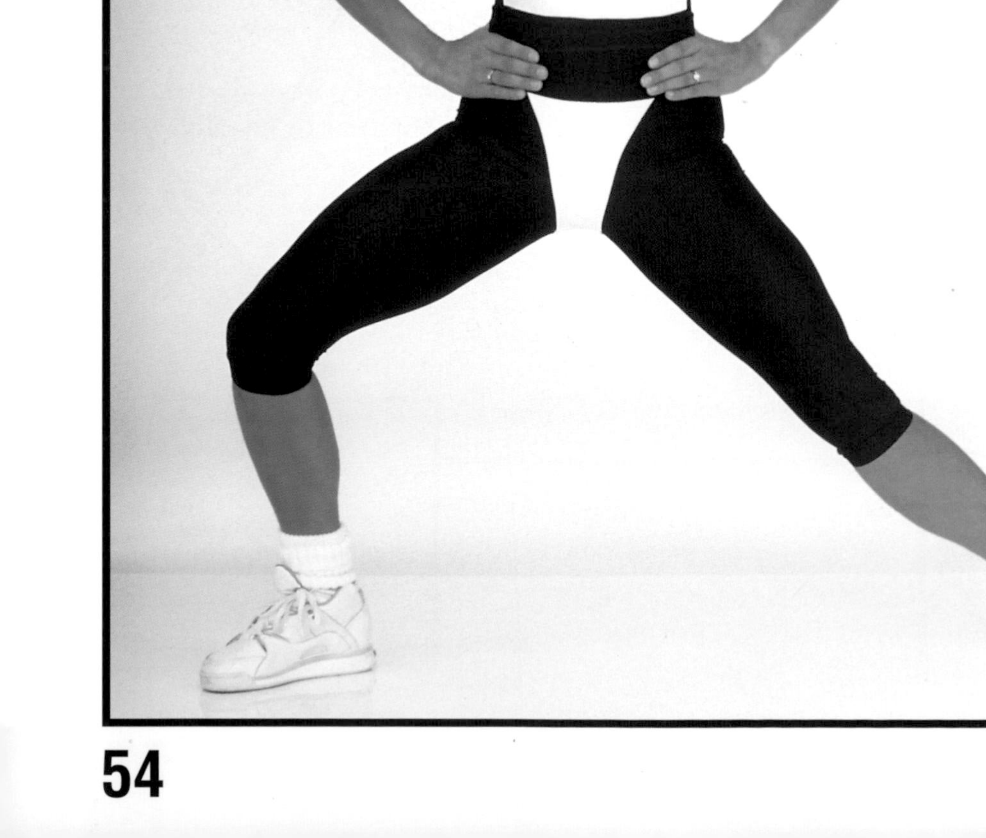

EXERCISE 10

STANDING HAMSTRING STRETCH

PURPOSE:
To stretch the hamstrings (back of the thigh)

- Stand with your legs hip-width apart and your feet parallel, your left leg slightly bent and your hands on your left thigh for support.

- Sticking your bottom backwards and pulling your shoulders back to keep your back straight, bend forwards from the hips until you feel a stretch in the back of your right leg.

- Hold for a count of 8, then repeat on the other side

If you feel a stretch in your back recheck your position. If this stretch continues to cause discomfort, try the lying hamstring stretch explained in cool-down (page 66).

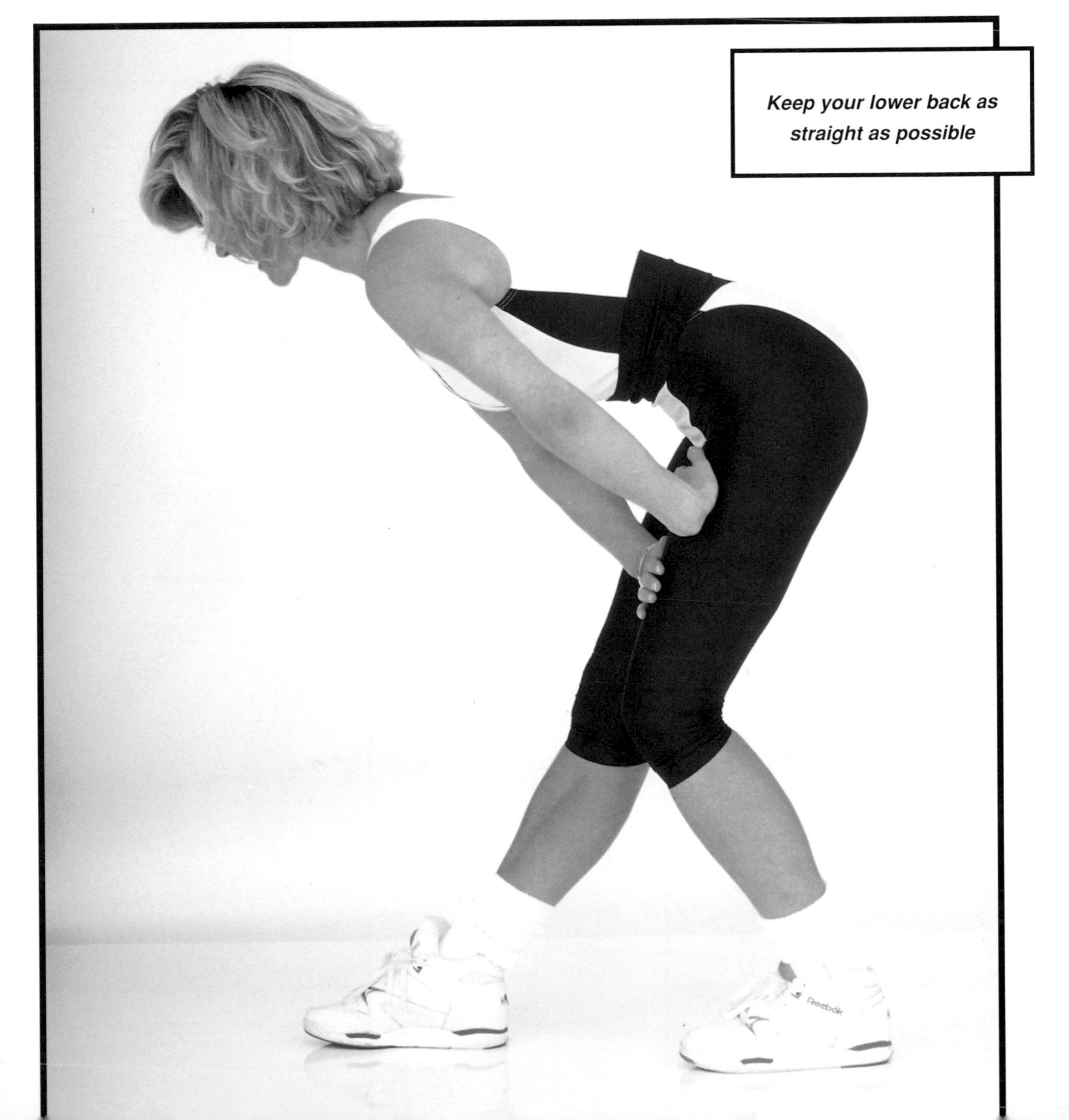

Keep your lower back as straight as possible

EXERCISE 1

STANDING SIDE LEG RAISES

REPETITIONS
3 x 6 Right 3 x 6 Left
PURPOSE:
To tone the abductors (hips)

- Holding on to a chair on your left side for support, stand with your weight on your left leg, left knee slightly bent, pelvis correctly tilted and your right hand on your hip.

- Keeping your hips still and level and squeezing your buttocks tight, slowly raise your right leg out to the side as far as possible, hold for a short moment, then close.

- Do this 6 times with the right leg, rest it and shake out.

- Repeat this twice more with the right leg, then turn round and repeat the whole exercise on the other side.

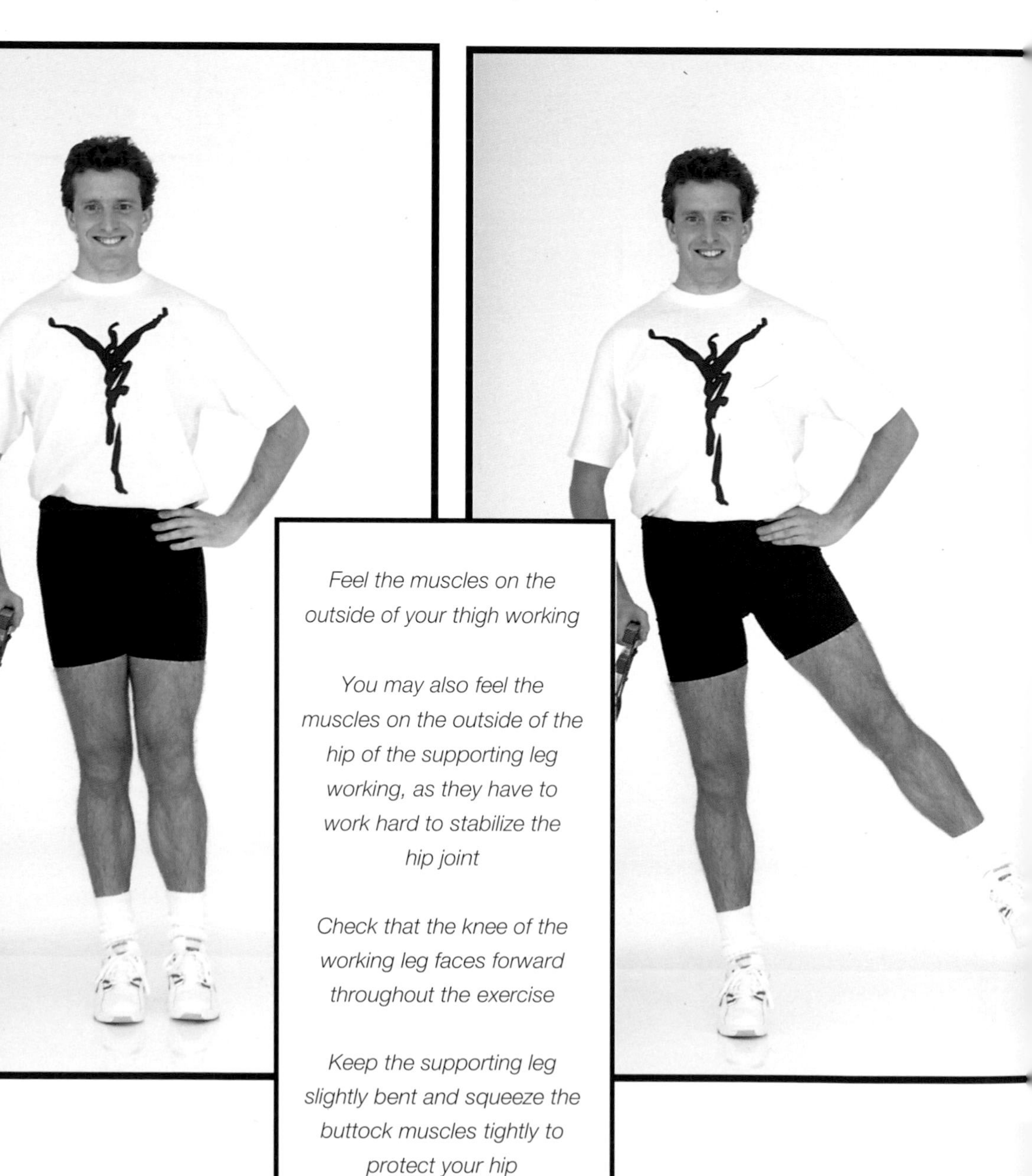

Feel the muscles on the outside of your thigh working

You may also feel the muscles on the outside of the hip of the supporting leg working, as they have to work hard to stabilize the hip joint

Check that the knee of the working leg faces forward throughout the exercise

Keep the supporting leg slightly bent and squeeze the buttock muscles tightly to protect your hip

These toning exercises are specifically for your hips and thighs. To gain the maximum benefit from them, perform each repetition with control and effort. Your muscles should ache a little by the end of each set (if they don't then it is probably because you are not doing them well enough!). If you find some of the exercises advocate too many repetitions for you to achieve comfortably at first, give your muscles a little rest when you feel they begin to ache, then continue working them again.

EXERCISE 2

STANDING REAR LEG RAISES WITH CURL

REPETITIONS
2 x 6 Right 2 x 6 Left
PURPOSE:
To tone the hamstrings (back of the thigh)

- Facing a chair, place your hands on it for stability, bend forwards very slightly from your hips, and extend one leg behind you, toes on the floor.

- Slowly raise this leg to the back, until it continues the line of your trunk then, keeping the thigh still, curl your heel in towards your buttocks, extend it and then lower it to return it to the start position.

- Do this 6 times, rest and repeat again with the same leg. Repeat whole exercise with the other leg.

Feel the muscles at the back of your thigh and your buttocks working

Keep your hips level and your tummy pulled in to keep your pelvis correctly tilted

To make the exercise harder squeeze your heel in towards your buttocks on the curl and check that your thigh is held as far back as is comfortable

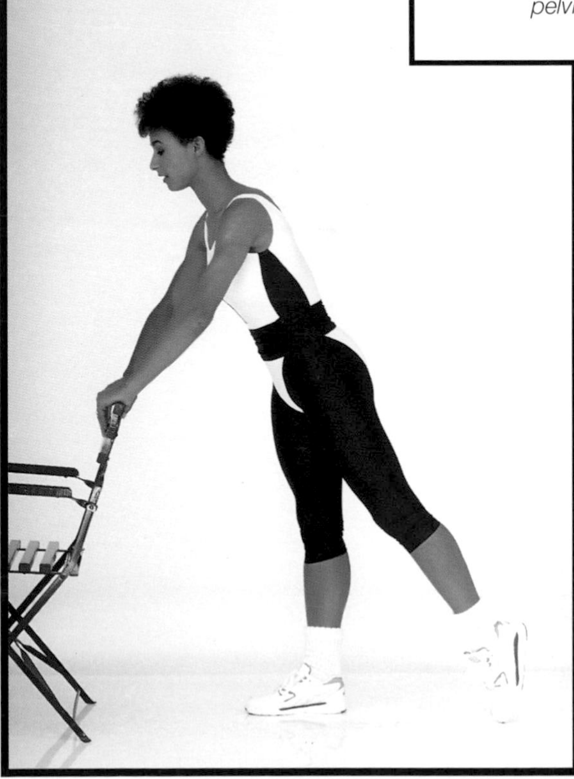

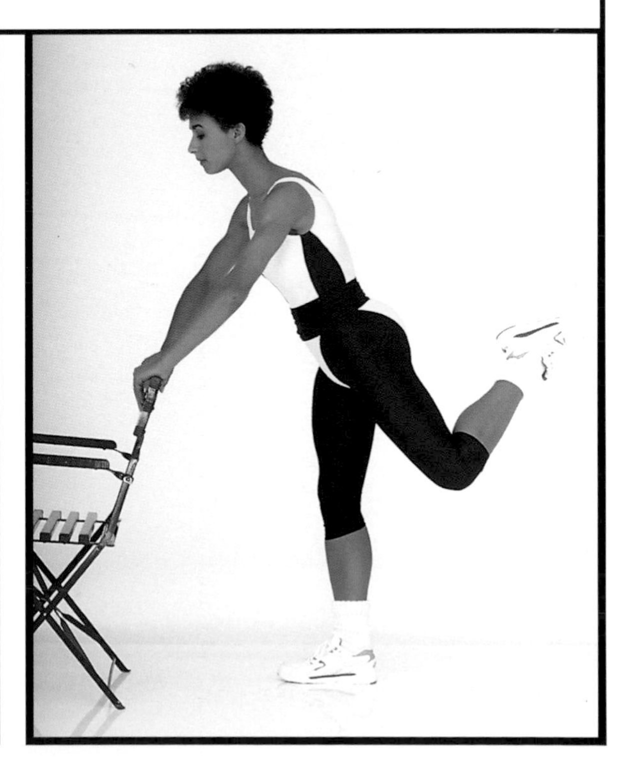

Exercise 3

HEEL RAISES

REPETITIONS *6*
PURPOSE:
To tone the calf muscles (back of the lower leg)

- Stand tall with your feet hip-width apart and parallel, one hand on a support if you need it.
- Raise up onto your toes then lower to the start.
- Do this exercise 6 times.

Feel your calf muscles working

Keep your weight over the ball of your foot, not out towards your little toe

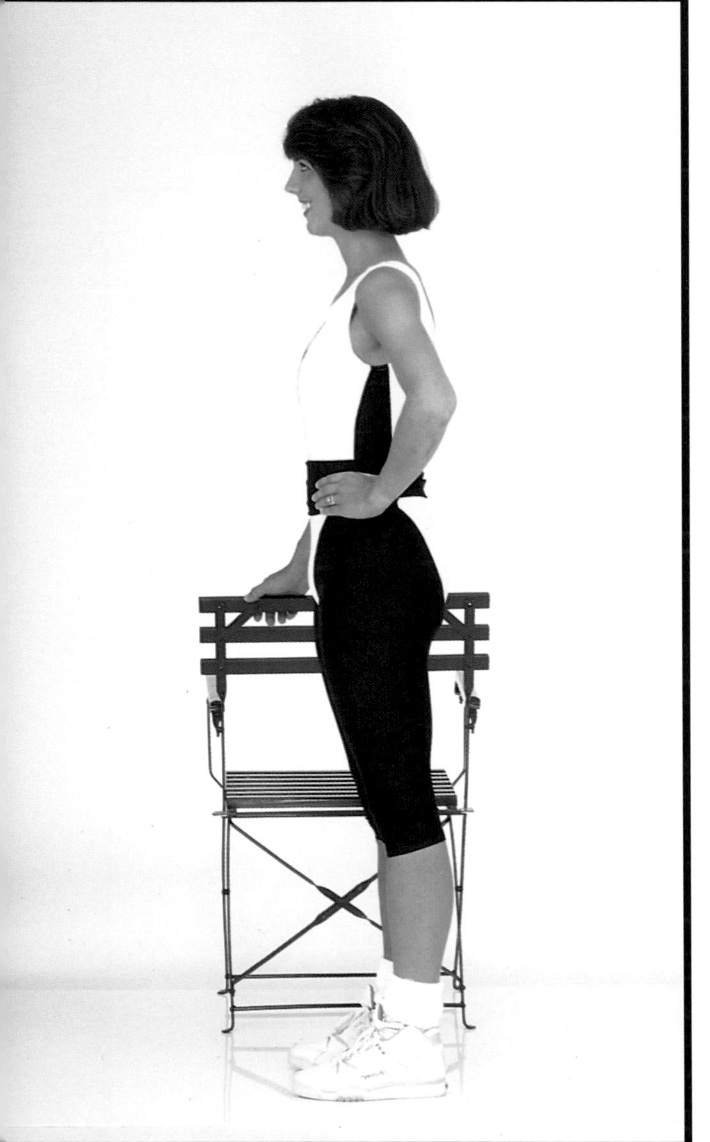

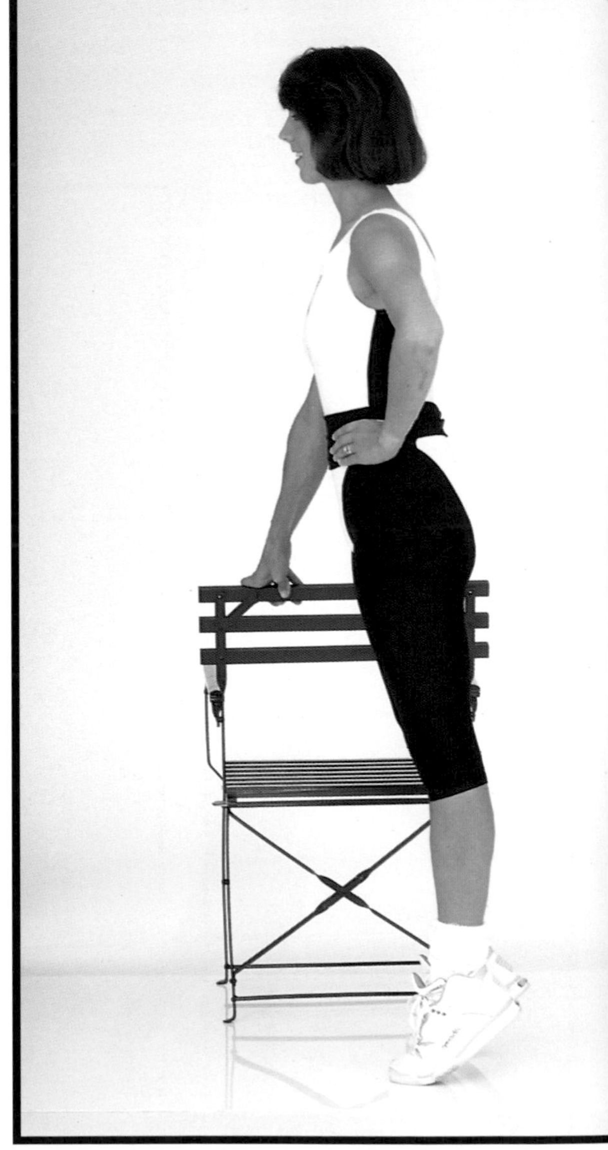

EXERCISE 4

ALTERNATING KNEE LIFTS

REPETITIONS *8*
PURPOSE:
To tone the quadriceps and hip flexors (front of thigh)

- Stand side on to a support, hand on for stability. Your feet should be hip-width apart and your posture correct.
- Keeping the supporting leg slightly bent, lift one knee up towards your chest then lower. Repeat with the other leg.
- Do this alternating the legs 4 times.

Feel the muscles at the top of your thighs working

Keep your back upright and still

To make the exercise harder, as you lift your knee, try to squeeze it right up towards your chest

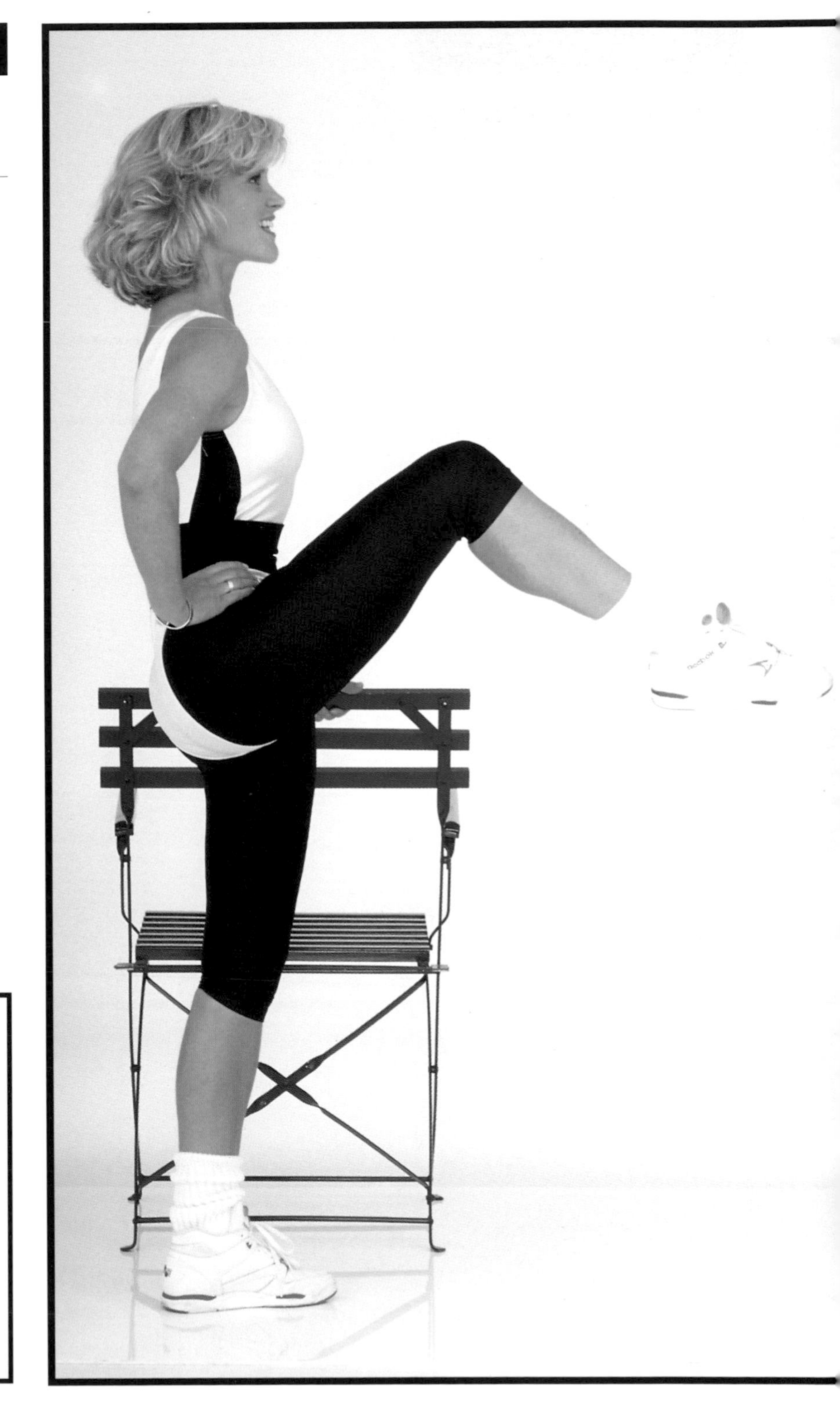

Level 1a Hips and Thighs

EXERCISE 5

STRAIGHT LEG RAISES ON ELBOWS

REPETITIONS
8 Right 8 Left
PURPOSE:
To tone the quadriceps and hip flexors (front of the thigh)

- Lie on your back propped up on your elbows, one knee bent and one leg straight.
- Tilt your pelvis, feeling the lower back pushing into the floor.
- Raise the straight leg up to the height of the bent knee so the thighs are parallel, then lower.
- Do 8 times. Repeat with other leg.

Feel the thigh muscle of the straight leg working

Keep your lower back pressed into the floor throughout the exercise

Check the leg is firm and straight throughout the movement

Don't let your back or bottom rock

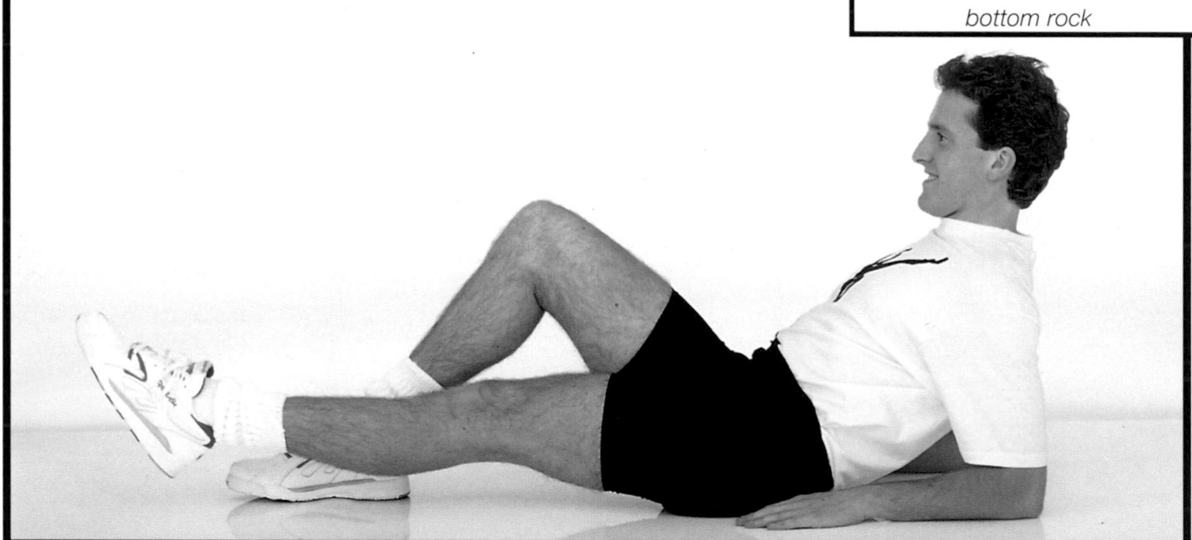

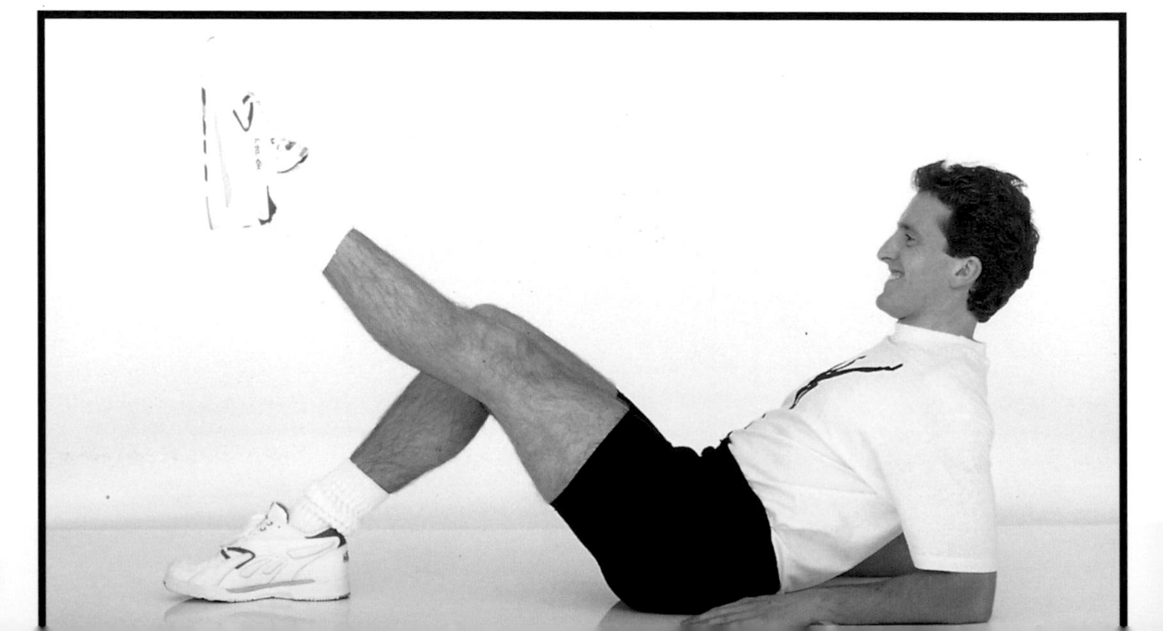

EXERCISE 6

KNEE CROSSES

REPETITIONS *2 x 12*
PURPOSE:
To tone the adductors (inner thigh)

- Lie flat on your back or propped up on your elbows with your knees slightly bent and up over your tummy.

- Keeping one knee firmly over your trunk, cross your knees by taking one in front of the other and squeezing your thighs together.

- Uncross your knees and then cross them again taking the other one back this time.

- Do this 12 times in total, rest then repeat 12 more times.

Feel the inner thigh muscles working

Check your knees stay over your tummy throughout the exercise

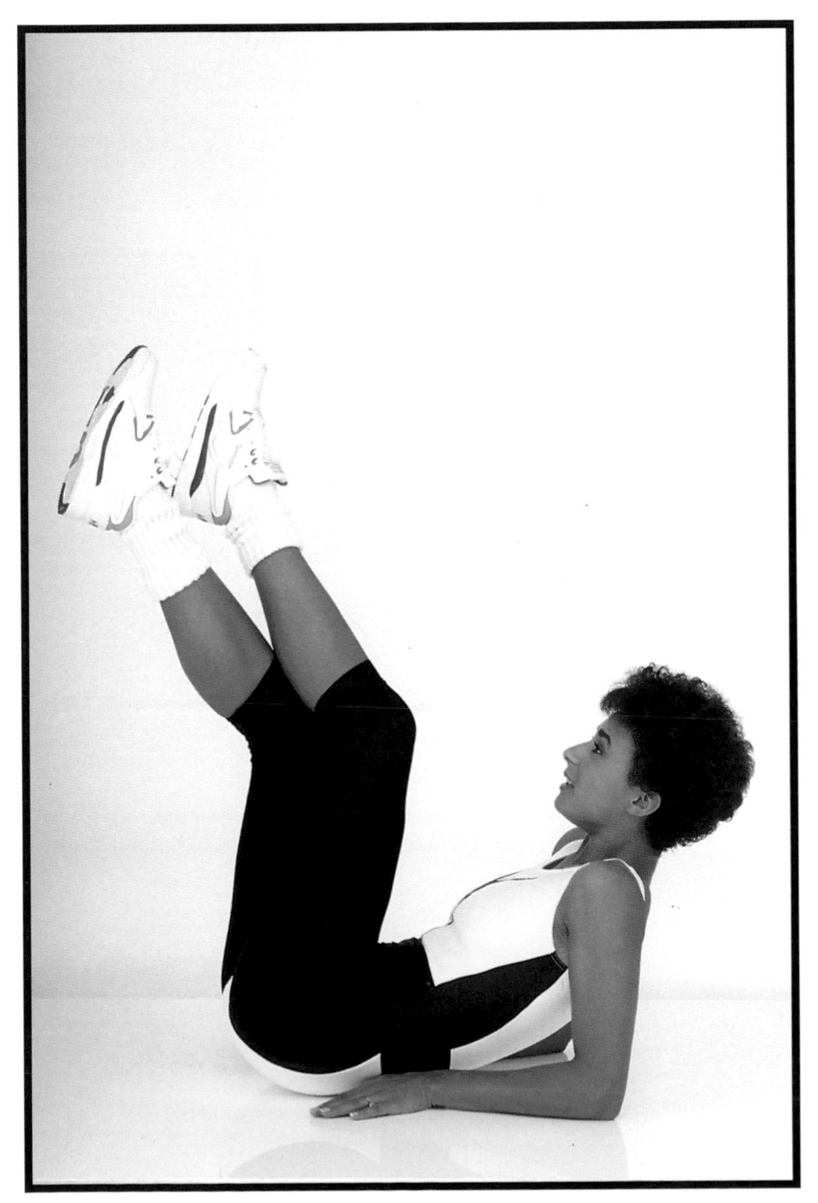

You may find it easier and more comfortable to maintain the correct position for your legs if you lie flat on your back rather than propped up on your elbows.

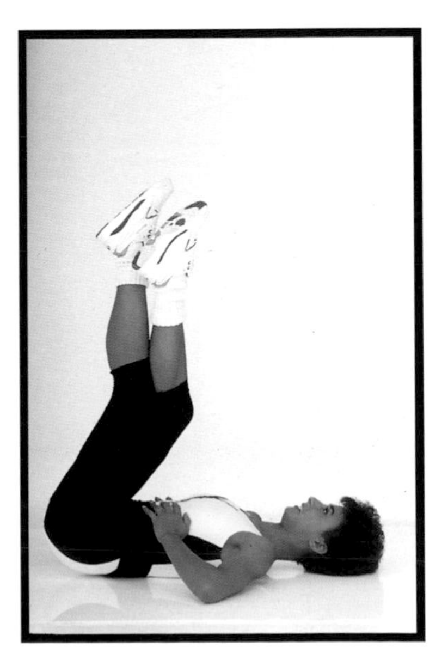

Exercise 7

LEG EXTENSIONS ON ELBOWS

REPETITIONS
4 Right 4 Left
PURPOSE:
To tone the quadriceps and hip flexors (front of the thigh)

- Lie on your back propped up on your elbows, lower back pressed into the floor, left leg bent, foot flat on the floor and the right leg held straight out in front parallel with the thigh of other leg.

- Bend the right leg in towards your chest then gently extend it forwards and out until the knees are level and the thighs parallel.

- Do this 4 times then repeat using the other leg.

Feel the thigh muscles working

Keep your lower back pressed into the floor throughout the exercise

To make the exercise harder, tense the thigh muscles as you extend the leg

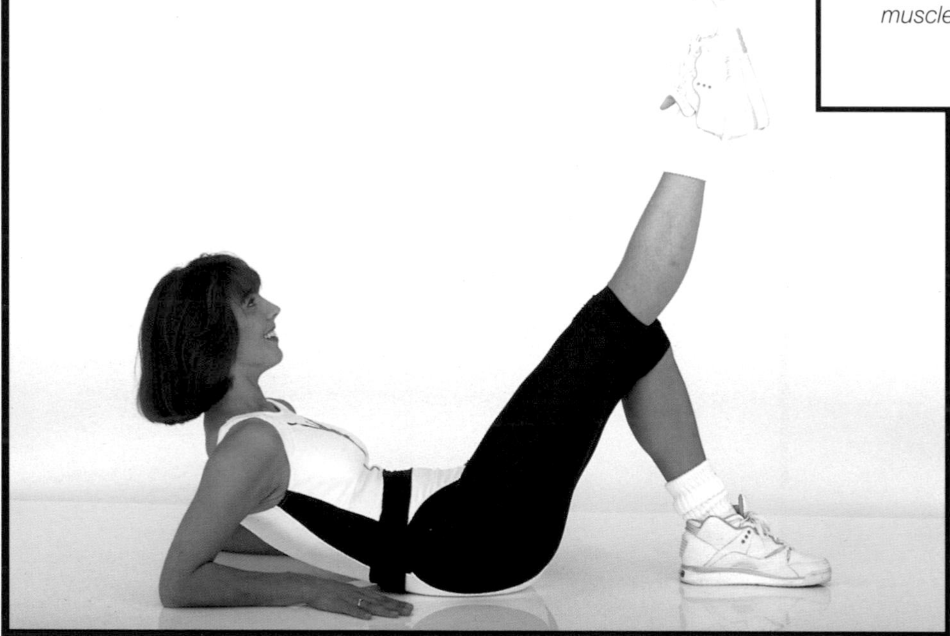

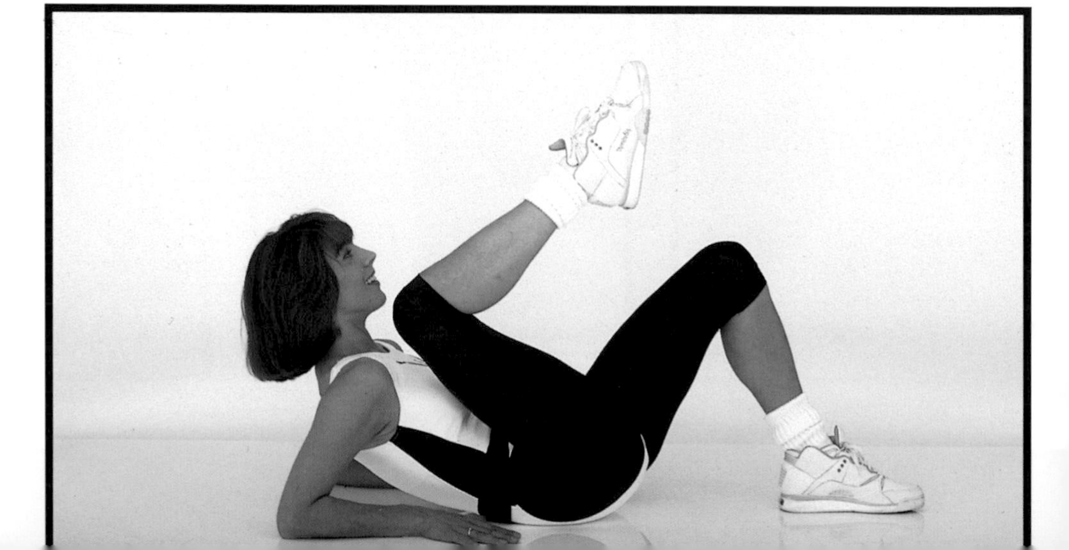

Exercise 8

KNEE SQUEEZES

REPETITIONS *8*
PURPOSE:
To tone the adductors (inner thighs)

- Sit up with your knees bent and together - you can rest back on your hands for comfort.
- Squeeze your knees together with as much effort as possible and hold for a count of one, relax.
- Do this 8 times.

Feel the muscles of your inner thighs working

Keep breathing throughout the movement

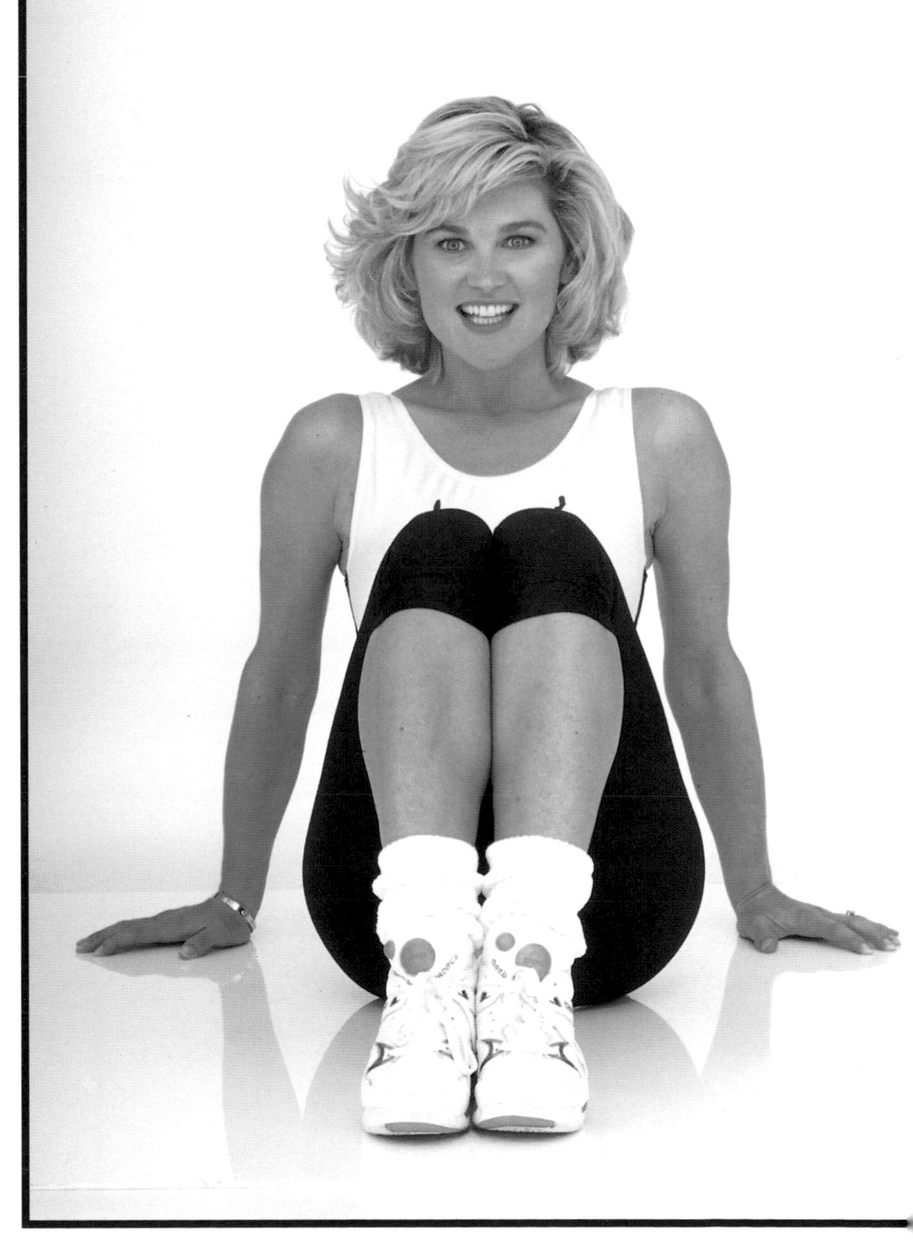

You may find it more comfortable to place a cushion or something else padded and soft between your knees.

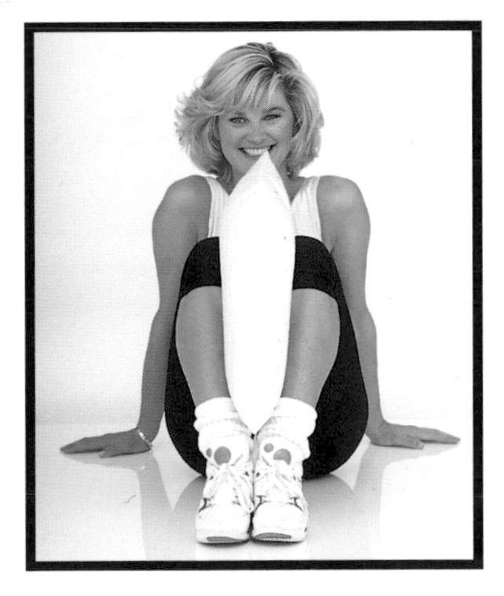

Level 1a Hips and Thighs

These cool-down stretches are aimed to relax the hip and thigh muscles that you have just been working and also to improve the suppleness in your hip joints (an area in which most people are too stiff). Refer to page 29 for a reminder of how to improve suppleness.

Keep breathing throughout the stretch and ensure that you are comfortable in all the stretches. If not relax and start again, checking your position carefully. Ease into the stretches gently and develop them to improve flexibility.

EXERCISE 1

SEATED INNER THIGH STRETCH

PURPOSE:
To stretch the adductors (inner thighs)

- Sit on the floor with your legs bent and the soles of your feet together, holding an ankle with each hand and the feet as close to your body as possible, allowing your knees to flop apart.
- Use your elbows to press your knees towards the floor until you feel a stretch in the inner thigh.
- Hold for a count of 16, relaxing the muscles to develop the stretch.

Keep your back as straight as possible

Keep your shoulders down and relax your body in general

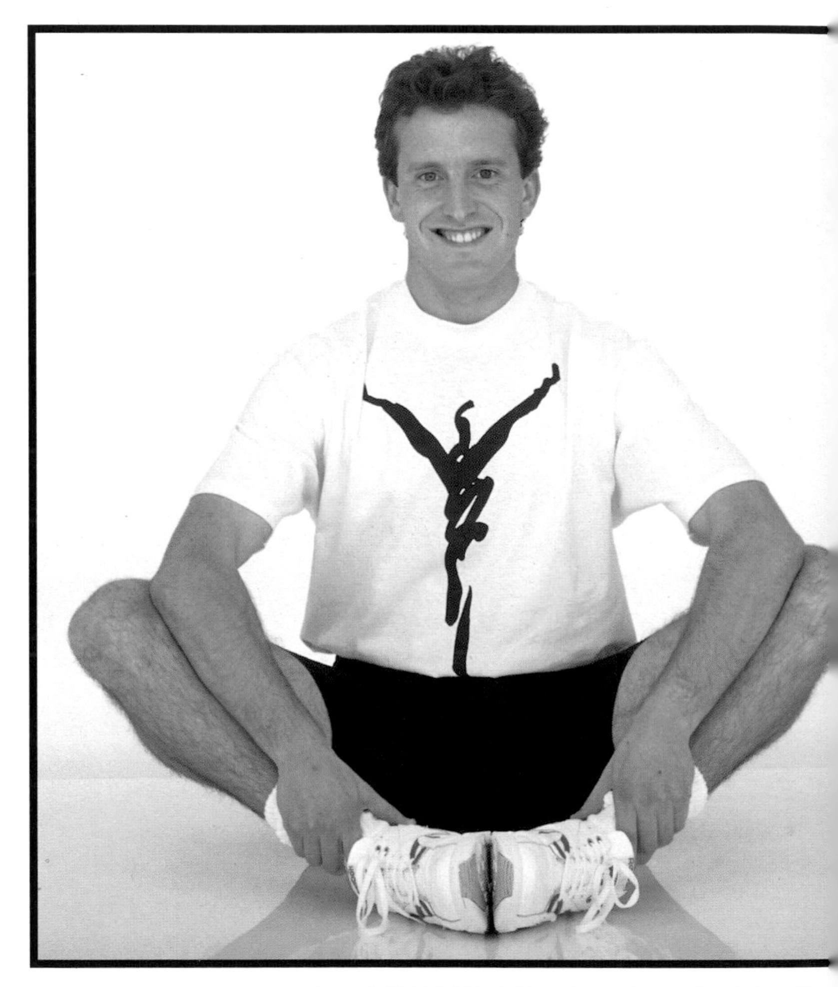

You may find it more comfortable to rest on your hands to support your back. Let the weight of your legs bring about the stretch.

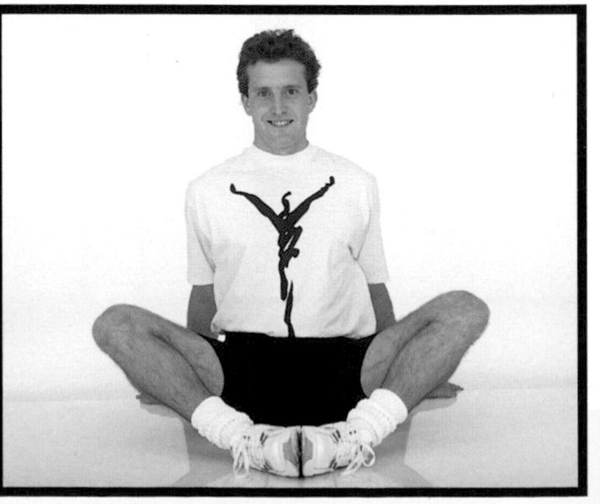

EXERCISE 2

SEATED BUTTOCK TWIST

PURPOSE:
To stretch the abductors (hips)

- Sit up tall with your left leg extended in front of you along the floor. Bend your right leg, take it over your left leg and place your right foot flat on the floor to the outside of your left leg.

- Sitting up tall and clasping the bent knee with your hands, pull it in towards your chest as you twist your body to the right until you feel the stretch in your right buttock.

- Hold this for a count of 8, then repeat on the other side.

Keep your back straight and sit up out of your hips

Feel the muscles below your shoulder blade working to assist the twist

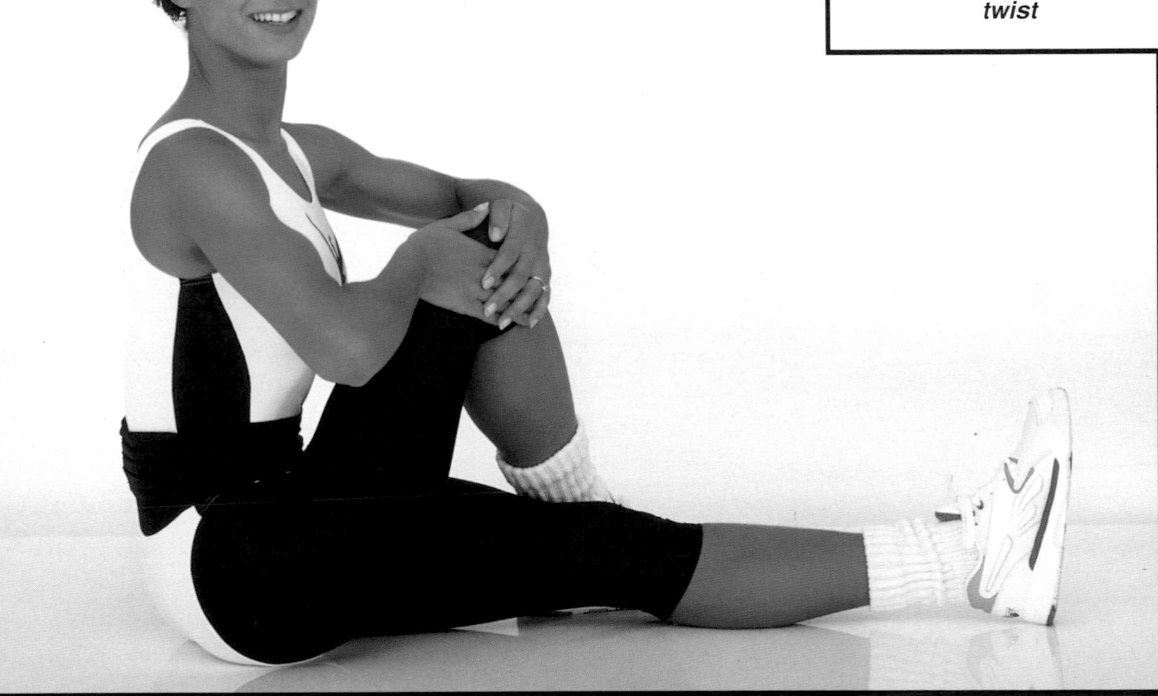

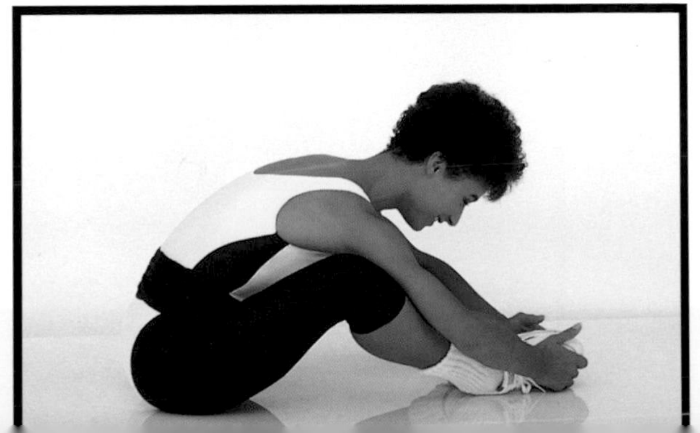

If you find this exercise uncomfortable, place the soles of your feet together and a little way out in front of you, knees apart, then lean forward to stretch the buttocks.

EXERCISE 3

LYING HAMSTRING STRETCH

PURPOSE:
To stretch the hamstrings (back of the thigh)

- Lie on your back with one leg bent and foot flat on the floor for stability.
- Bend the other leg into your chest and place your hands around the back of the lower leg.
- Keeping the knee still, very gently raise the lower leg until you feel a stretch down the back of that leg.
- Hold for a count of 16, relaxing the muscles and trying to develop the stretch. Repeat with other leg.

Relax your head and shoulders and keep the base of your spine on the floor

Keep your body straight, don't allow it to twist

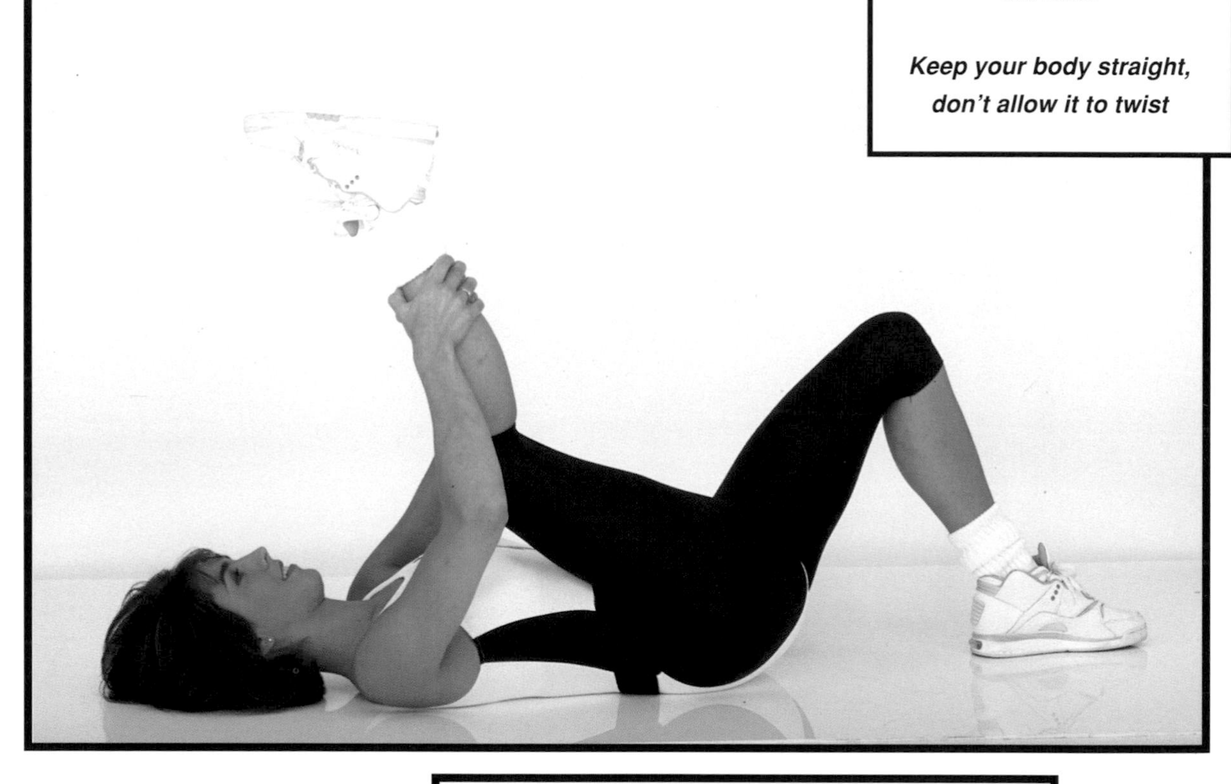

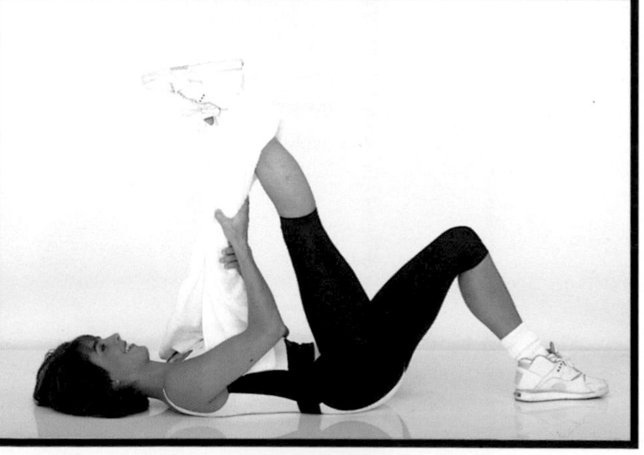

You may find it more comfortable to keep the leg straight and use a towel looped around the ankle to assist the stretch.

EXERCISE 4

SIDE LYING QUAD STRETCH

PURPOSE:
To stretch the quadriceps (front of the thigh)

- Lie on your left side with your head resting in your left hand and bend your left leg for balance, keeping the thigh in a straight line with your trunk.

- Keeping your thighs parallel and your pelvis correctly tilted, bend your right leg and clasp your ankle with the right hand. Gently ease the heel in towards your buttock until you feel a stretch down the front of the thigh.

- Hold for a count of 16, trying to relax your muscles and develop the stretch. Roll over and repeat with the other leg.

Take care not to twist or hollow your back

If your knee feels uncomfortable try pushing against your hand with your foot as you stretch the thigh

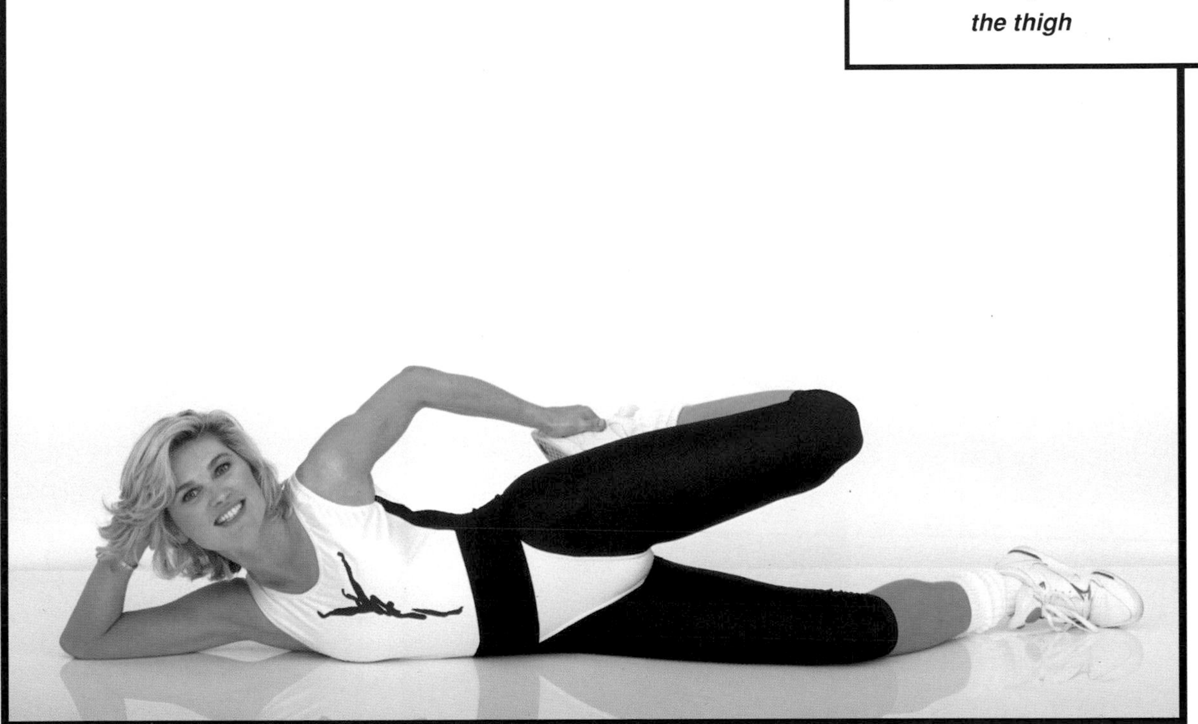

If you have difficulty with this exercise, try it lying flat on your front and perhaps use a towel looped around your ankle to assist the stretch.

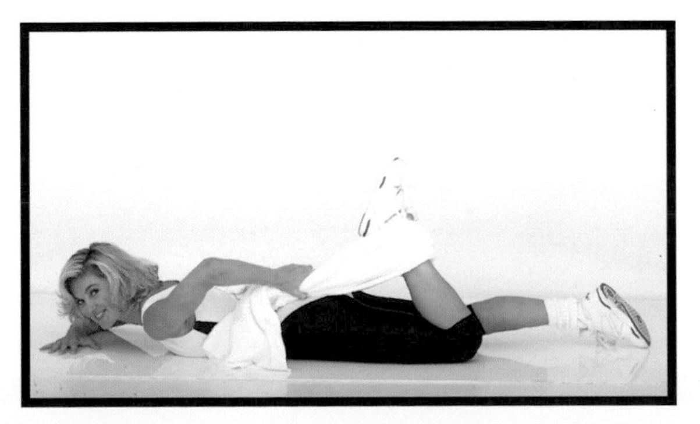

Level 1b Tums, Bums & Arms

Try to develop a rhythm for these warm-up exercises, so that as they become familiar to you they will become even more effective in warming and loosening your muscles. The stretches are aimed at preparing the muscles and joints for the tums, bums and arms workout that follows.

EXERCISE 1

TAP LEG OUTS

REPETITIONS
2 x 4 Right, 2 x 4 Left
PURPOSE:
To warm the muscles

- Standing with your weight on your left leg, your left knee slightly out and your right leg extended to the side, bend slightly forwards from the hips and extend your arms down but slightly out to the sides.

- Keeping your weight over your left leg, bring the right leg in to tap the foot on the floor next to the left foot and at the same time swing your arms to cross in front of your body.

- Do this 4 times with the right and left leg and then repeat.

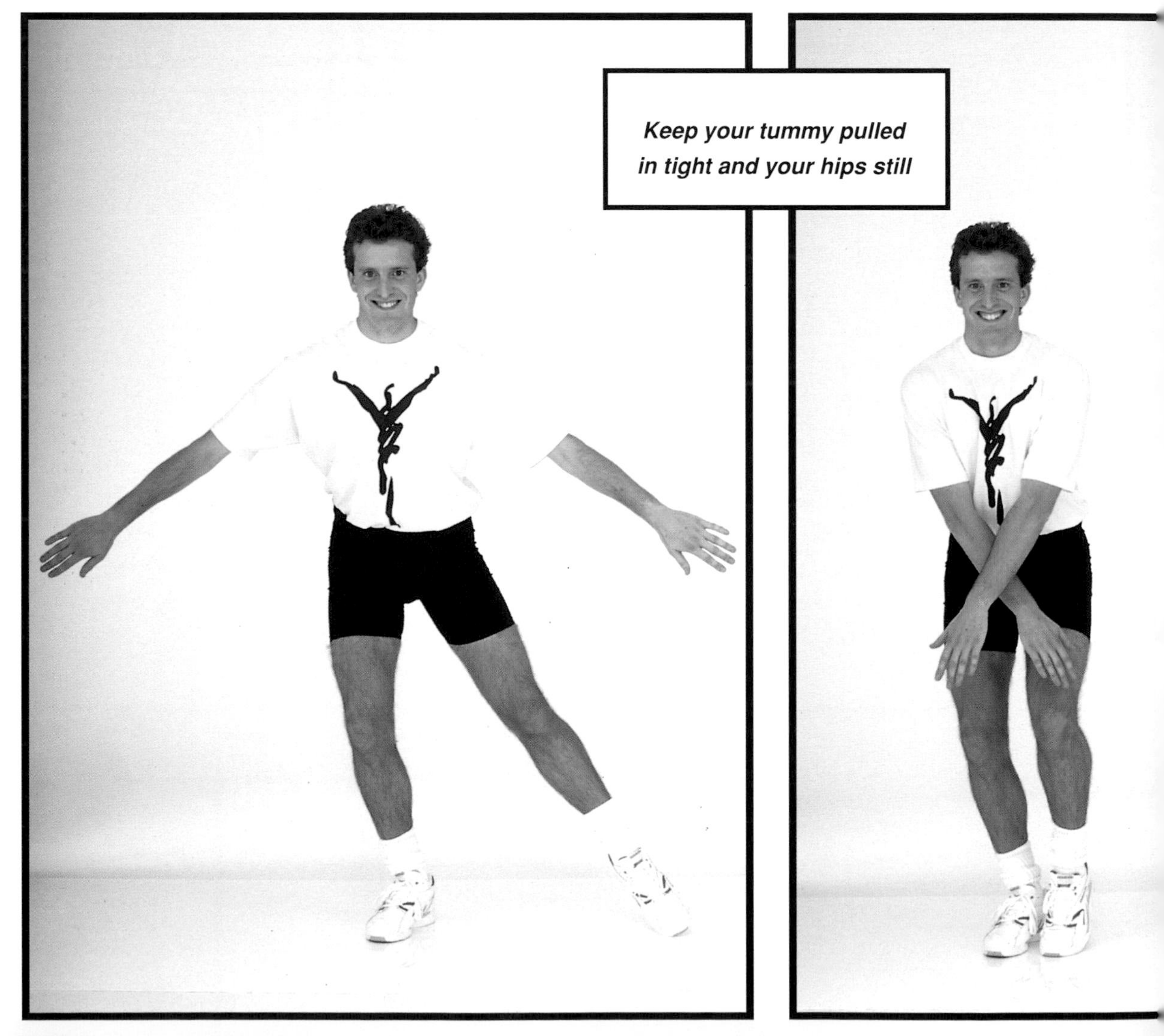

Keep your tummy pulled in tight and your hips still

EXERCISE 2

SIDE SPRINGS

REPETITIONS *8*
PURPOSE:
To warm the muscles

- Stand with your feet together and your arms held up in front of you, elbows bent and fists towards the ceiling.

- With a slight spring and transferring your weight, step out sideways on to your right leg, at the same time open your arms out to the side. Having arrived there and absorbed the movement with a slight knee bend, immediately return to the start position with feet together again.

- Repeat this stepping to the left, then continue until you have done 8 in total.

Keep your knees in line with your feet every time they bend

Find a rhythm for the exercise that suits you

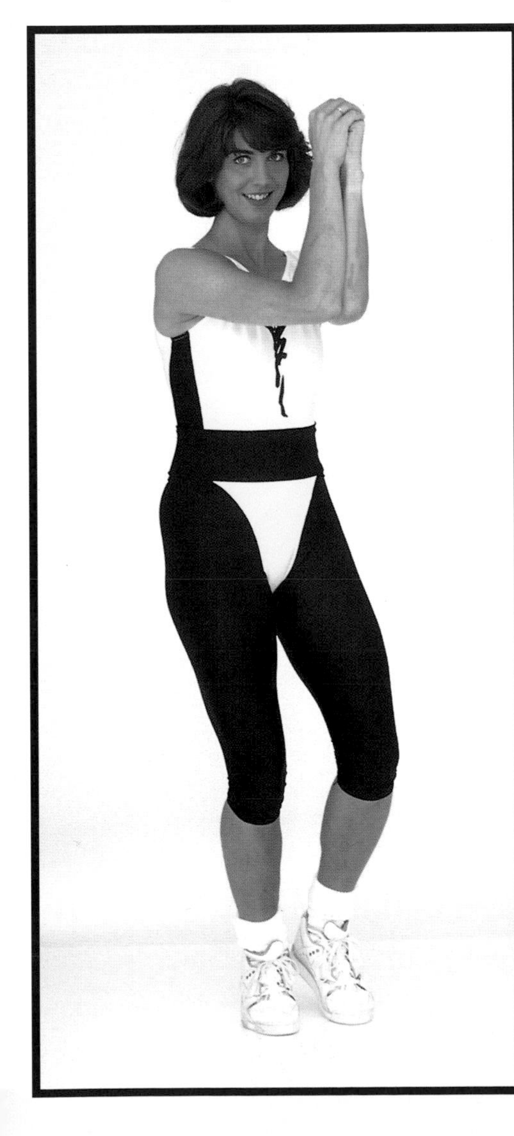

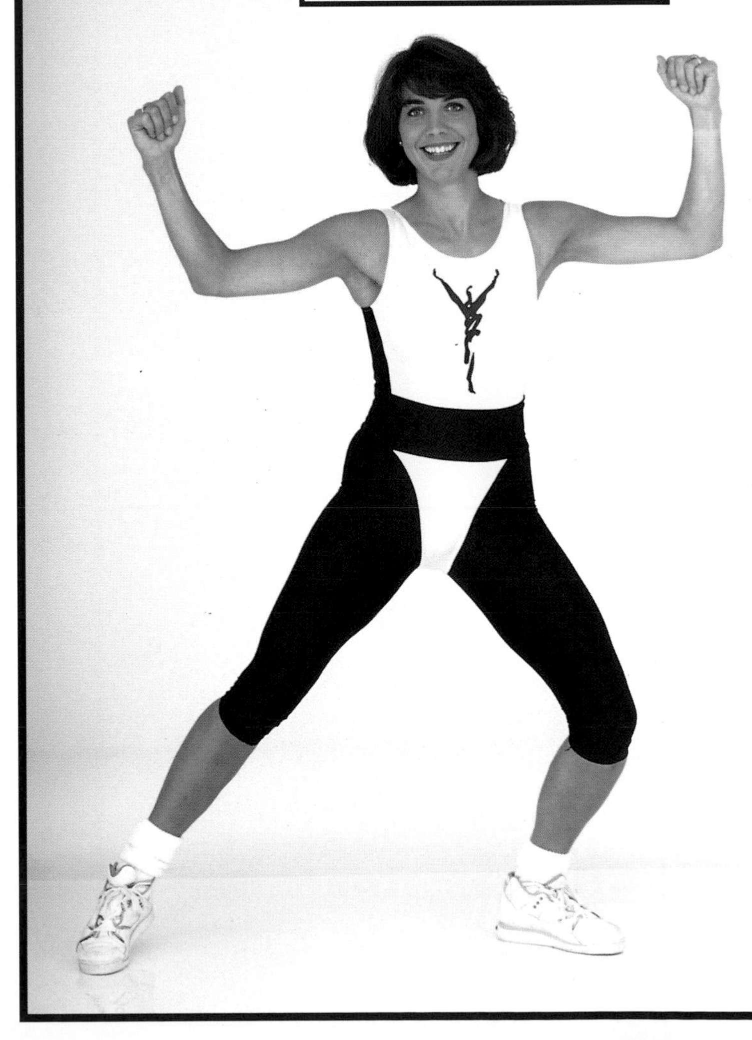

EXERCISE 3

KNEE LIFTS WITH ARM PULL DOWN

REPETITIONS *8*
PURPOSE:
To warm the muscles and mobilize the hip joints

- Stand tall with good posture, your feet hip-width apart and your arms extended above your head.
- Lift one knee up towards your chest and at the same time bend your arms and pull them down to an open position at the side. Lower your foot to the floor and extend the arms up again.
- Repeat, using the other leg and then continue until you have done 8 knee raises in total.

Hold your tummy muscles in tightly to stabilize your lower back

Keep the supporting leg straight as you lift the other knee

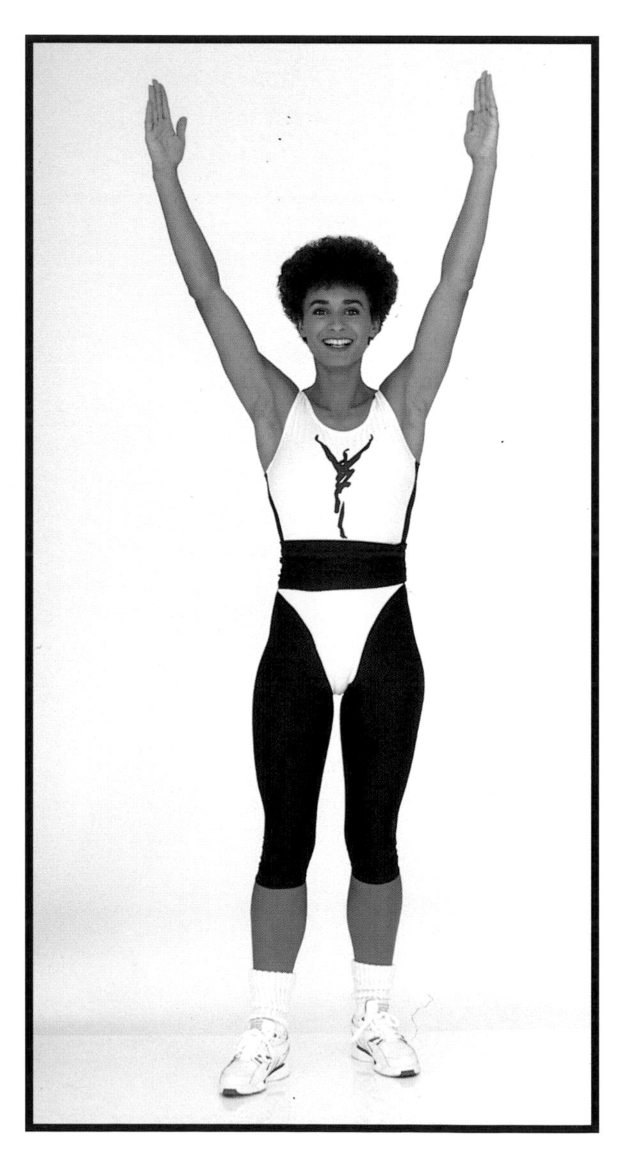

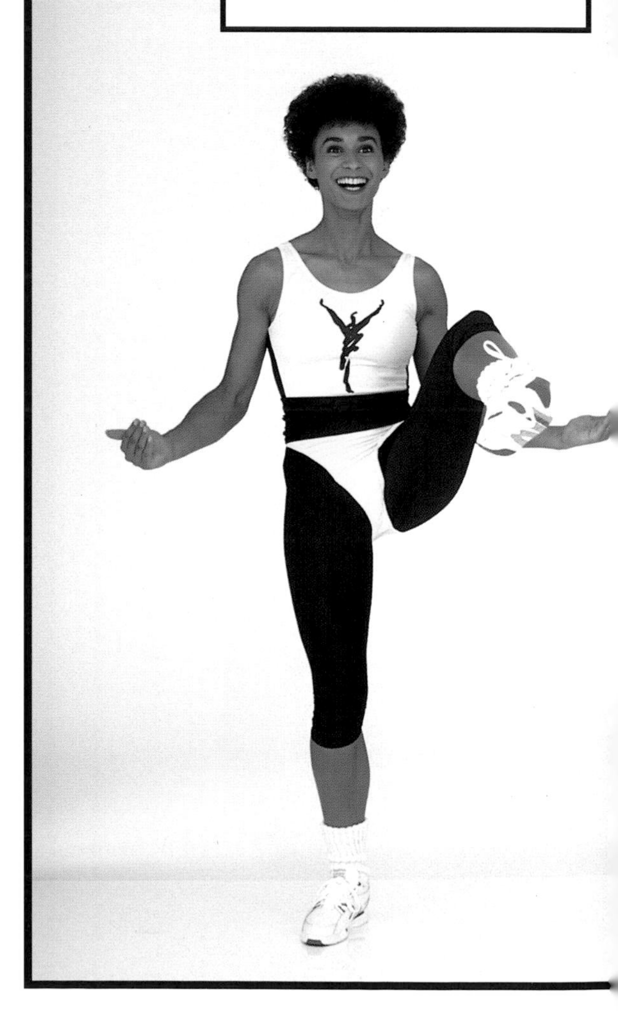

EXERCISE 4

REACHES

REPETITIONS *4*
PURPOSE:
To loosen the sides of the body and warm the muscles

- Stand with your feet shoulder-width apart and a good pelvic tilt.
- Extend your right arm above your head and reach for the ceiling. Drop your left shoulder and ease up with your right hand until you feel a full extension down your right side.
- Relax, then repeat to the other side. Do the whole exercise once more.

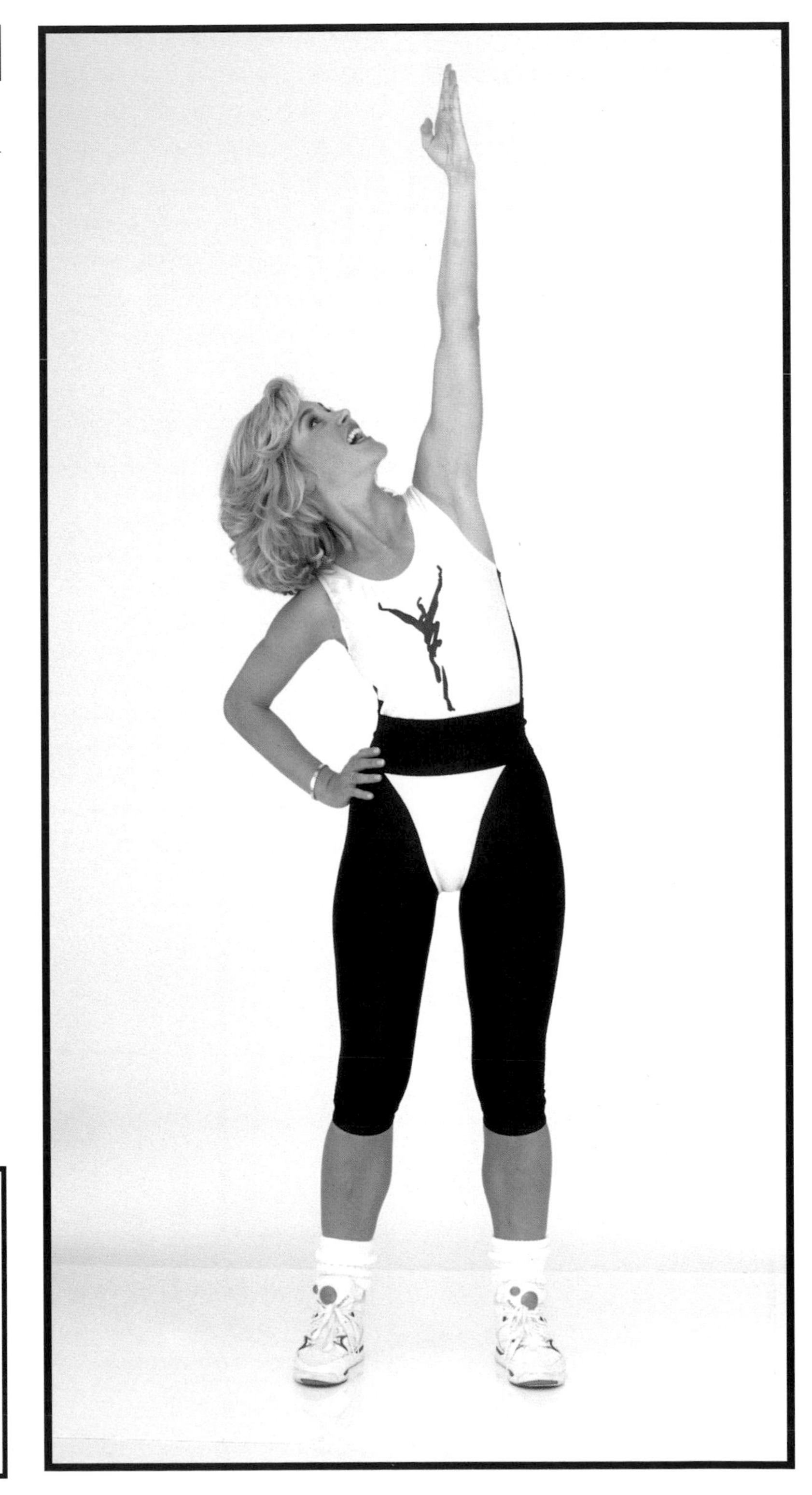

Look up towards your hand and take a deep breath in as you reach up

Check that you don't twist or bend to the side

EXERCISE 5

STANDING PELVIC TILTS

REPETITIONS 4
PURPOSE:
To mobilize the lower back

- Stand with your feet shoulder-width apart, toes pointing very slightly outwards, knees slightly bent and your hands on your hips.

- Tilt your pelvis forwards by pulling in your tummy muscles as much as you can, and, rounding your back slightly as you tuck your buttocks under, feel your lower back extend.

- Then tilt your pelvis backwards by relaxing your tummy muscles and tightening your lower back muscles, trying to hollow your back very gently and slowly.

- Do the whole exercise 4 times.

If your back feels uncomfortable you may find it better to miss out the backwards pelvic tilt and return to the start position instead.

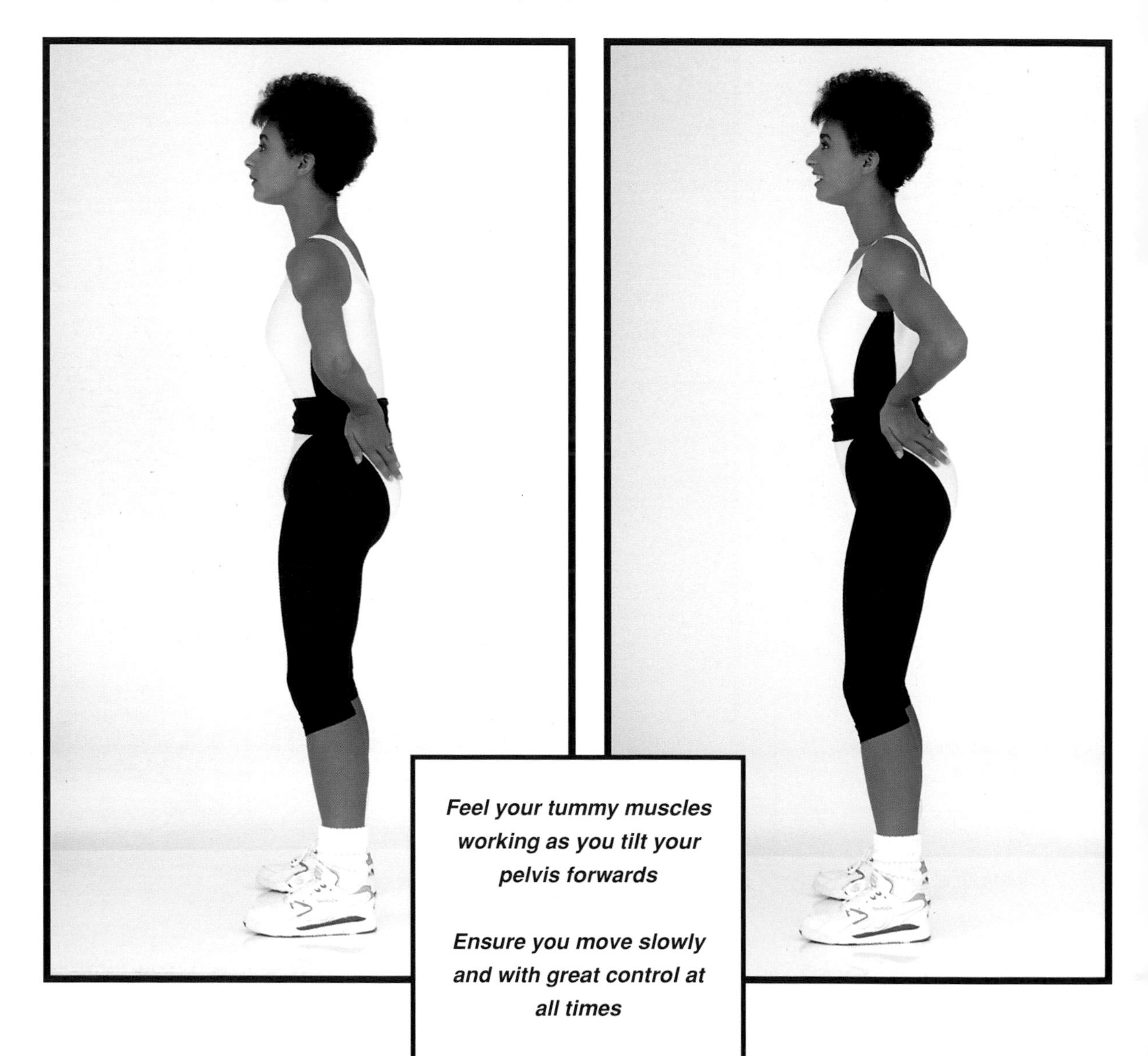

Feel your tummy muscles working as you tilt your pelvis forwards

Ensure you move slowly and with great control at all times

EXERCISE 6

STANDING HOLLOW AND HUMPS

REPETITIONS *4*
PURPOSE:
To mobilize the lower back

- Stand with your feet shoulder-width apart and your legs slightly bent. Bend slightly forwards from the hips, rest your hands on your thighs and lean on them.

- As in the pelvic tilts opposite, pull in your tummy muscles and tuck your bottom under as you slowly tilt your pelvis forwards and round your back.

- Relax and slowly hollow your back, sticking your bottom out.

- Do this whole exercise 4 times.

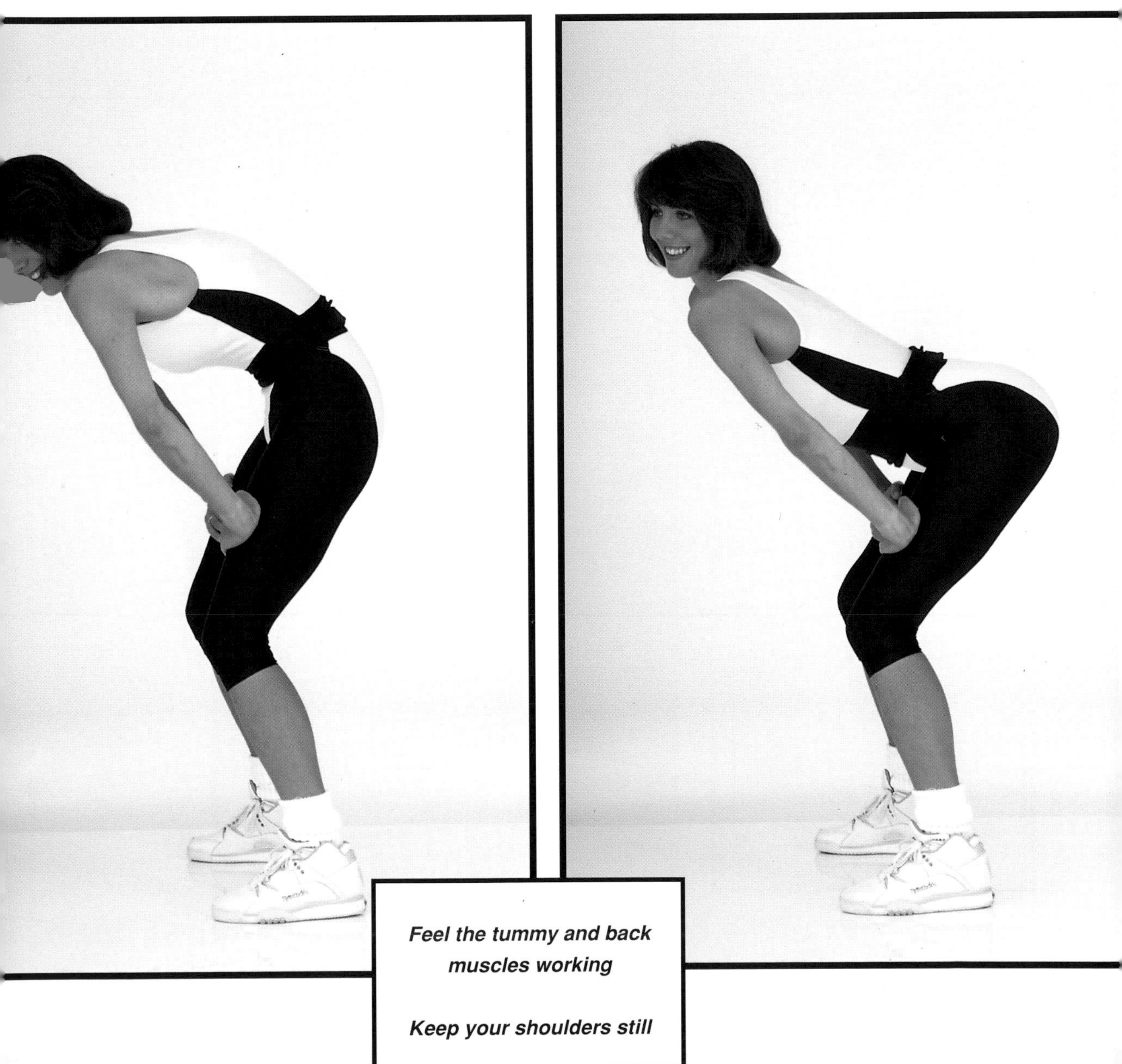

Feel the tummy and back muscles working

Keep your shoulders still

EXERCISE 7

ARM CIRCLES ACROSS BODY

REPETITIONS
2 Right 2 Left
PURPOSE:
To mobilize the shoulder joints

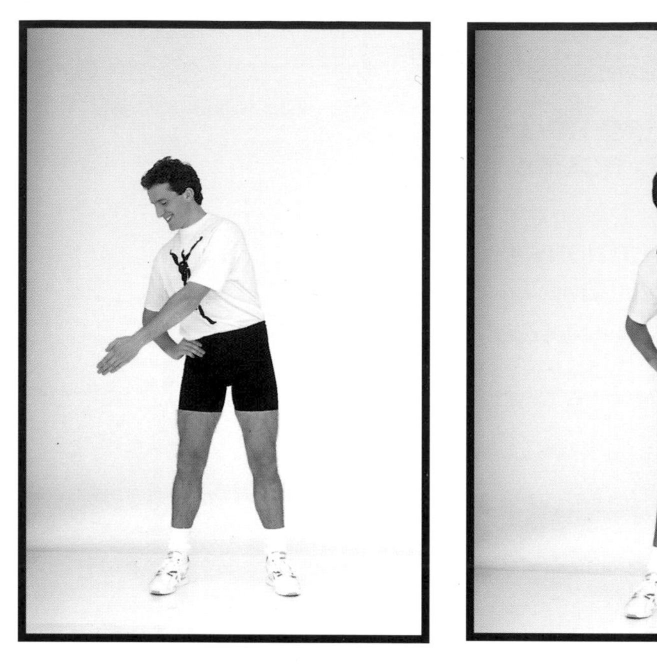

- Stand with your feet shoulder-width apart and good centre control.
- Circle your right arm across your body keeping it as straight as possible and drawing an imaginary circle as large as possible with your longest finger.
- Do this twice with the right arm and then repeat with the left arm.

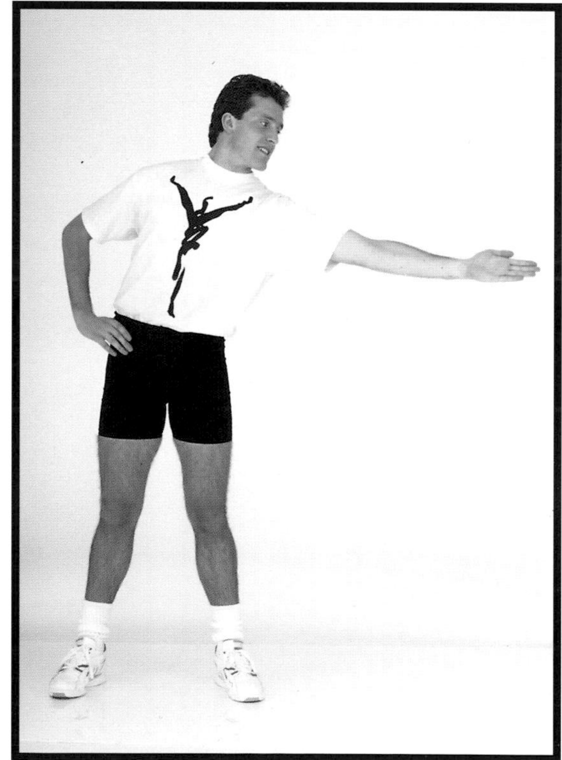

Feel the movement loosening your shoulder joint

Keep your hips and shoulders facing forwards

Now go back to the beginning and repeat each exercise again, before moving on to the following warm-up stretches.

Exercise 8

SIDE STRETCH

REPETITIONS
1 Left 1 Right
PURPOSE:
To stretch the obliques (waist muscles)

- Stand with your feet shoulder-width apart or a little wider, knees slightly bent and your left hand on your left hip for support. Reach up to the ceiling with your right arm.

- Tilt your pelvis to straighten your lower back then breathing out, bend sideways to the left, reaching up and over with the extended arm until you feel a stretch down the side of your body.

- Hold for a count of 4 then repeat for the other side.

Keep your tummy muscles pulled in to support your back and keep it straight

Don't lean forwards or backwards

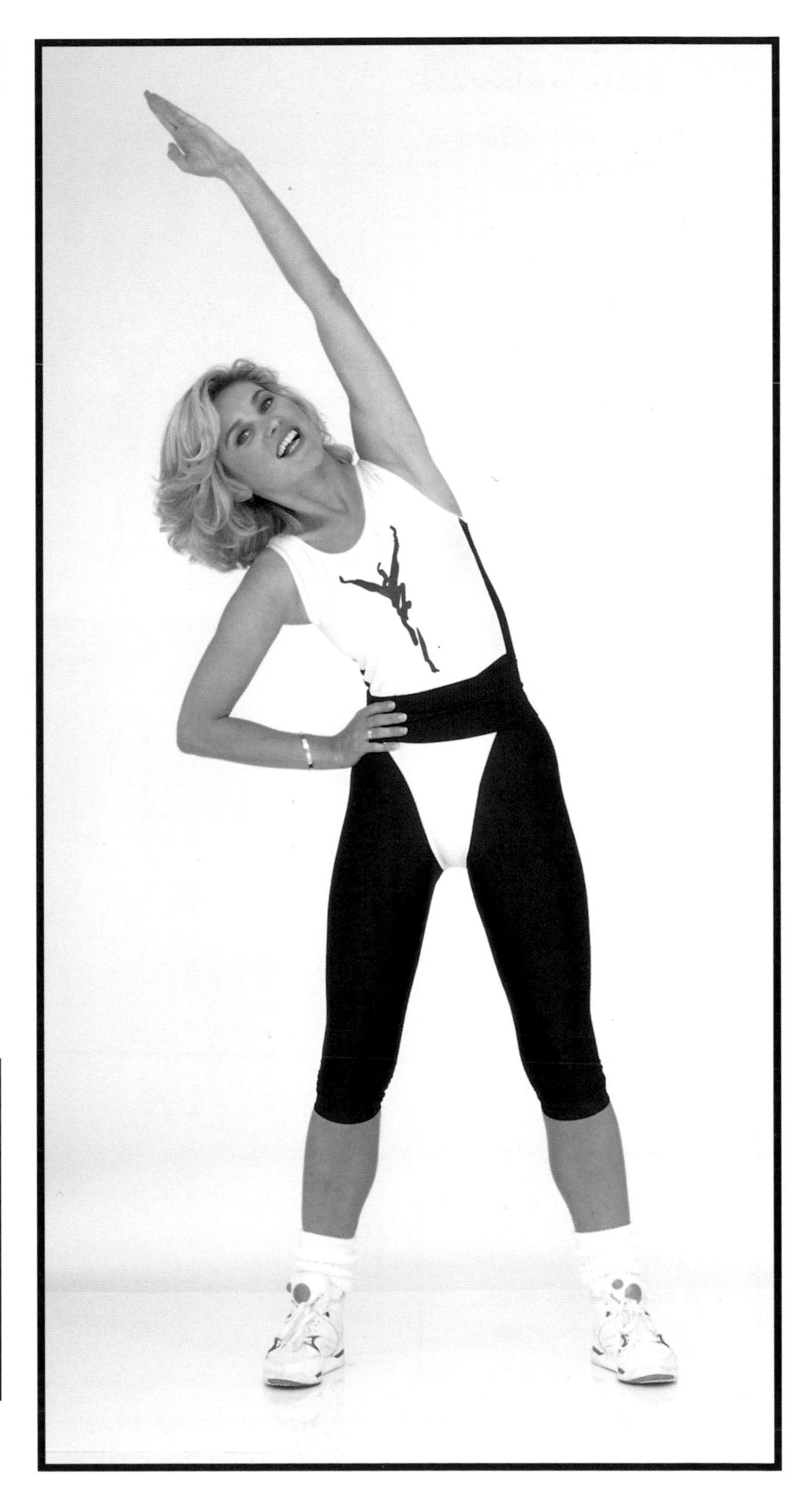

EXERCISE 9

STANDING TRICEPS STRETCH

PURPOSE:
To stretch the triceps (back of the upper arm)

- Stand with good posture, feet hip-width apart and your knees slightly bent.

- Take your right hand over your head and place your palm on to the top of your back, grasp your right elbow with your left hand.

- Using the left hand to assist the stretch, gently pull the right elbow across and behind the head until you feel a stretch down the back of the right arm.

- Hold for a count of 4 then repeat for the left arm.

Check your back does not arch

Aim to reach your fingers down between your shoulder blades

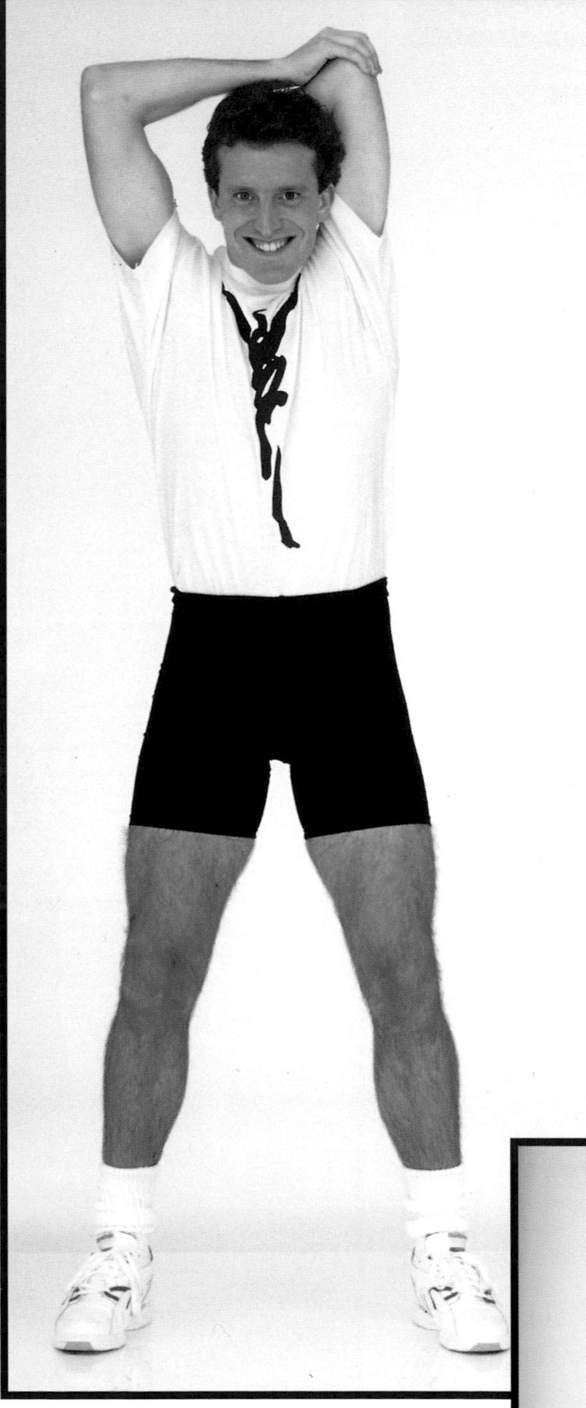

You may find it suits you better to assist the stretch by pushing the front of the arm with the other hand, rather than pulling the elbow across.

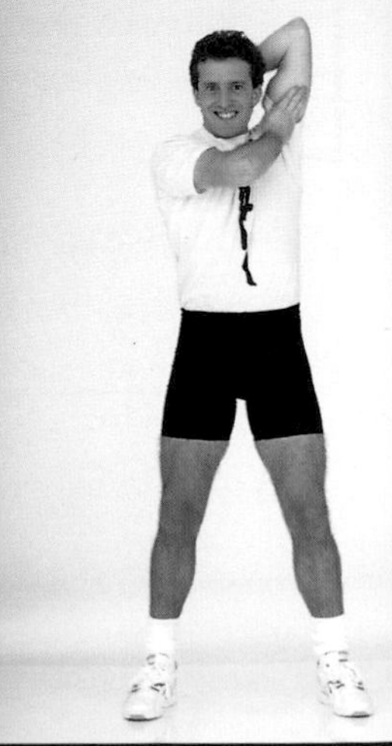

Exercise 10

STANDING SHOULDER STRETCH

PURPOSE:
To stretch muscles around the shoulders

- Stand with good posture and your feet hip-width apart.
- Clasp your hands together and, keeping your pelvis correctly tilted, pull in your tummy muscles and extend your arms above your head, reaching them back until you feel the stretch around your shoulders.
- Hold for a count of 4, rest and repeat.

Keep breathing

Try to squeeze your ears with your upper arms

Don't allow your back to arch

Repeat these warm-up stretches again before moving on to the toning exercises.

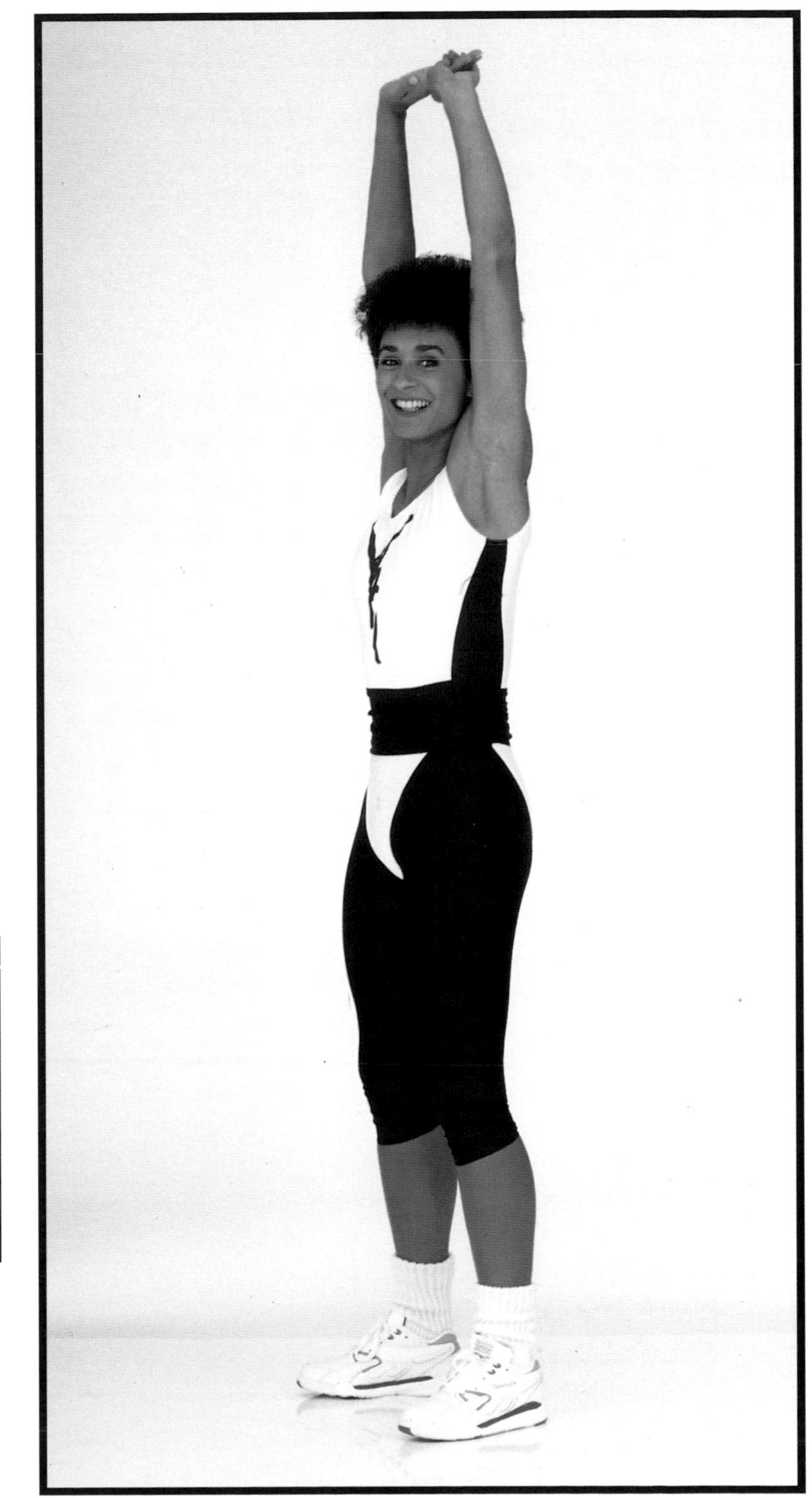

These exercises are designed to make the selected muscles ache a little by the end of each set. Remember that each exercise must be performed correctly to be most effective, and in all the exercises for your tum, holding it in is the key to achieving a flatter, firmer shape. After each exercise allow yourself a little rest before moving on to the next exercise, and listen to your body so that you do not overdo it at first.

EXERCISE 1

PELVIC TILTS

REPETITIONS 4
PURPOSE:
To tone the abdominals (tum)

● Lie on your back with both knees bent, legs slightly apart and feet flat on the floor. Place your hands on your tummy or on the floor by your sides.

● As in the warm up, tilt your pelvis forwards by pulling in your tummy muscles and curling your bottom slightly off the floor against the downward pressure of your tummy muscles. Relax. Feel your lower back come off the floor.

● Repeat until you have done the exercise 4 times.

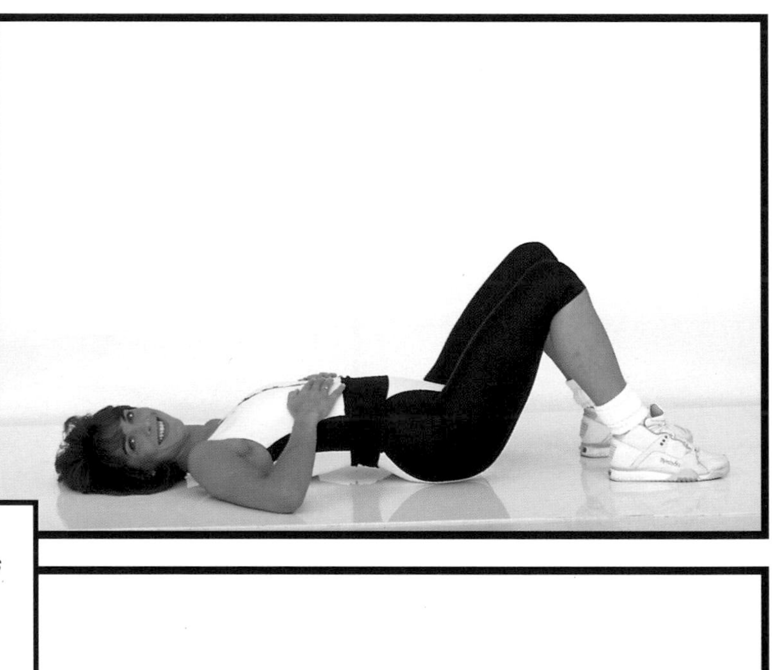

Feel your tummy muscles working

Think of shortening your abdomen

Keep your chin towards your chest

EXERCISE 2

STARTERS CURL-UPS

REPETITIONS
8 Right 8 Left
PURPOSE:
To tone the abdominals (tum)

● Lie on your back, both knees bent, your feet flat on the floor and hip-width apart, your head resting in your left hand and your right hand on the right thigh.

● Tilting your pelvis and pulling in your tummy muscles, slowly curl your head and shoulders off the floor to reach your right hand up over the knee. Relax.

● Do this 8 times, rest, change arms and repeat another 8 times.

Feel your tummy muscles working and breathe out as you curl up

Keep your tummy flat throughout the movement

Look at the tops of your knees as you curl up

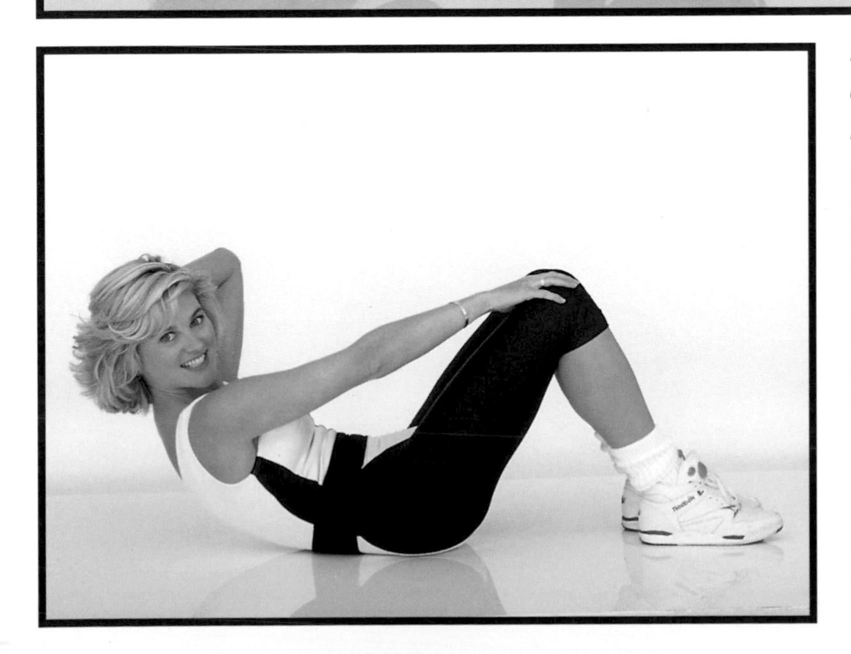

If this curl-up causes any discomfort, try the Alternative Reverse Curl (see page 36).

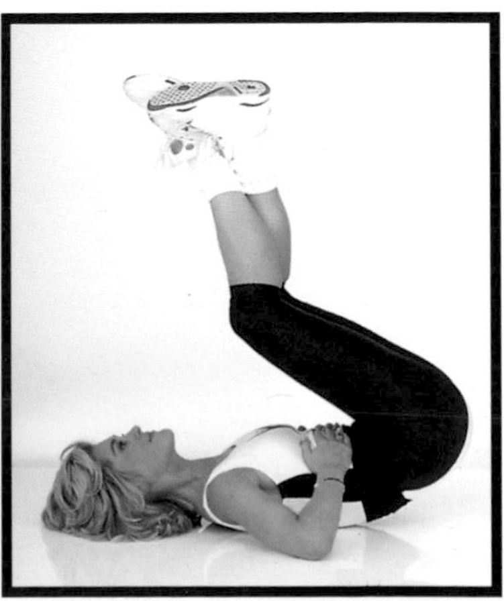

Exercise 3

BUTTOCK SQUEEZES

REPETITIONS *12*
PURPOSE:
To tone the gluteals (bum)

- Lie on your back, flatten your tummy and tilt your hips towards you as in the pelvic tilt.
- Raise your hips off the floor to make a straight line from your knees to your chest.
- Keeping your body still, tighten then relax your buttocks.
- Do this 12 times.

Feel the buttock muscles working

Take care to keep your upper back (shoulder blades) in contact with the floor

Ensure you do not arch your back

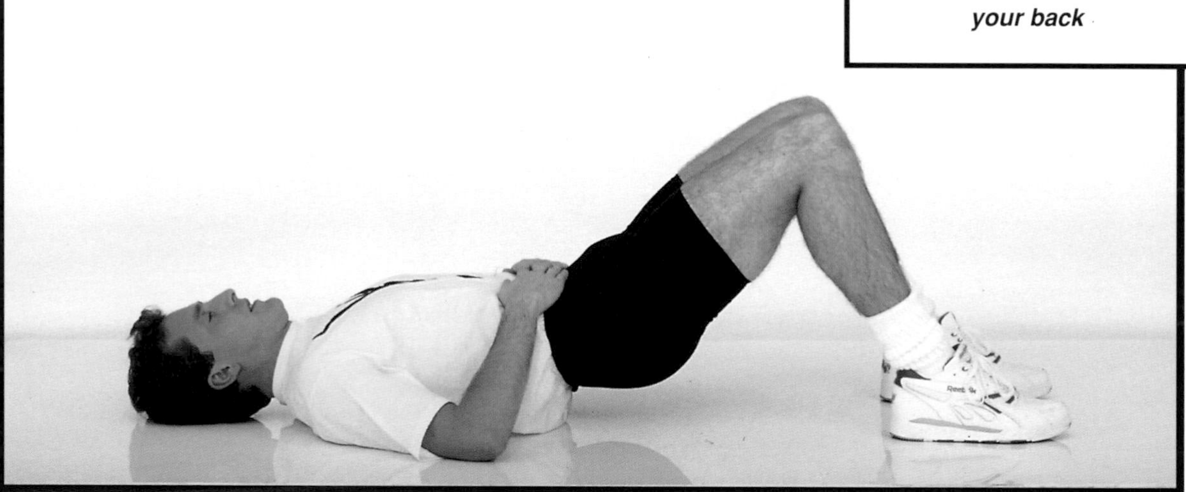

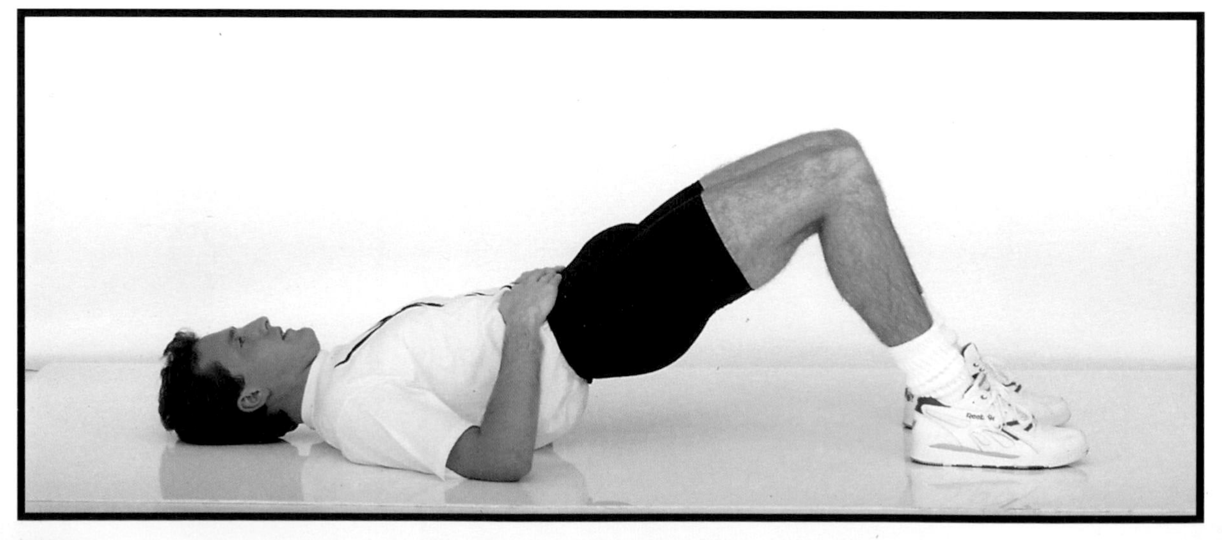

EXERCISE 4

CURL-UP WITH KNEE IN

REPETITIONS
8 Right 8 Left
PURPOSE:
To tone the abdominals (tum)

- Lie on your back, knees bent and your feet flat on the floor. Place your fingertips behind your head for support.

- Keeping your elbows back and your tummy muscles held in firmly, curl up off the floor bringing your right knee in to meet your face. Relax.

- Do this 8 times with the right knee, then repeat another 8 times using the left leg.

Remember, if any type of curl-up causes discomfort, find an alternative that suits you.

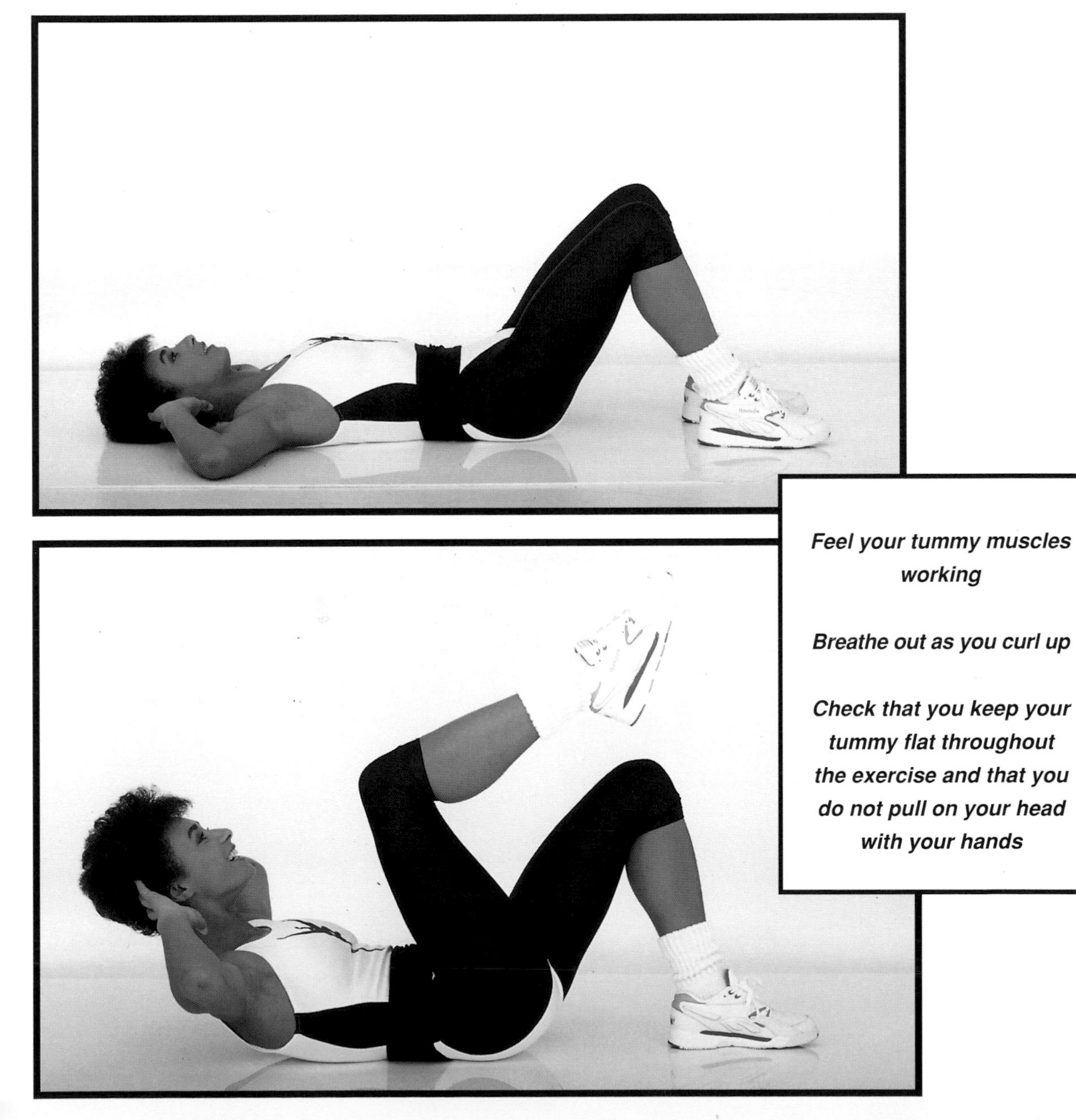

Feel your tummy muscles working

Breathe out as you curl up

Check that you keep your tummy flat throughout the exercise and that you do not pull on your head with your hands

EXERCISE 5

BUTTOCK WORKER

REPETITIONS *16*
PURPOSE:
To tone the gluteals (bum)

- Lie on your back as for buttock squeezes, feet flat on the ground, hips off the ground, this time placing your arms on the floor down by your sides.

- Keeping the hips still, bring your right knee in towards your chest, then place your foot back on the ground and repeat, using the other leg.

- Do this entire exercise 8 times.

Feel the buttock muscles of the supporting side working hard to hold you in position (keep your hips still)

Use your hands on the floor to help balance

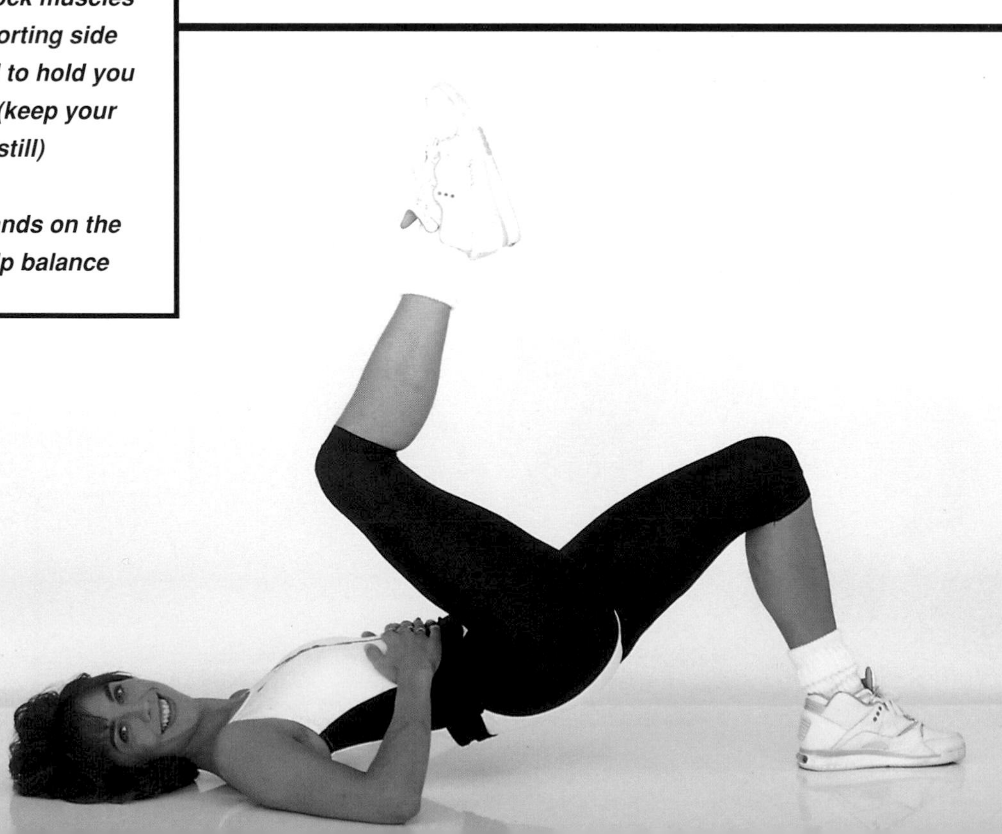

EXERCISE 6

CURL-UPS

REPETITIONS *2 x 8*
PURPOSE:
To tone the abdominals (tum)

- Lie on your back as for curl-ups, legs bent and feet flat on the floor. Rest your head in your fingertips and keep your elbows back.

- Tightening your tummy muscles to pull in your tummy as much as possible, slowly curl your head and shoulders off the floor, supporting your head by your fingertips. Relax.

- Do this 8 times, rest and repeat.

You may prefer to do two more sets of the Starters Curl-ups (see page 79).

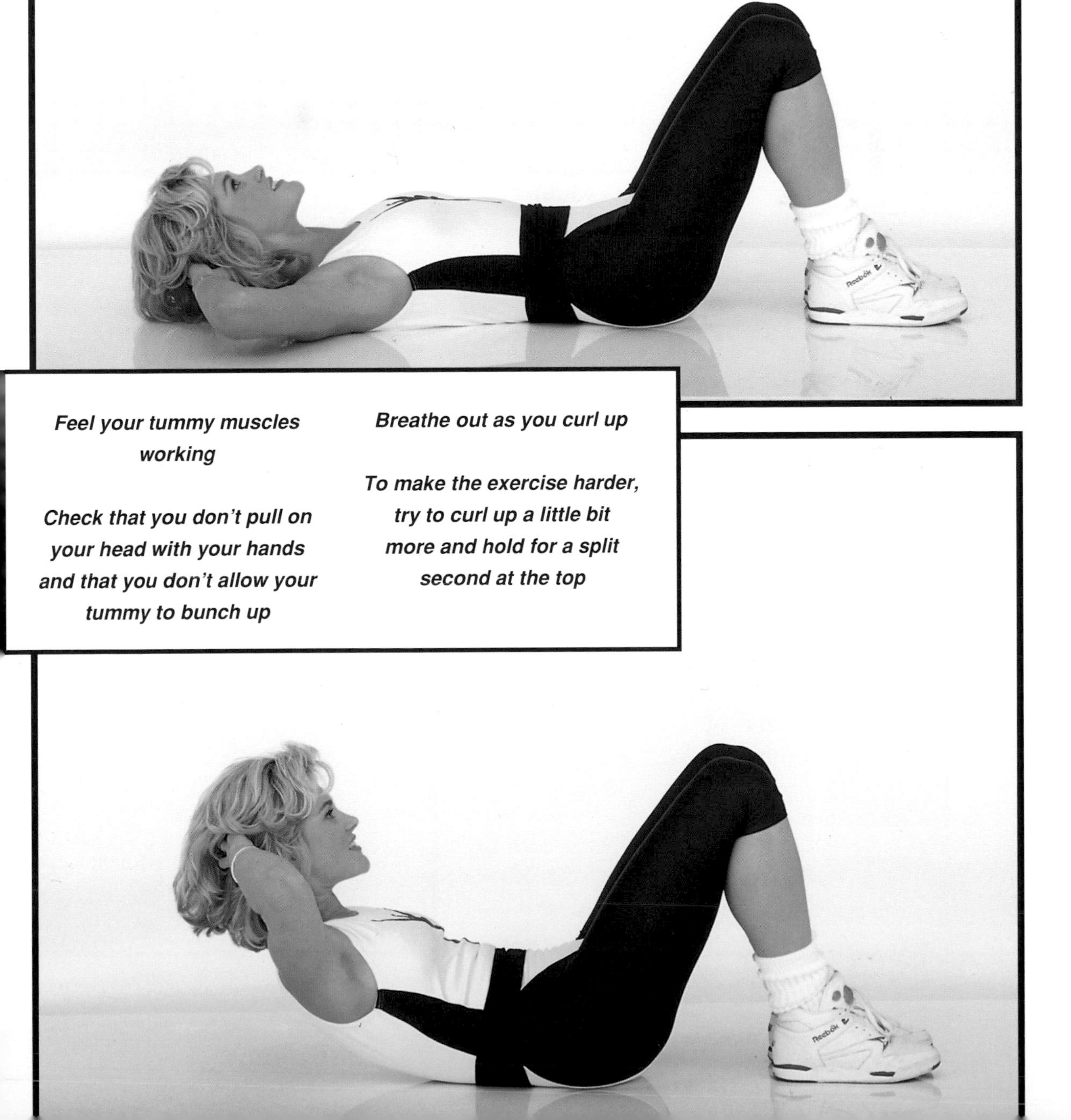

Feel your tummy muscles working

Check that you don't pull on your head with your hands and that you don't allow your tummy to bunch up

Breathe out as you curl up

To make the exercise harder, try to curl up a little bit more and hold for a split second at the top

EXERCISE 7

BOX PRESS-UPS

REPETITIONS *2 x 8*
PURPOSE:
To tone the pectorals (chest), and triceps (back of the upper arms)

- Adopt a position on all fours with your hands directly under your shoulders and your knees under your hips. Pulling in your tummy and tilting your pelvis to keep your back flat, shift your weight, taking your shoulders forwards slightly in front of your hands.

- Bend your elbows, lowering your forehead to touch the floor just in front of your hands. Push up slowly to return to the start.

- Do this 8 times then rest. Repeat 8 more times.

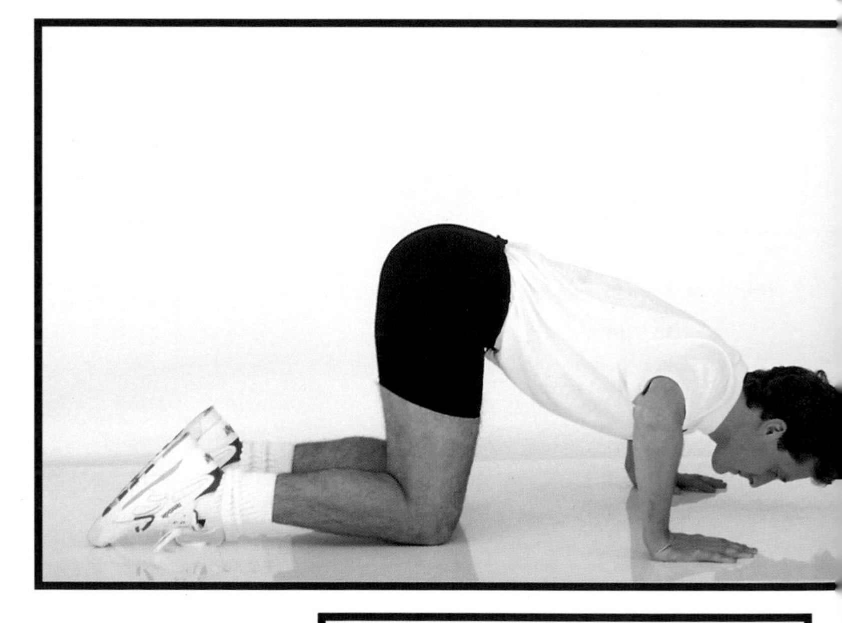

Feel the muscles of your chest and arms working

Breathe out as you push up

Don't allow your back to dip

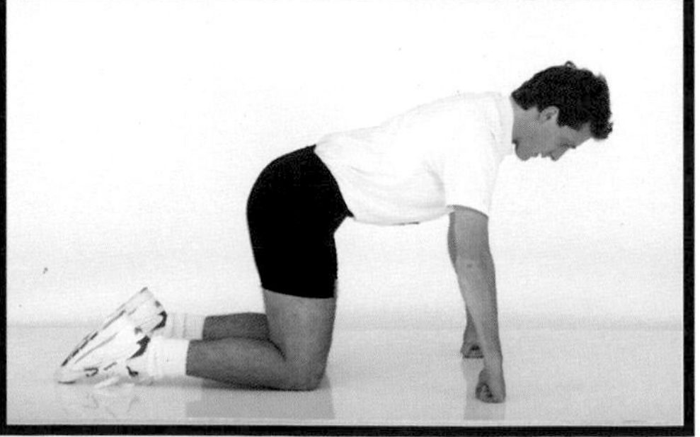

If your wrists are uncomfortable, try leaning on your fists instead.

EXERCISE 8

HIP HITCHES (TAIL WAGS!)

REPETITIONS *2 x 16*
PURPOSE:
To tone the obliques (waist)

- Adopt an all-fours position as for press-ups with your pelvis correctly tilted to keep your back flat.

- Wag your bottom from side to side, squeezing your waist muscles and drawing your hip up towards your ribs on one side then the other.

- Do this 8 times, rest and repeat.

Feel your waist muscles working

Think of shortening the distance between your hips and your ribs

Try to keep your arms straight and your shoulders still

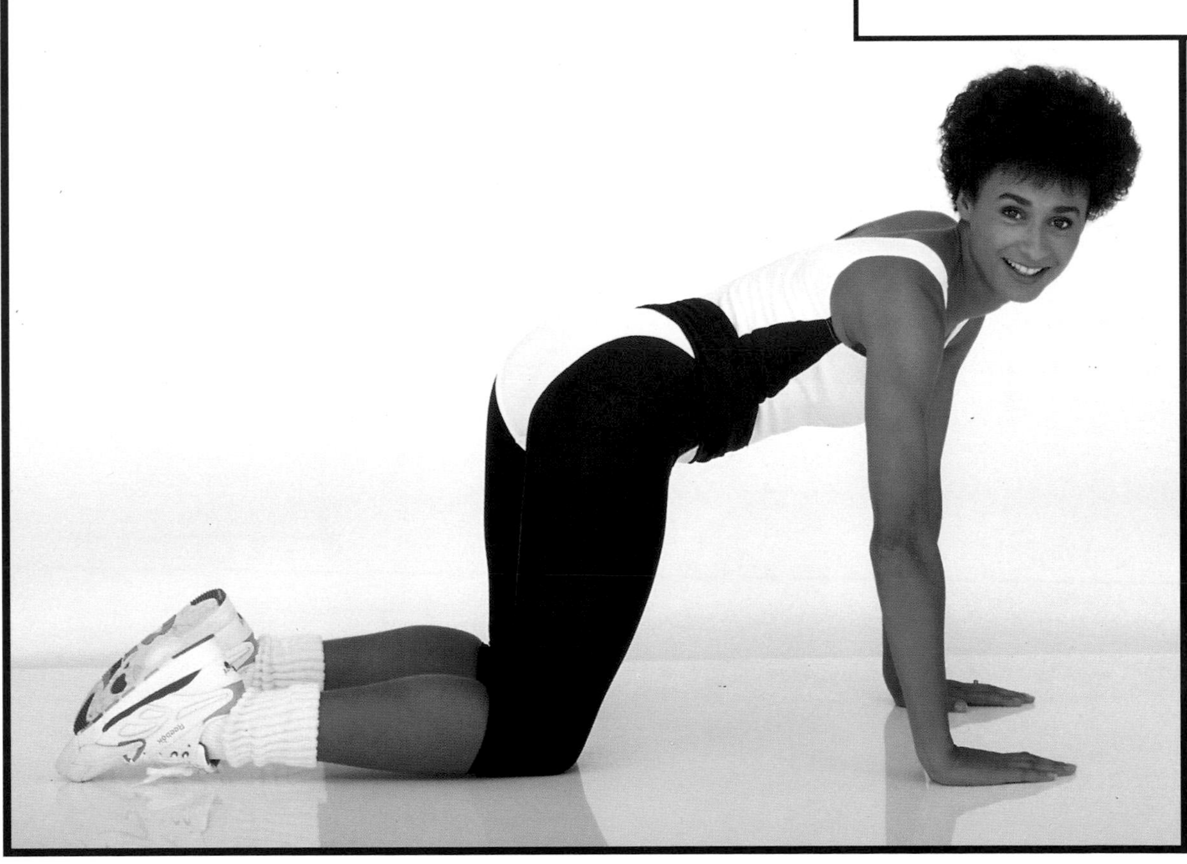

Try to think of relaxing the muscle into the stretches. You do not need to hold most of these stretches for as long as you held those in Level 1a because the positions are not as comfortable and improvement in suppleness in most of these areas is not as profound or as necessary.

EXERCISE 1

KNEELING SHOULDER STRETCH

PURPOSE:
To stretch the muscles around the shoulder joints

- Adopt a kneeling position with your buttocks on your heels, your arms extended out in front of you, your hands on the floor with your thumbs close together, and your chest resting on your thighs.
- Keeping your chest low, slide your hands and hips forwards, raising your buttocks up off your heels until your hips are directly above your knees.
- Keeping your hips high, push your chest down towards your knees until you feel the stretch in your shoulders.
- Hold for a count of 8.

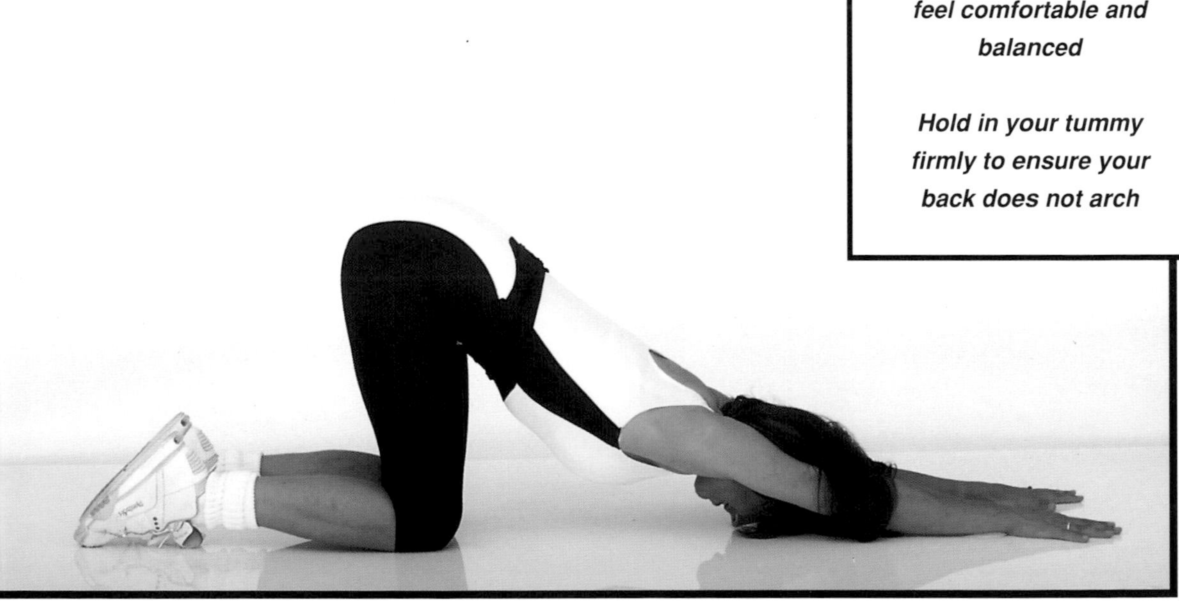

Check your hips are not in front of or behind your knees - you should feel comfortable and balanced

Hold in your tummy firmly to ensure your back does not arch

To make the exercise easier keep your buttocks on your heels and simply press your chest towards the floor, keeping your arms as extended as possible.

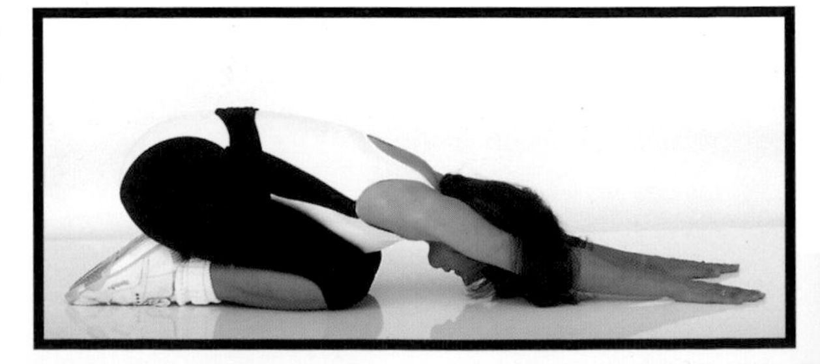

EXERCISE 2

HOLLOW AND HUMP

REPETITIONS *4*
PURPOSE:
To mobilize the spine and relax the back muscles

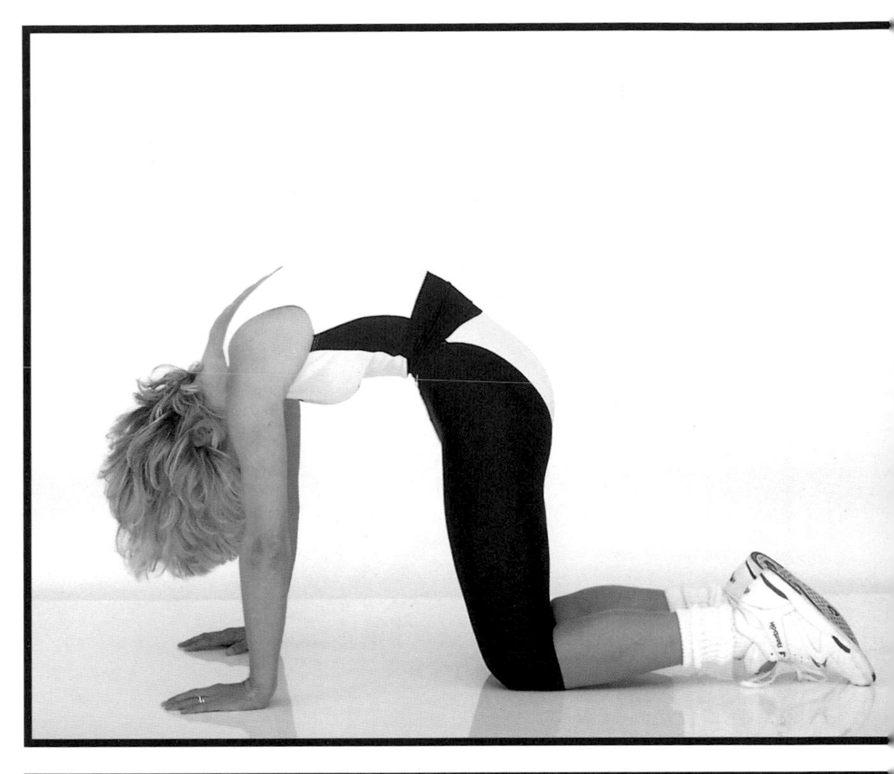

- Adopt an all-fours position with your hands under your shoulders and your knees under your hips.
- Slowly and gently round your back by lifting it up, looking at your tummy and pulling it in at the same time. Hold for a count of two then slowly relax, letting your back dip into a hollow.
- Do this 4 times.

Feel the stretch across the shoulder blades as well as in the lower back

Think of making a hump with your back and separating your shoulder blades as much as possible

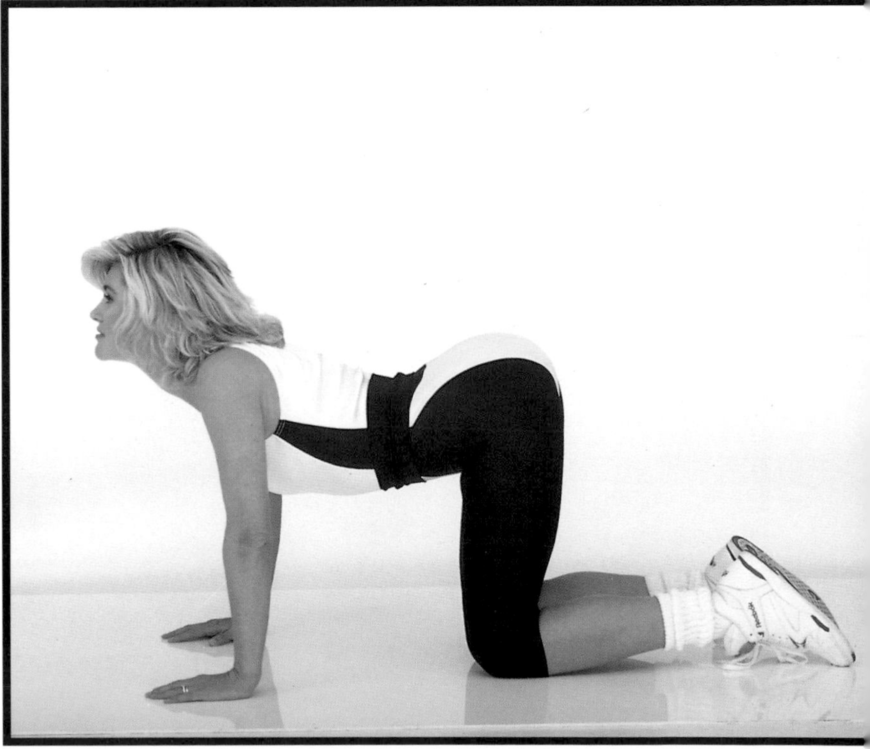

If your back feels uncomfortable, relax to a flat rather than a hollow position.

Exercise 3

SEATED TRICEP STRETCH

PURPOSE:
To stretch the triceps (back of the upper arm)

- Sit up tall with your legs in any position that's comfortable.

- As in the back of the arm stretch in the warm-up, place the palm of your right hand on to the top of your back and grasp your right elbow with your left hand.

- Using your left hand to assist the stretch, gently pull the right elbow across behind your head until you feel a stretch down the back of your right arm.

- Hold for a count of 8, then repeat for the left arm.

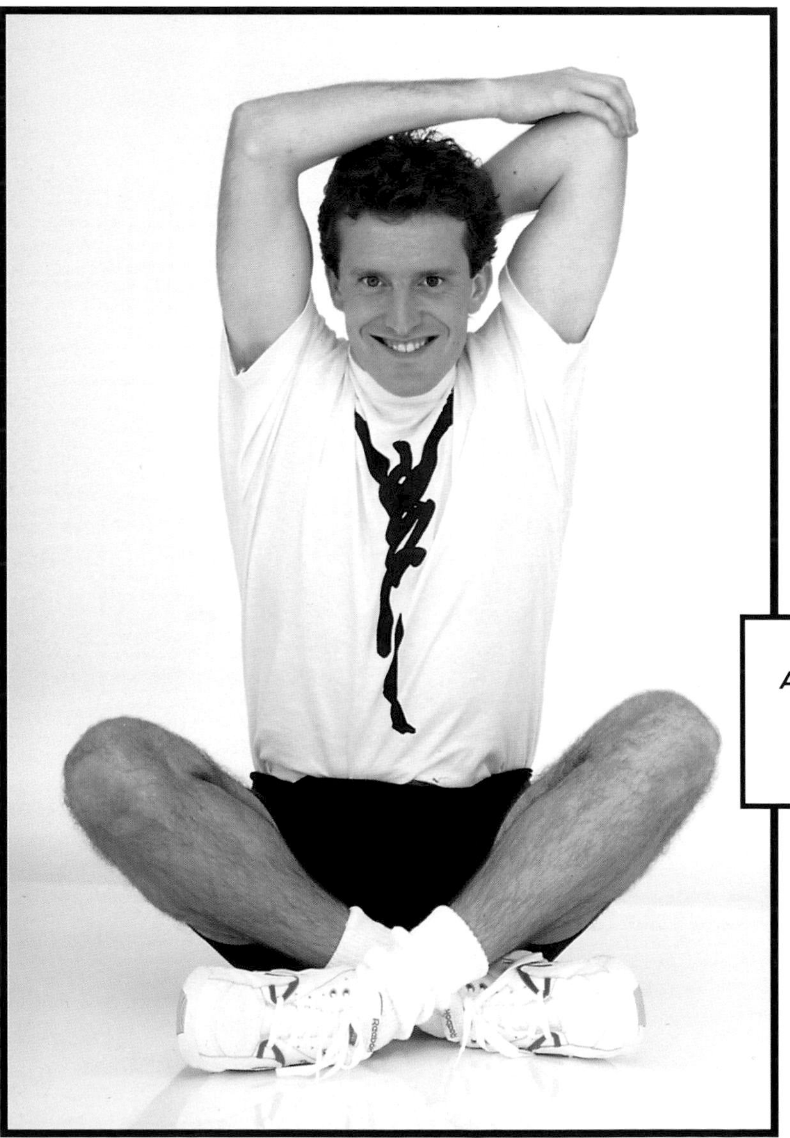

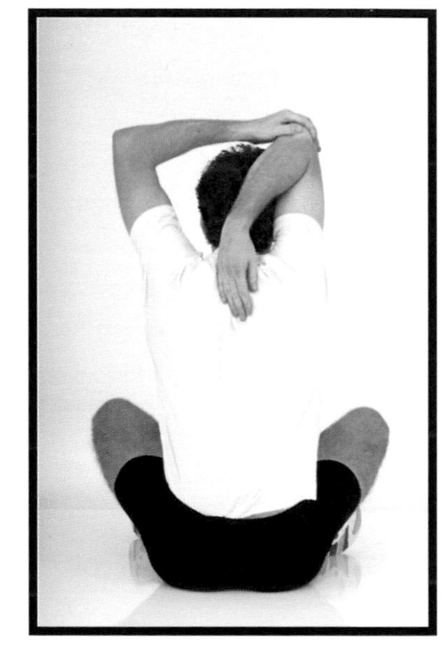

Aim to reach your fingers down between your shoulder blades

You may be more comfortable standing for this stretch, as in the warm-up on page 76.

EXERCISE 4

SEATED HAMSTRING STRETCH

PURPOSE:
To stretch the hamstrings (back of the thigh)

- Sit on the floor with one leg straight out in front and the other leg slightly to the side, bent out of the way.

- Sit up tall and place your hands on the floor either side of the straight leg.

- Pull in your tummy muscles and, trying to keep your back straight, bend forwards from the hips over the straight leg until you feel the stretch down the back of this leg.

- Hold for a count of 16, relaxing the muscles and developing the stretch. Repeat with other leg.

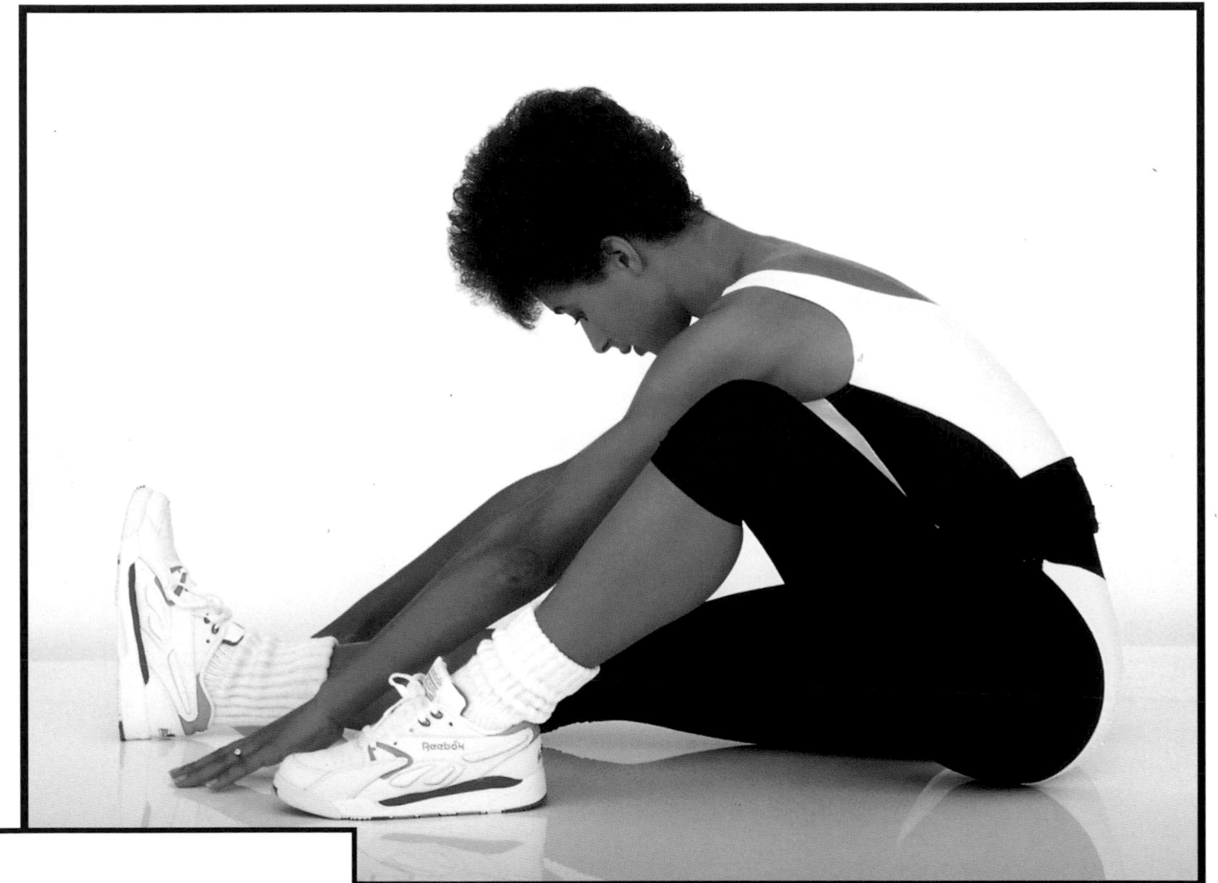

Keep the hips square and your back as straight as possible

Be content not to reach your nose to your shin!

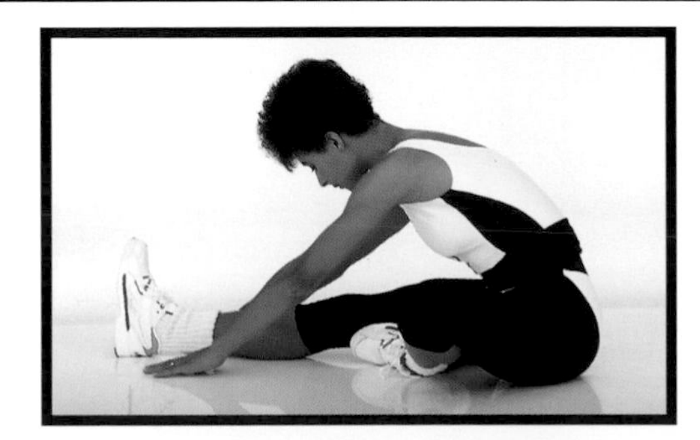

If you feel a pull in your back try adjusting the position of the bent leg or try the Lying Hamstring Stretch on page 66 .

Level 2a Hips and Thighs

You will now be familiar with the Level 1a warm-up exercises and should be able to perform them effectively and safely without instructions. For Level 2a repeat the warm-up exercises and incorporate the two new ones (opposite and page 93) into your routine. Remember the aim is to be warm and loose before you stretch.

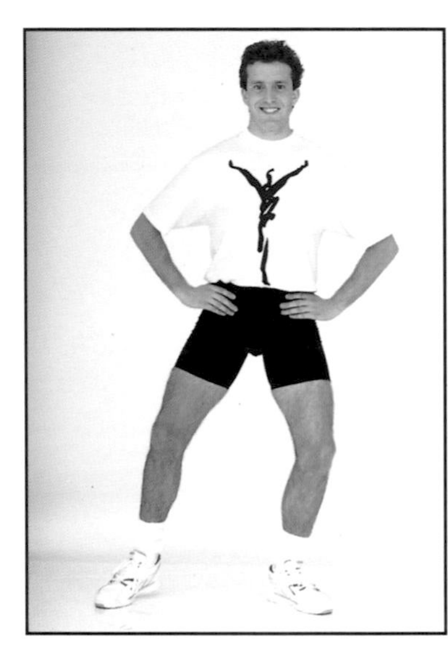

SWAYS x 8

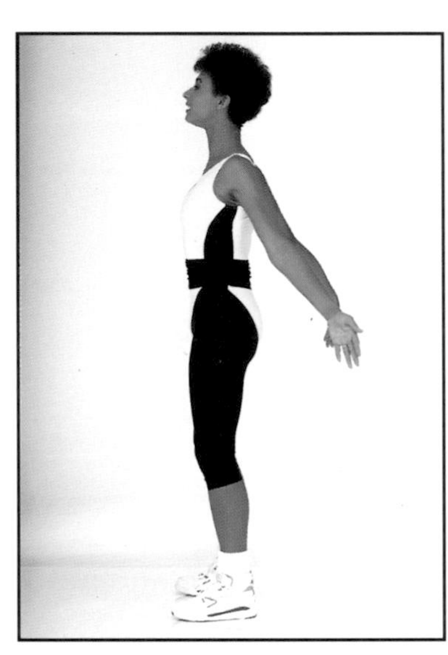

SHOULDER SQUEEZES x 4

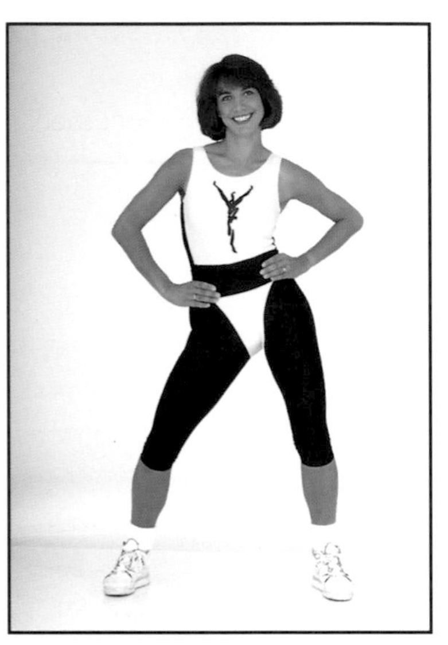

HIP CIRCLES x 2 Right 2 Left

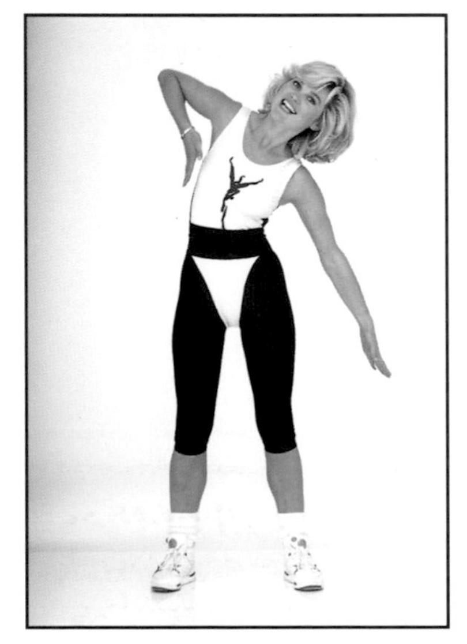

SIDE BENDS x 4

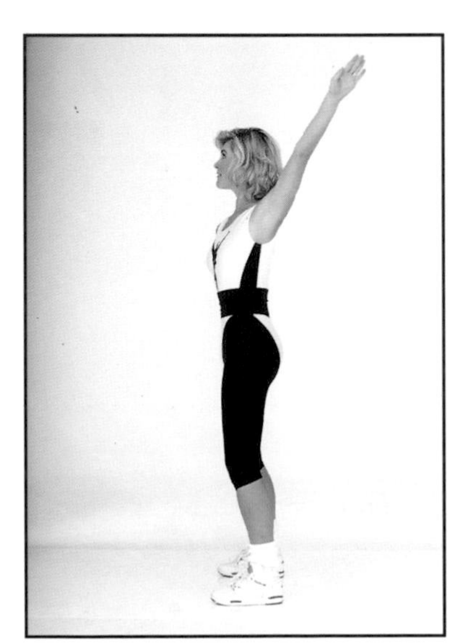

FORWARD ARM CIRCLES x 2 Right 2 Left

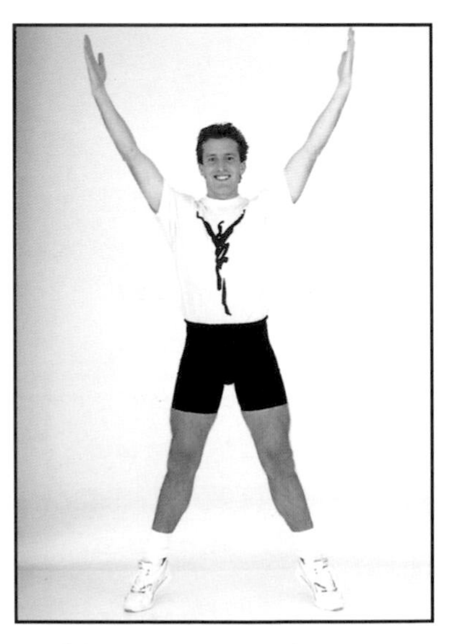

SQUAT AND REACH WITH HEEL RAISE x 4

EXERCISE 1

FULL CIRCLE SWINGS

REPETITIONS *8*
PURPOSE:
To warm the muscles

- Stand with your weight evenly over both feet, arms extended to one side and good centre control.

- Bending your knees as for knee bends in Level 1A, begin to circle your arms down across in front of your body. As your arms begin to rise straighten your legs and rise up on to your toes as your arms reach up above your head. Continue to complete the circle with your arms while lowering your heels back to the floor so that both your arms and legs are back to the start position.

- Do this 4 times, circling the arms in one direction, then repeat the circles the other way.

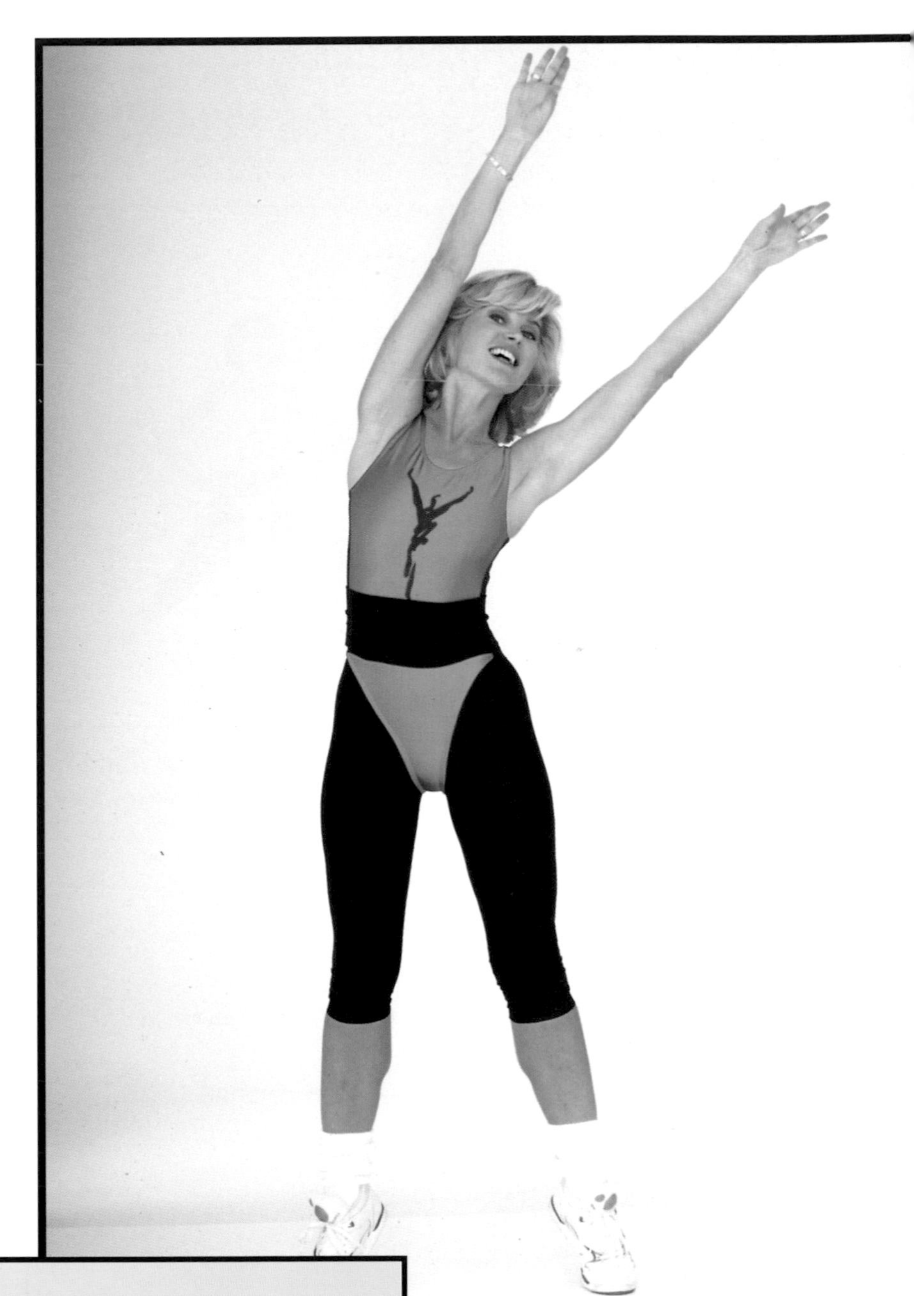

Develop a flowing and comfortable rhythm that suits you

Make the circles as large but controlled as possible

Maintain good centre control throughout and keep your weight over your big toe joint during the heel raise

Check your posture and legs are correctly positioned during the knee bends

Repeat all of these mobility and pulse raising exercises before moving on to the warm-up stretches.

After completing the mobility and pulse-raising exercises on the previous two pages, repeat the stretch exercises below and the new one opposite.

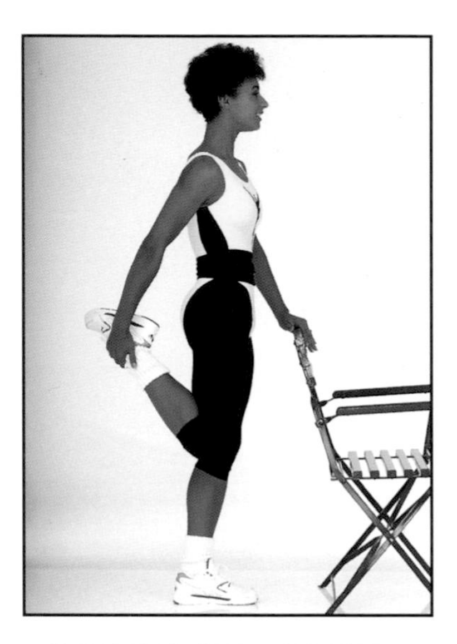

STANDING QUAD STRETCH: 8 counts each leg

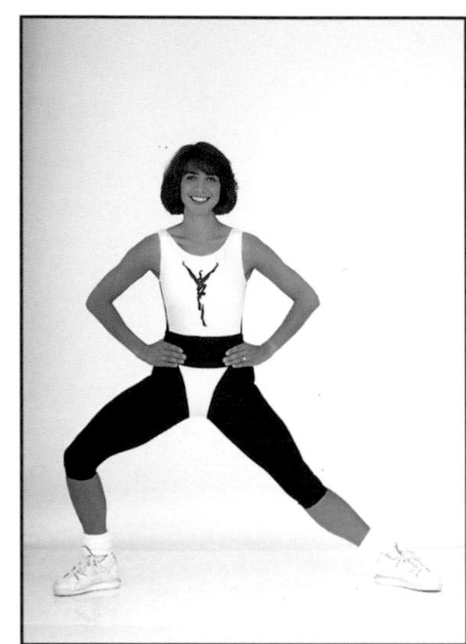

STANDING INNER THIGH STRETCH: 8 counts each side

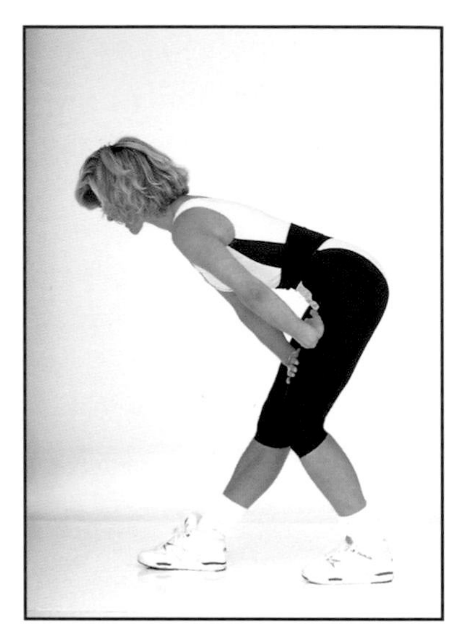

STANDING HAMSTRING STRETCH: 8 counts each leg

EXERCISE 2

STANDING BUTTOCK STRETCH

PURPOSE:
To stretch the gluteals (buttocks)

- Face a chair and, holding it for support, transfer your weight on to your left leg, bend it slightly and rest the ankle of your right leg on the left knee.

- Sticking your bottom backwards and keeping your back as straight as possible, bend forwards from the hips until you feel a stretch in your right buttock.

- Hold for a count of 8 then repeat for the other side.

You may find this easier to do sitting down *(see page 65).*

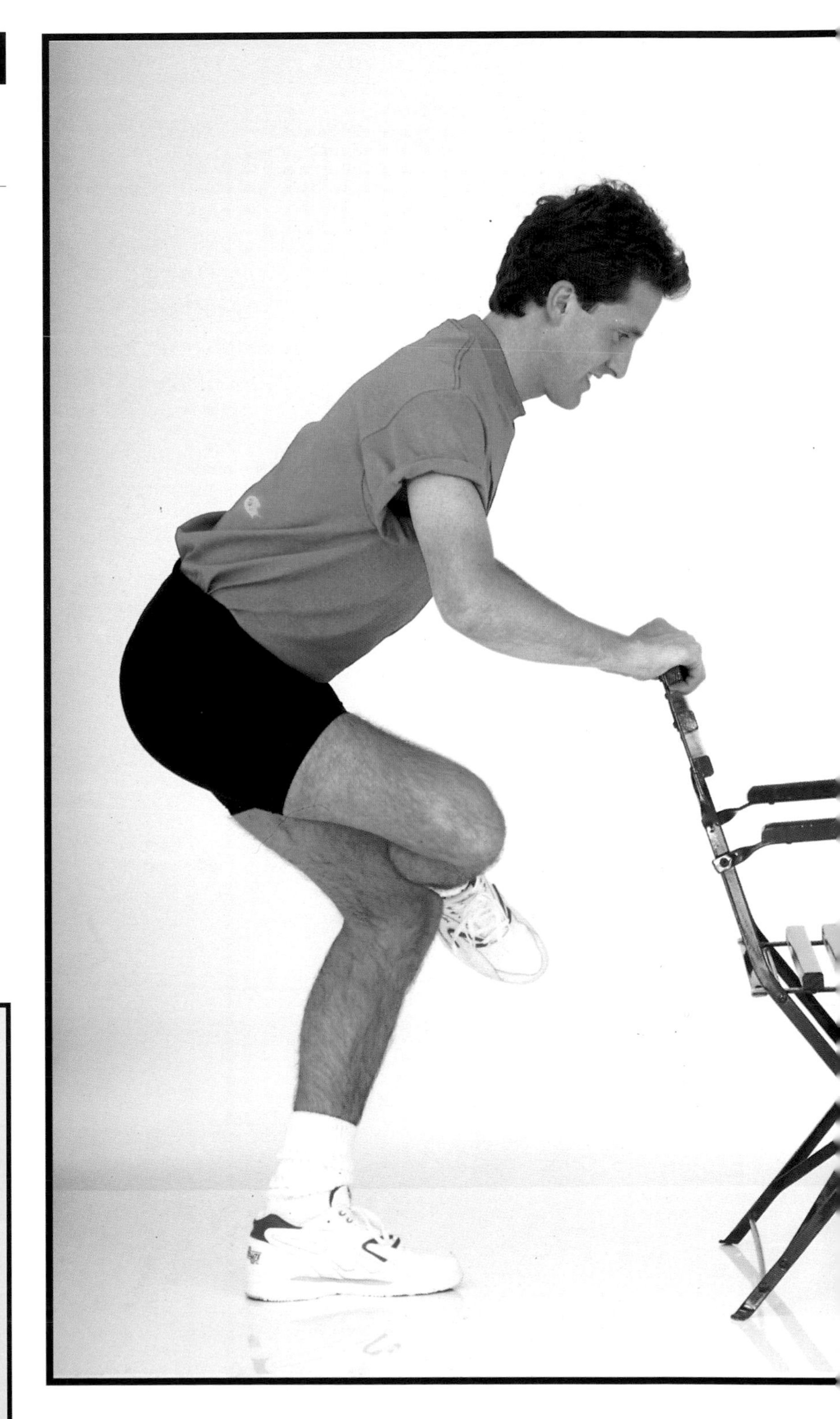

Keep your back as straight as possible

To achieve a greater stretch, try to stick your bottom out further and imagine that you are trying to sit on a chair

Check that you are resting your ankle or lower leg on the knee

Level 2a Hips and Thighs

Having prepared your joints and muscles you can move on to this toning section for the hips and thighs. At first take time to learn the new exercises thoroughly as correct technique is important for safety as well as effectiveness. Listen to your body and always rest if your muscles feel very tired. A short rest can be quite reviving, and it's amazing how you can then continue exercising safely and effectively.

EXERCISE 1

STANDING FRONT LEG RAISES

REPETITIONS
8 Right 8 Left
PURPOSE*:*
To tone the quadriceps (front of thigh)

- Stand side on to a chair and hold on to it for support.
- Extend one leg out in front of you and very slightly bend the supporting leg.
- Keeping your back and supporting leg still, slowly raise the front leg as high as you can.
- Do this 8 times then repeat with the other leg.

Feel your thigh muscles working and keep the working leg straight throughout the exercise

Tighten your tummy muscles to hold your back firm

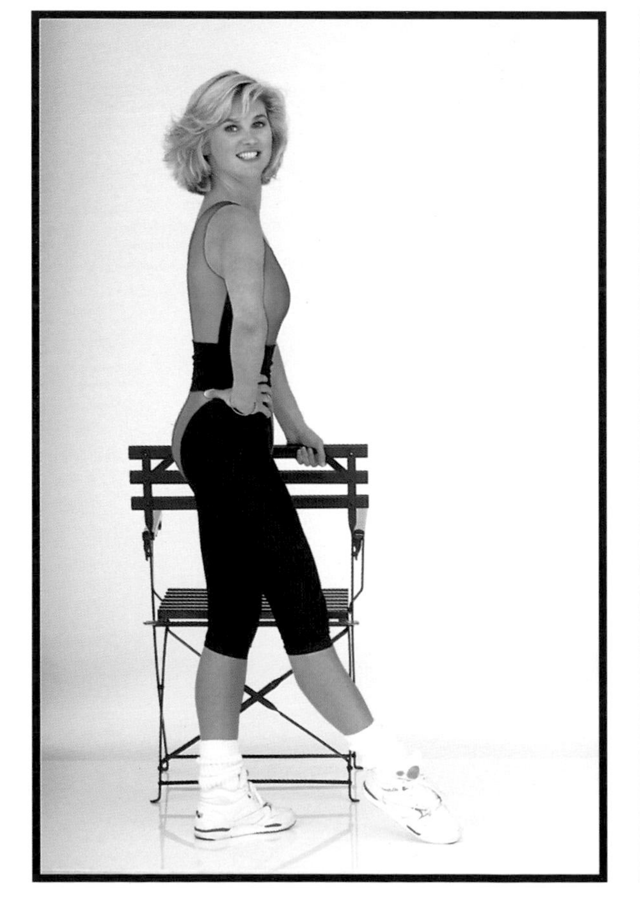

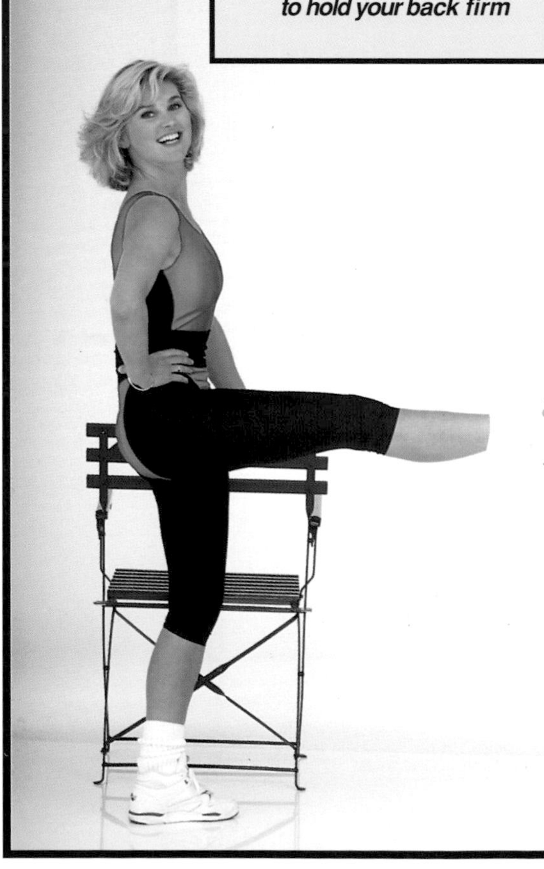

EXERCISE 2

STANDING SIDE LEG RAISES

REPETITIONS
8 Right 8 Left
PURPOSE:
To tone the abductors (hips)

- Stand with your left side leaning on a chair for support, with your weight on your left leg, left knee slightly bent, pelvis correctly tilted and your right hand on your hip.

- Keeping your hips still and level and squeezing your buttocks tight, slowly raise the right leg out to the side as far as possible, hold for a short moment, then close.

- Do this 8 times, turn around to change legs, then repeat.

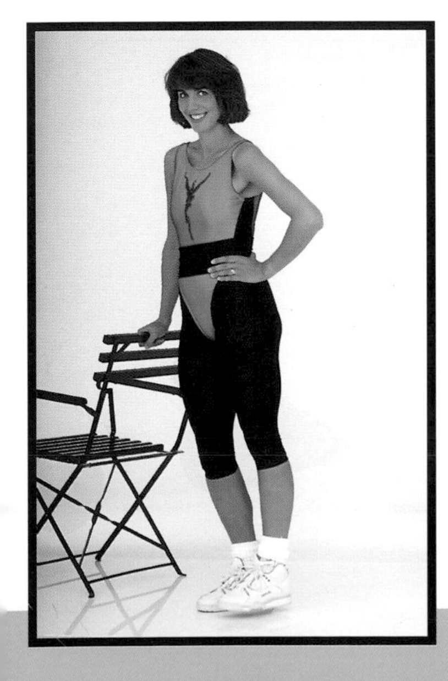

Feel the muscles on the outside of the hip and thigh working

You may also feel the muscles on the outside of the hip of the supporting leg working, as they have to stabilize the hip joint

Check that the knee of the working leg faces foward throughout the exercise

Keep the supporting leg slightly bent and squeeze the buttock muscles tightly to protect and support that hip

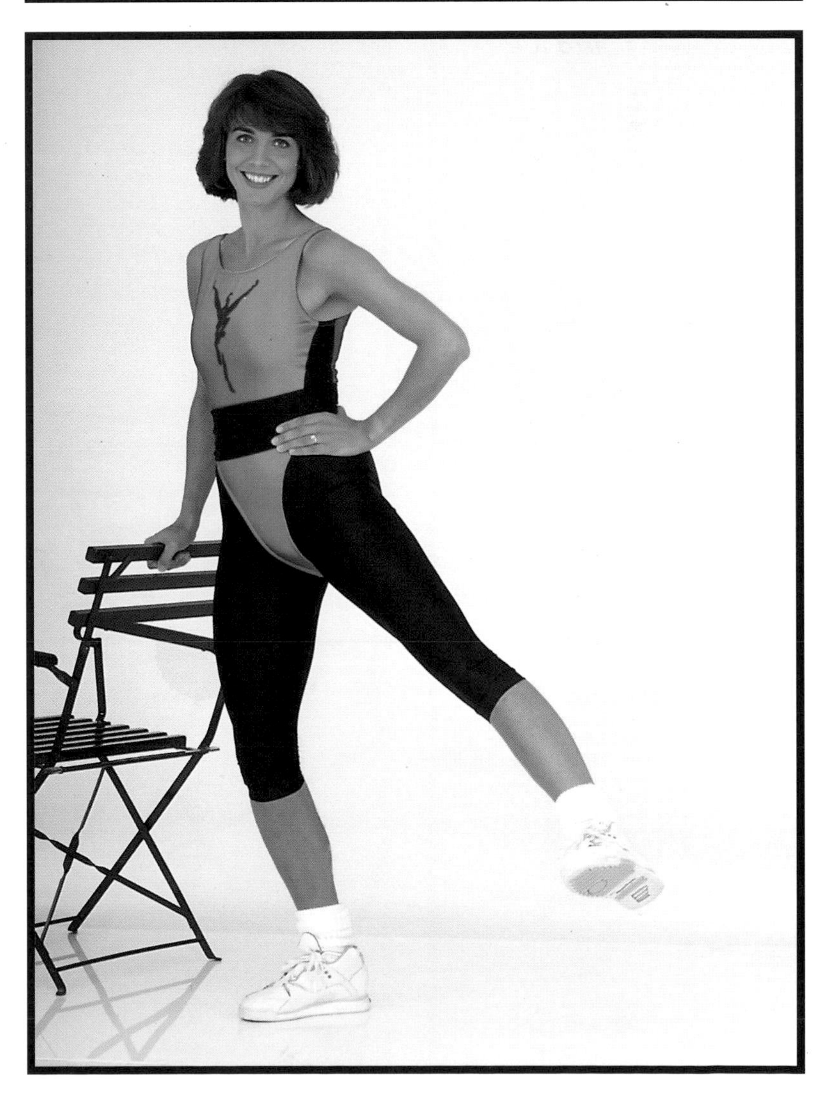

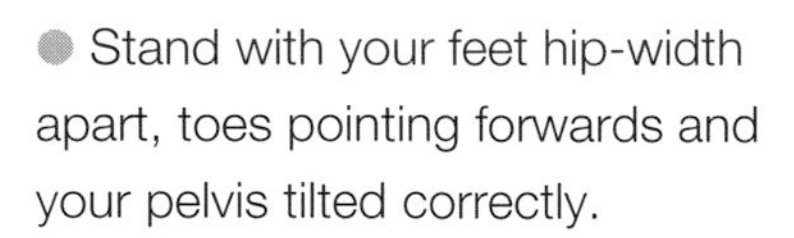

EXERCISE 3

SQUATS

REPETITIONS *24*
PURPOSE:
To tone the quadriceps (front of the thigh)

- Stand with your feet hip-width apart, toes pointing forwards and your pelvis tilted correctly.
- Leaning very slightly forwards from the hips and keeping your heels on the floor, bend your knees as far as possible without letting your hips drop below your knees. Recover.
- Do this 12 times, rest and repeat a further 12 times.

Feel your thigh muscles working

Keep your knees in line with your feet and your tummy held in firmly throughout

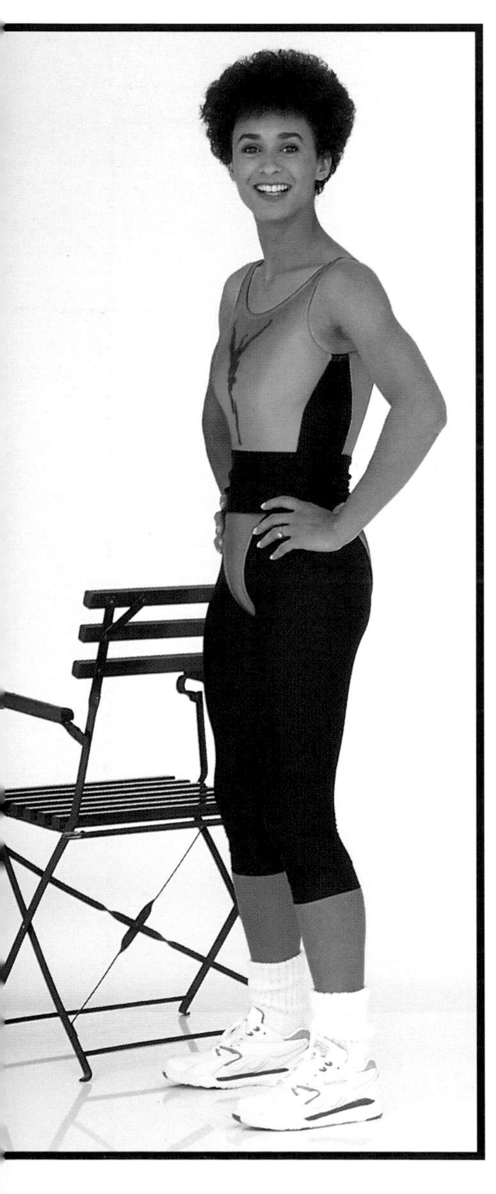

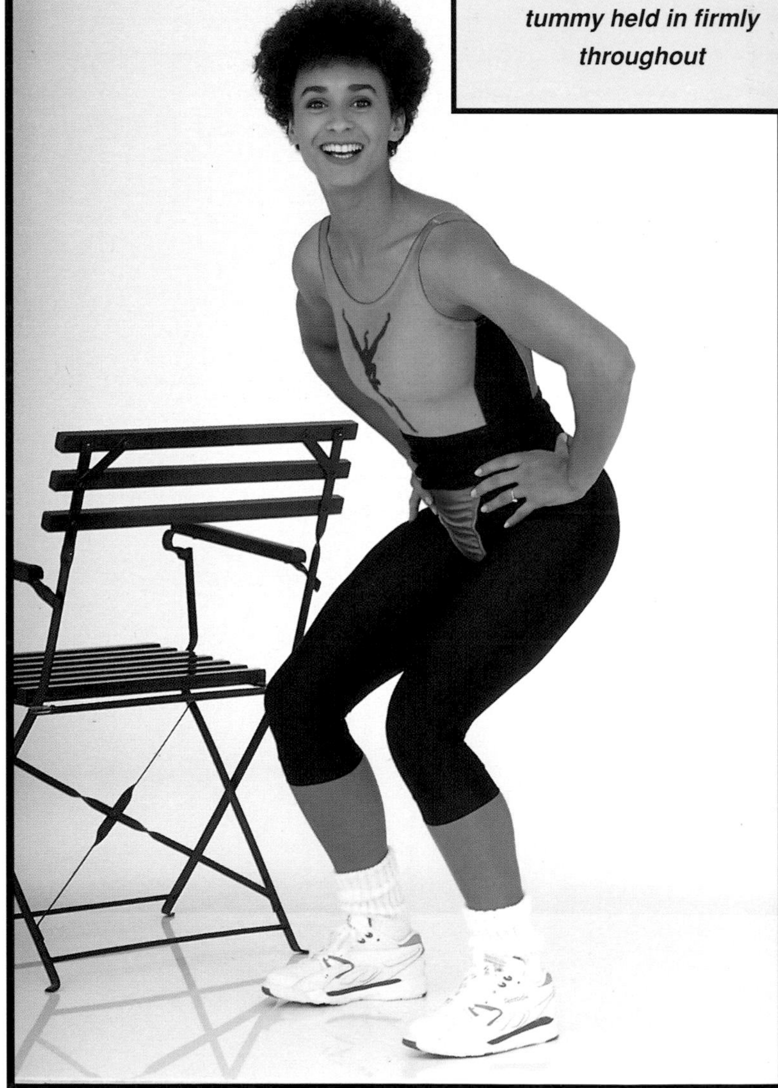

EXERCISE 4

STANDING SIDE LEG RAISES

REPETITIONS
16 Right 16 Left
PURPOSE:
To tone the abductors (hips)

- Stand facing a chair, with your weight on your left leg, left knee slightly bent, pelvis correctly tilted and your hands on the chair for balance.

- Keeping your hips still and level and squeezing your buttocks tight, slowly raise the right leg out to the side as far as possible, hold for a short moment, then close.

- Do this 16 times, change legs, and repeat with the left leg.

Feel the muscles on the outside of the hip and thigh working

You may also feel the muscles on the outside of the hip of the supporting leg working, as they have to stabilize the hip joint

Check that the knee of the working leg faces forward throughout the exercise

Keep the supporting leg slightly bent and squeeze the buttock muscles tightly to protect and support the hip

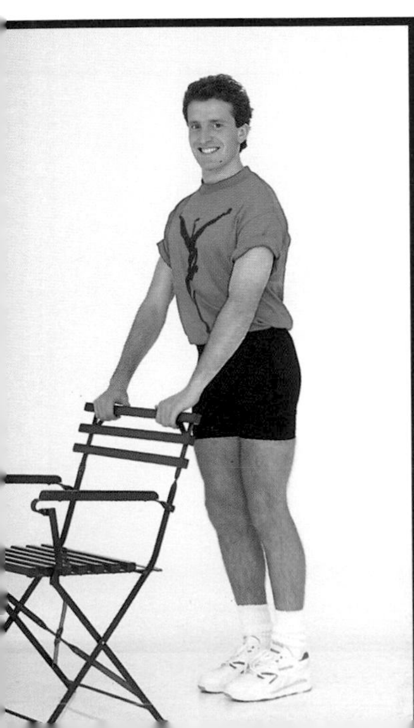

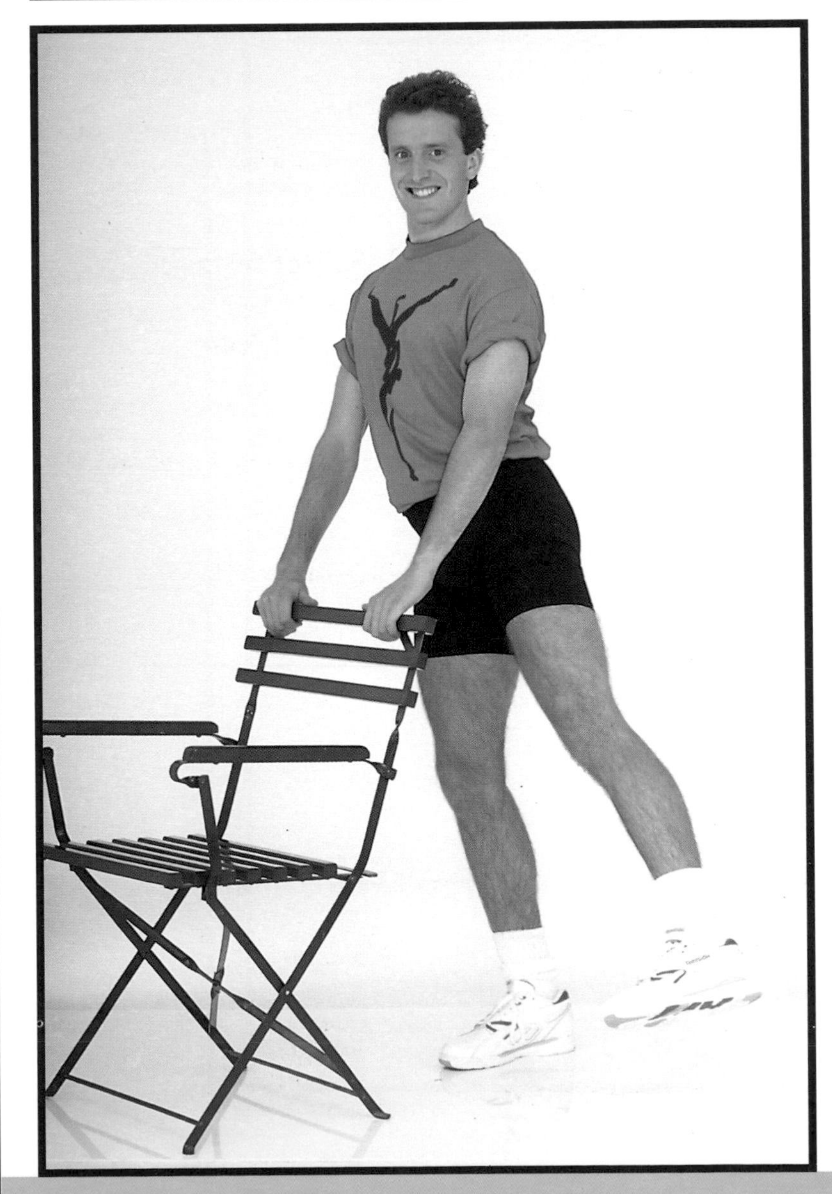

EXERCISE 5

TOE LIFTS AND HEEL RAISES

REPETITIONS *8*
PURPOSE:
To tone the shin and calf muscles (front and back of the lower leg)

- Stand with your feet hip-width apart and your pelvis tucked under for good posture. Hold on to a chair for balance.

- With your knees slightly bent and weight forwards over your toes, keeping your heels on the floor, lift your toes and the balls of your feet off the floor as much as possible. Recover, straighten your legs and rise up on to your toes, lifting the heels up off the floor.

Do this complete exercise 8 times.

Feel the muscles at the front of the shin and in the calf working alternately

Aim to raise your toes up at least 10 cm (4 ins) off the floor! Don't worry if you can't manage it at first

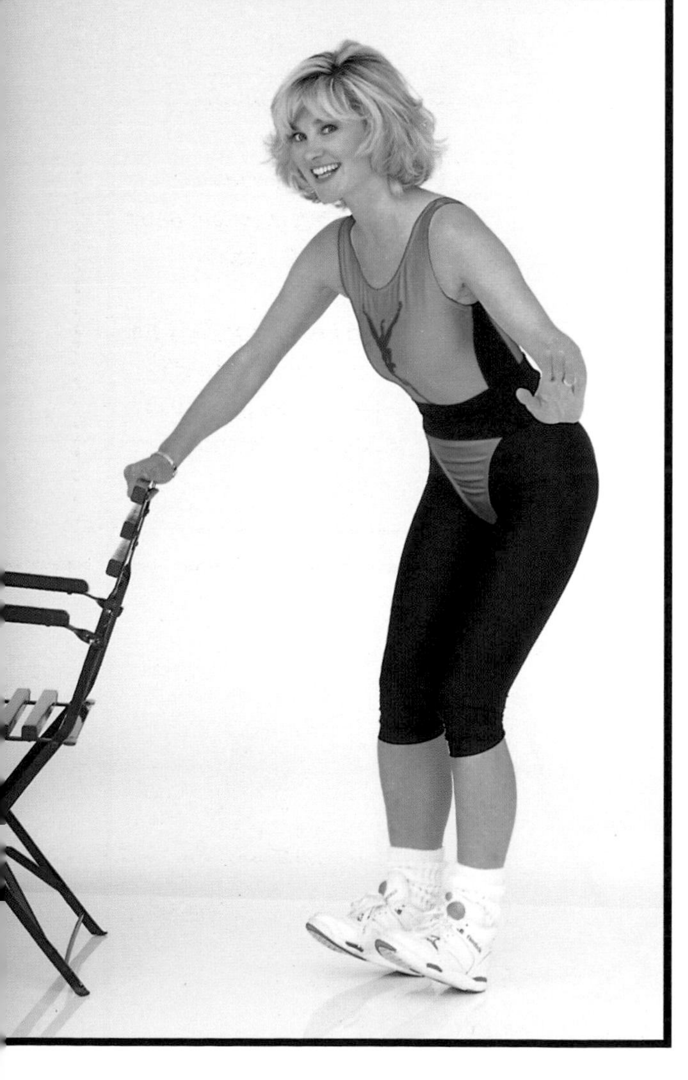

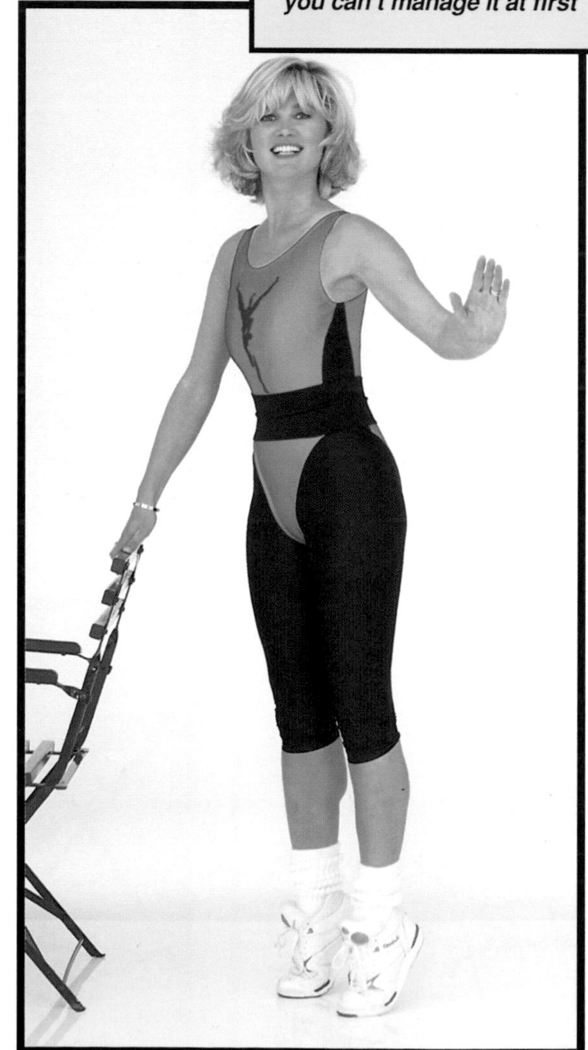

EXERCISE 6

LYING INNER THIGH RAISES

REPETITIONS
2 x 12 Right 2 x 12 Left
PURPOSE:
To strengthen the adductors (inner thighs)

- Lie on your left side, resting your head in your hand for comfort. Straighten the lower leg and bend the other one, placing the foot on the floor in front of the knee of the straight leg and placing your free hand on the floor in front of you for balance.

- Keeping your hips facing forwards and your hips and trunk still, raise and lower the lower leg.

- Do this 12 times, rest and repeat with the same leg.

- Roll over and repeat the complete exercise again using the other leg.

Feel the muscles of the inner thigh working

Think of squeezing the inner thighs together as you raise the leg

Relax the rest of your body but maintain good centre control

Don't expect to lift your leg very high – the exercise only requires a small range of movement

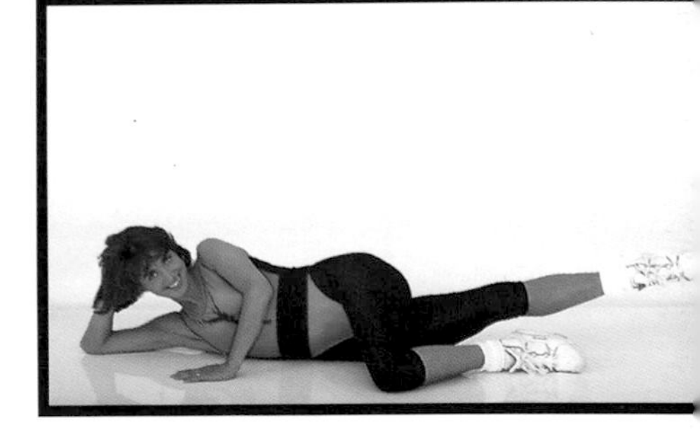

You may be more comfortable resting your knee and the side of your foot on the floor.

EXERCISE 7

BOX POSITION REAR LEG CURLS

REPETITIONS
12 Right 12 Left
PURPOSE:
To tone the hamstrings (back of the thigh)

- Adopt an all-fours position and then stretch one leg behind. Check that you are well balanced.

- Holding your back still and firm, raise the straight leg to the horizontal, slowly curl the leg in (squeezing the heel into your buttocks), extend the leg and then lower it again.

- Do this 12 times then repeat using the other leg.

Feel the muscles at the back of your thigh working

Check that your lower back does not dip

Keep your hips square to the floor, your arms straight and look between your hands

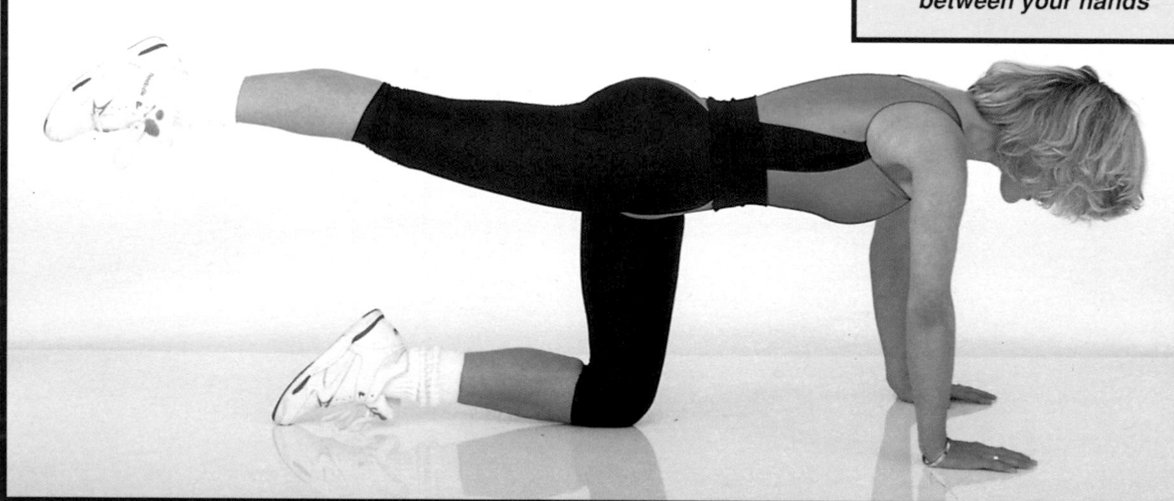

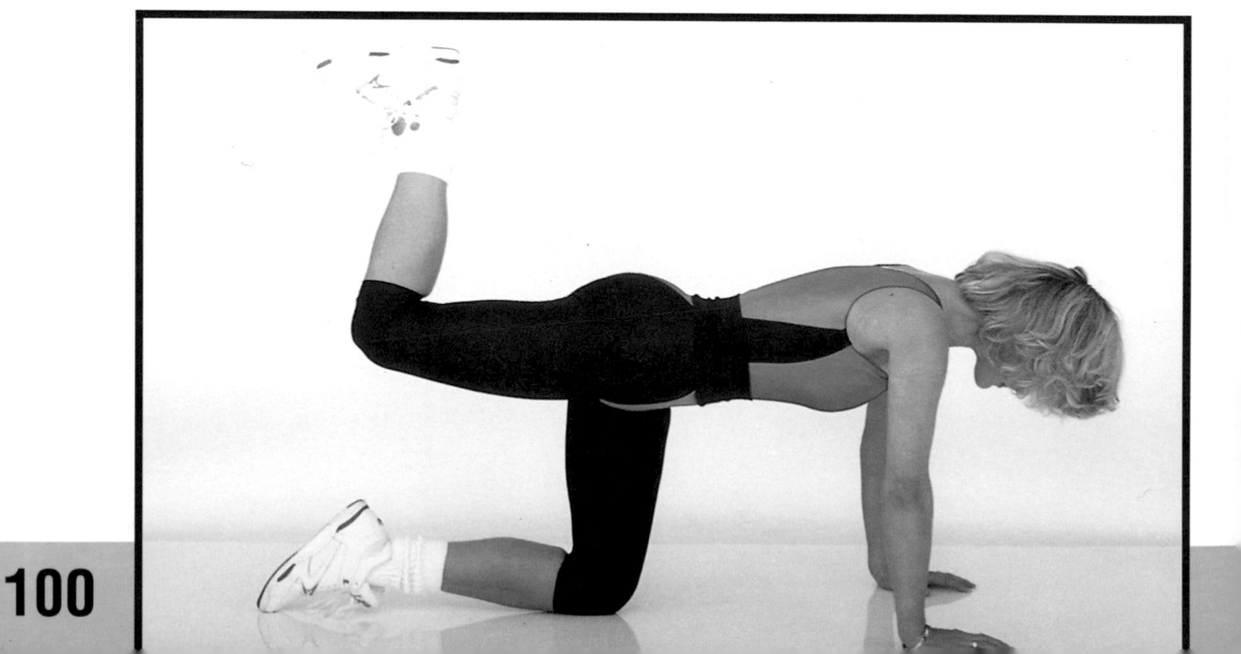

EXERCISE 8

DOGGIES

REPETITIONS
8 Right 8 Left
PURPOSE:
To tone abductors (hips)

- Adopt an all-fours position and transfer your weight very slightly over to the left leg.

- Keeping your hips level, your right leg bent at 90 degrees and the movement small, slowly raise your right leg out to the side, then lower.

- Do this 8 times with the right leg and repeat with the left.

If this exercise causes discomfort, do 8 side leg raises on each leg, either standing (see page 95) or lying (see page 126).

Feel the muscles on the outside of your hip working to raise the leg

You may feel the muscles of the other hip working to stabilize the position

Don't expect or try to lift your knee too high

Think of taking the knee slightly back as you lift it

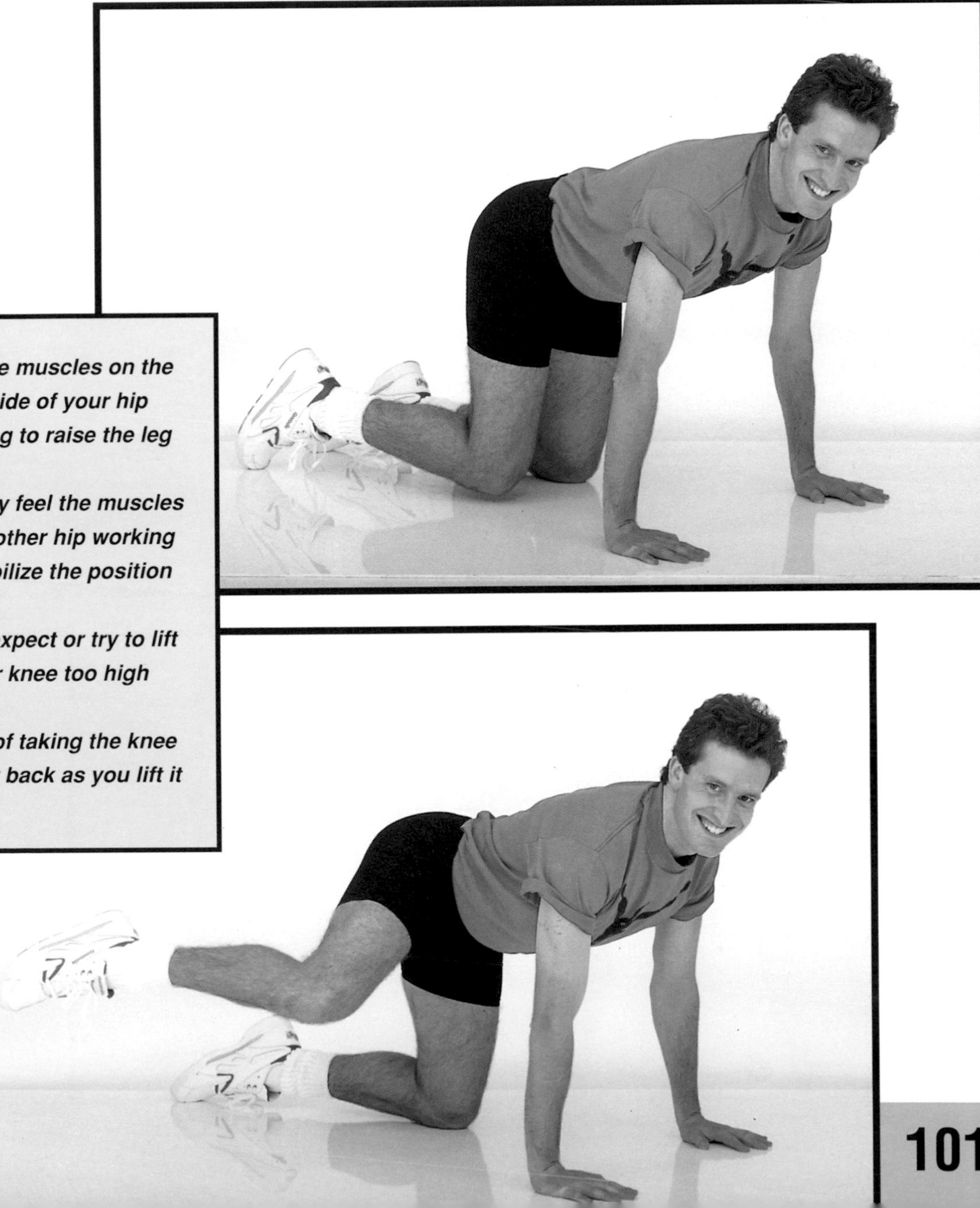

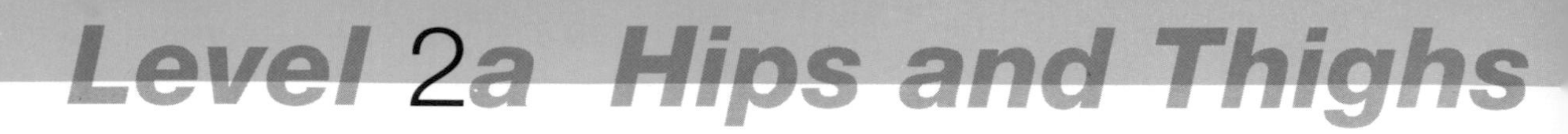

Level 2a Hips and Thighs

This cool-down repeats the cool-down exercises from Level 1a which continue to develop the stretches to improve your suppleness. You may feel that you now want to hold some of the stretches even longer, this will make them more effective providing you are comfortable. Do not bounce or jerk and aim to develop the stretch as you hold it there. As you are familiar with these exercises and can therefore work through the sequence a little more quickly, two new exercises are provided to develop the effectiveness of the session.

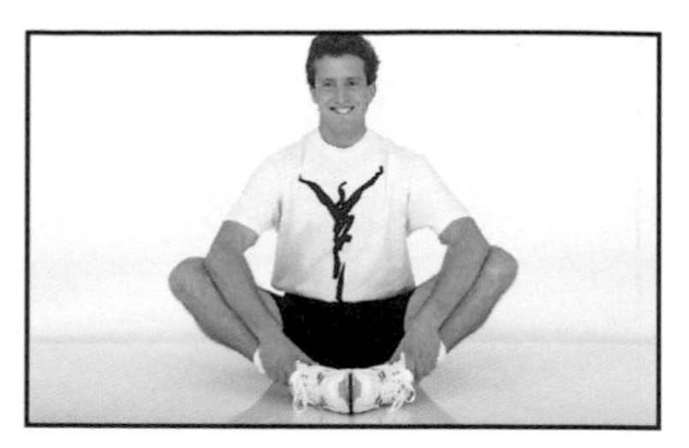

SEATED INNER THIGH STRETCH 16 counts

EXERCISE 1

KNEELING SIDE STRETCH

PURPOSE:
To stretch the obliques (waist)

- Adopt a position kneeling up, with your weight even over both knees. Extend your right leg out to the right side, bend over to the left to place your left hand on the floor level with your knees. Reach your right arm out beyond your head.

- Stretch your right arm over your head and down towards the floor until you feel a full stretch down the right side of your body.

- Hold for a count of 8, relax and repeat to the other side.

Check your body is in a flat plane and a straight line

Your supporting hand should be under your shoulder

Your supporting hand, knee and extended leg should all be in a straight line

Hold your tummy in tightly to keep your back straight

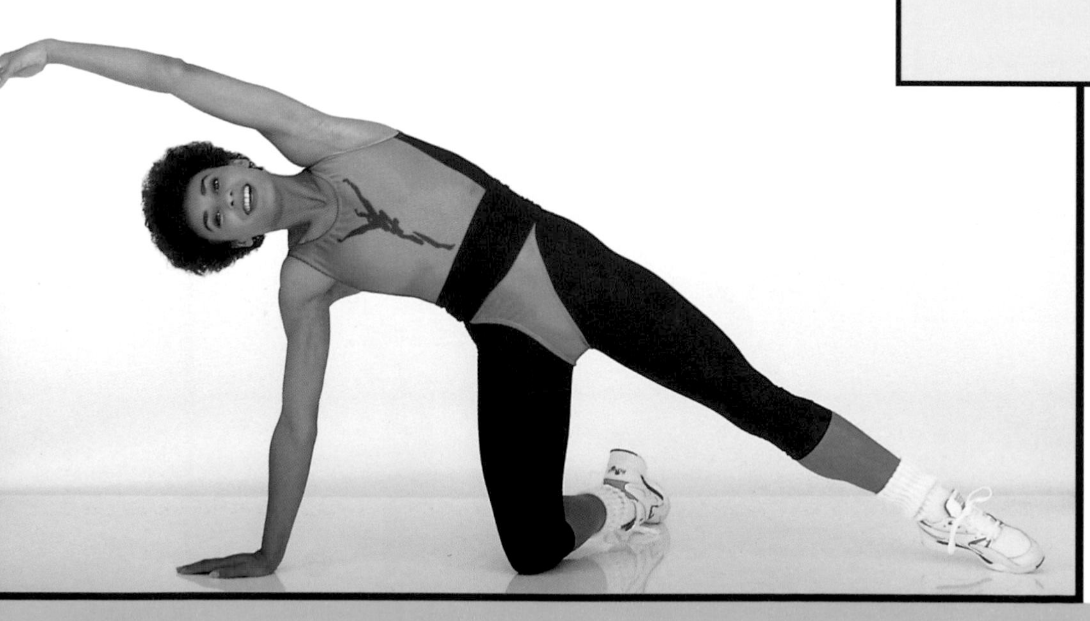

You may find the Standing Side Stretch on page 75 more comfortable.

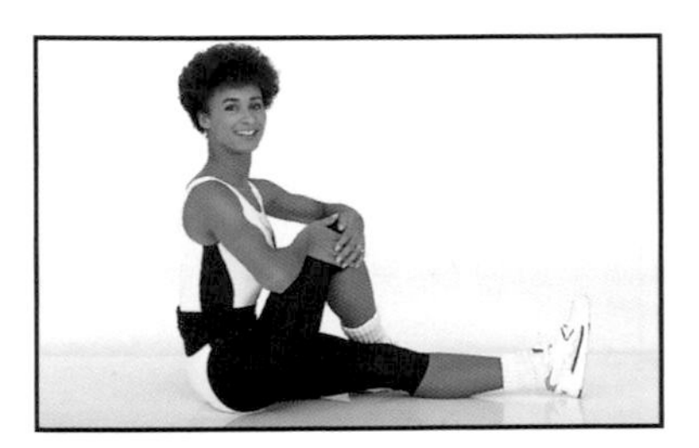

SEATED BUTTOCK TWIST
8 counts each side

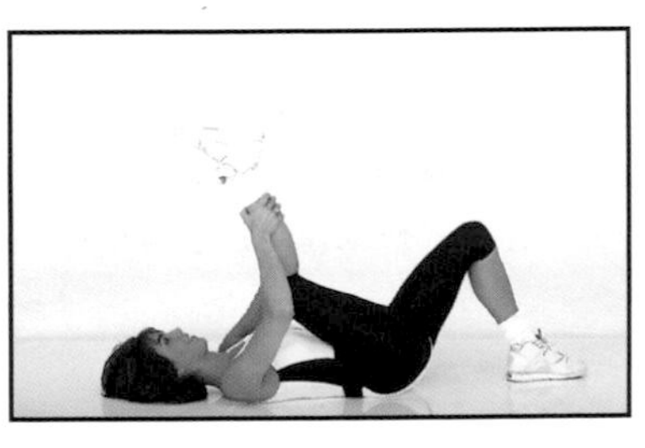

LYING HAMSTRING STRETCH
16 counts each leg

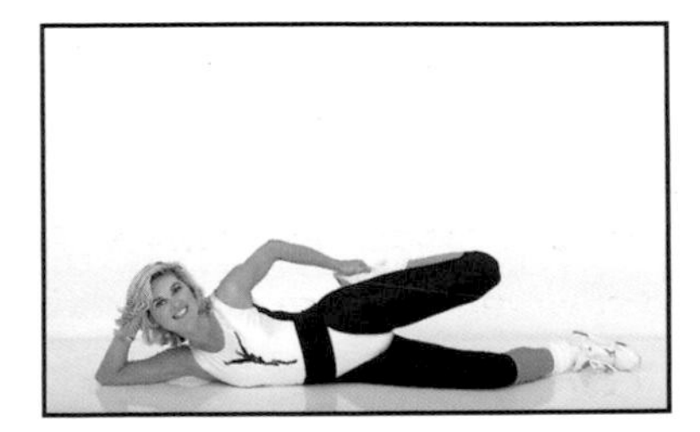

SIDE LYING QUAD STRETCH
16 counts each leg

EXERCISE 2

SITTING REACHES

REPETITIONS *4*
PURPOSE:
To loosen the sides of the body and warm the muscles

- Sit up tall with your legs in a comfortable position.

- Extend your right arm above your head and place your left hand on the floor by your side. Dropping your left shoulder and leaning on your left hand, reach up for the ceiling with your right hand, until you feel a full extension down your right side.

- Hold for a count of 1, relax, then repeat to the other side. Repeat the whole exercise once more.

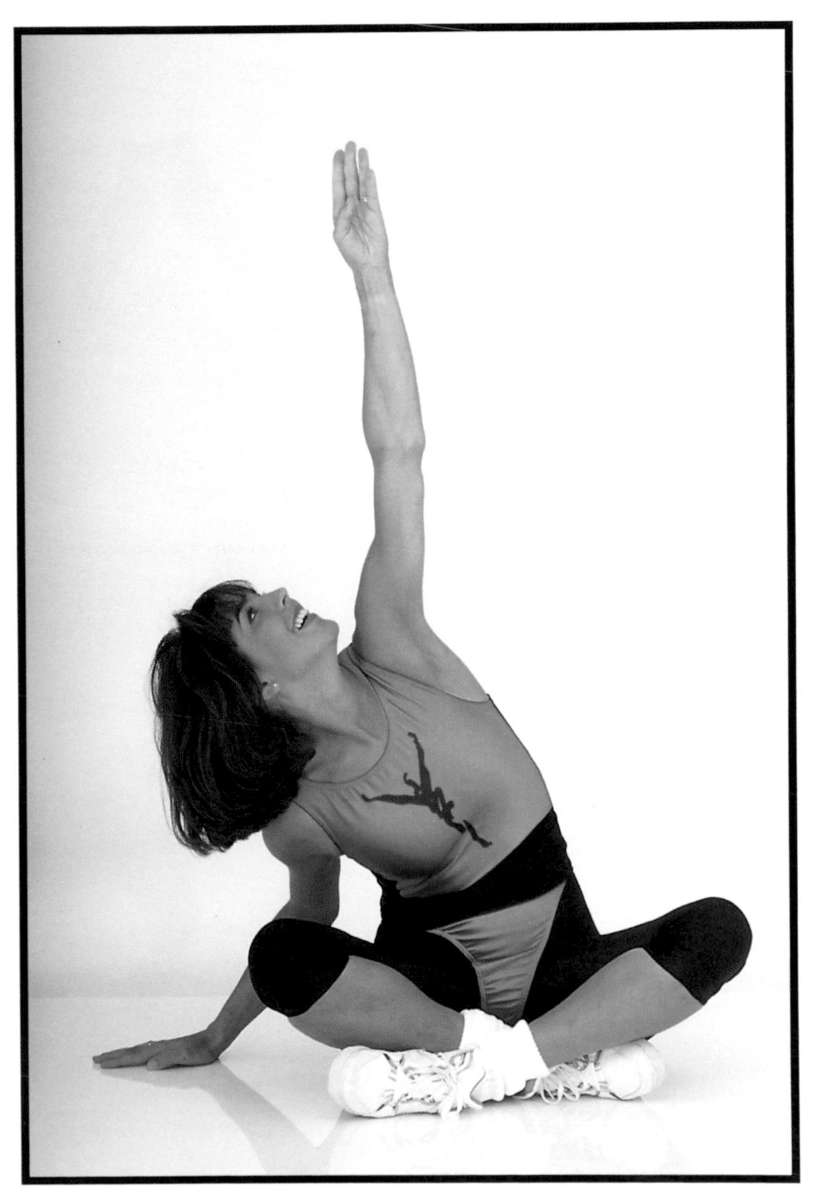

Look up towards your hand and take a deep breath in as you reach

Level 2b Tums, Bums & Arms

As for Level 2a, this warm-up adds to the exercises from Level 1b with which you are already familiar. Do not skimp on the time you allocate to this section and take time to learn the two new exercises thoroughly.

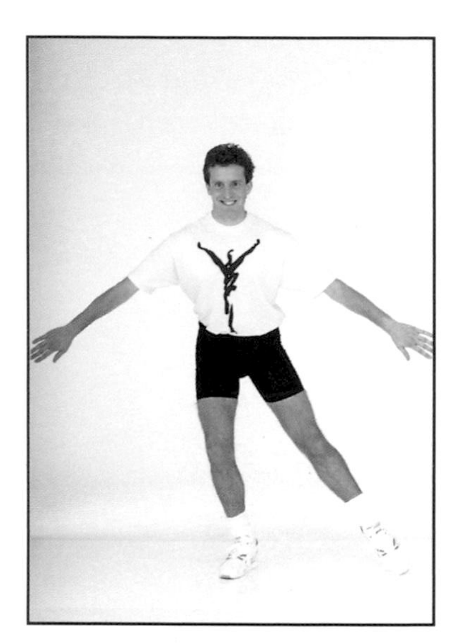

TAP LEG OUT x 4 Right 4 Left

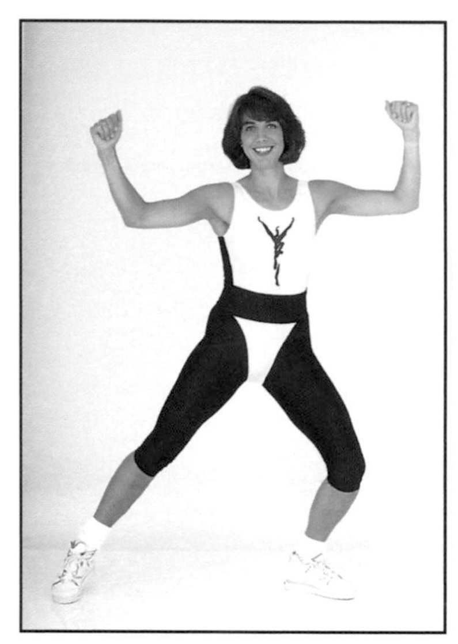

SIDE SPRINGS x 8

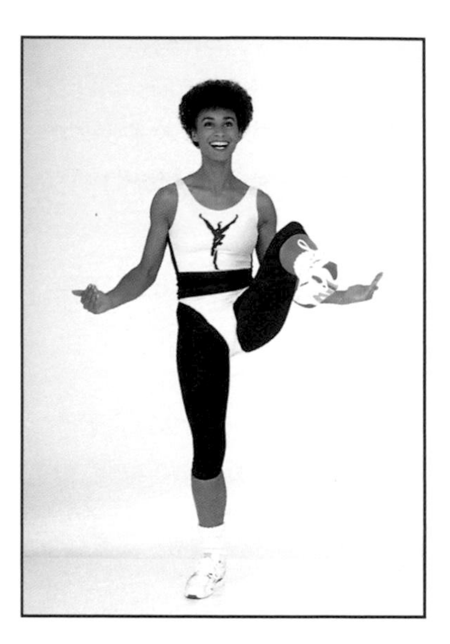

KNEE LIFTS WITH ARM PULL DOWNS x 8

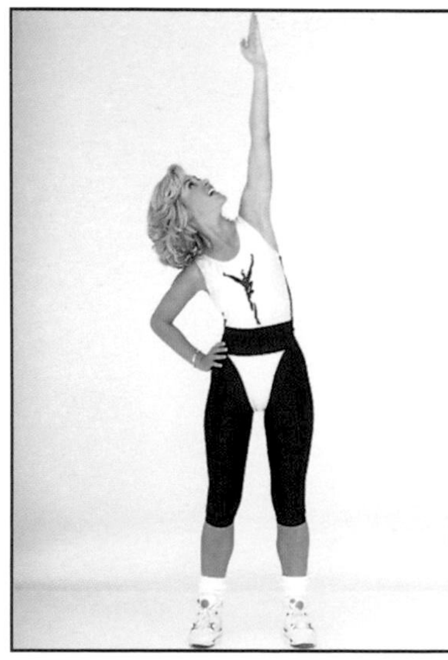

REACHES x 4

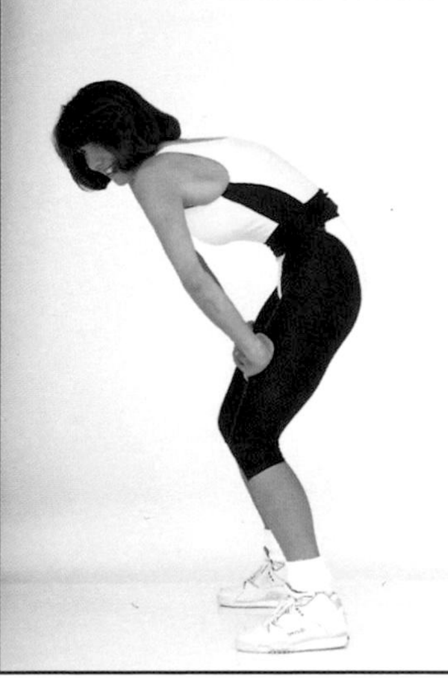

HOLLOW AND HUMP x 4

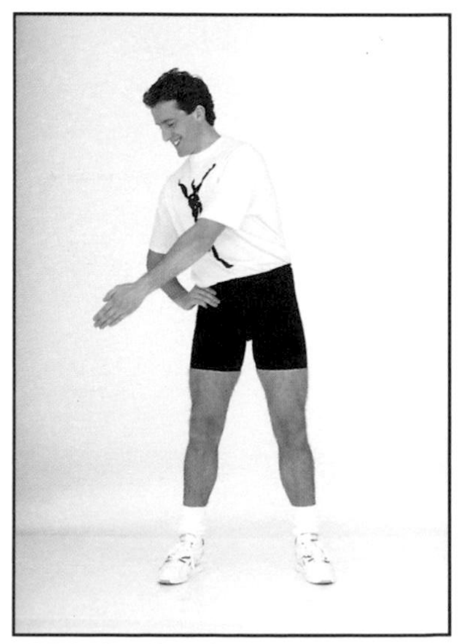

ARM CIRCLES ACROSS BODY x 2 Right 2 Left

EXERCISE 1

REACHES WITH KNEE BEND

REPETITIONS *8*
PURPOSE:
To warm the muscles and loosen the waist muscles

- Stand with your feet wider than shoulder-width apart as long as they are comfortable.

- Bending your right leg and keeping your left leg straight with the foot flat on the floor, slowly and with control reach your right arm up towards the ceiling, until you feel a stretch down your right side.

- Repeat this to the other side, then continue until you have done 8 reaches in total.

Feel the extension down the side of your rib cage

Keep your pelvis tilted correctly, your hips square and both feet flat on the floor

Look up towards your hand as you reach

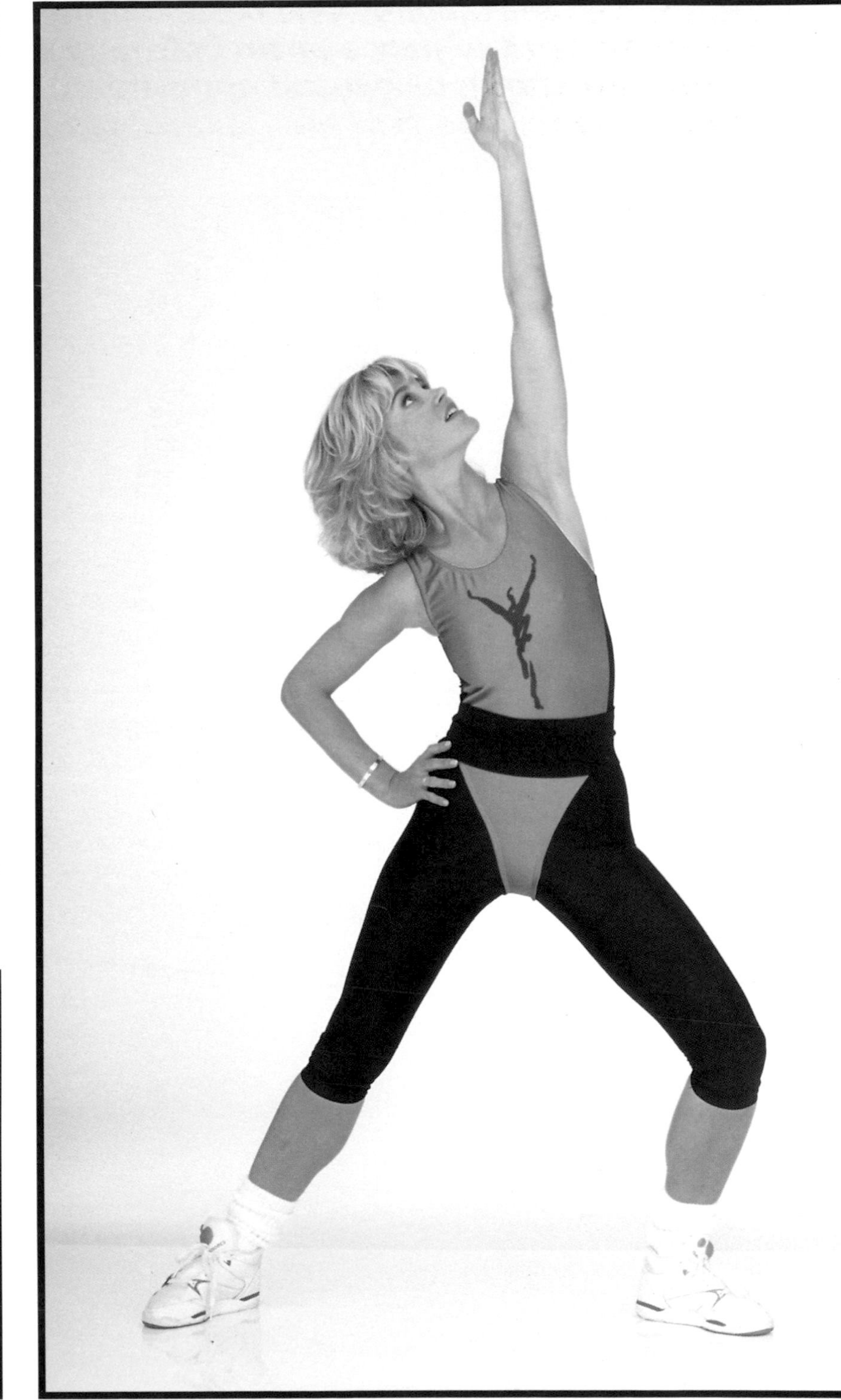

Repeat all the mobility and pulse-raising exercises listed on the previous two pages again before going on to the warm-up stretches shown below and opposite.

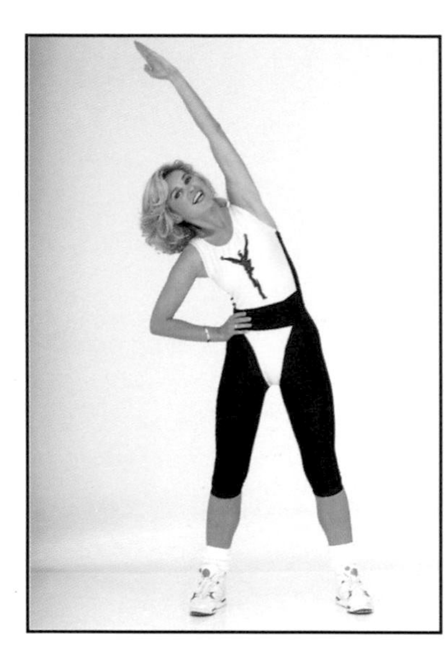

SIDE STRETCH
4 counts each side

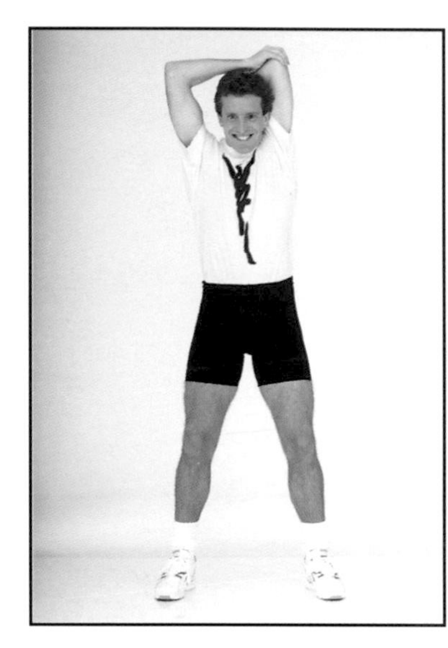

STANDING TRICEP STRETCH
4 counts each side

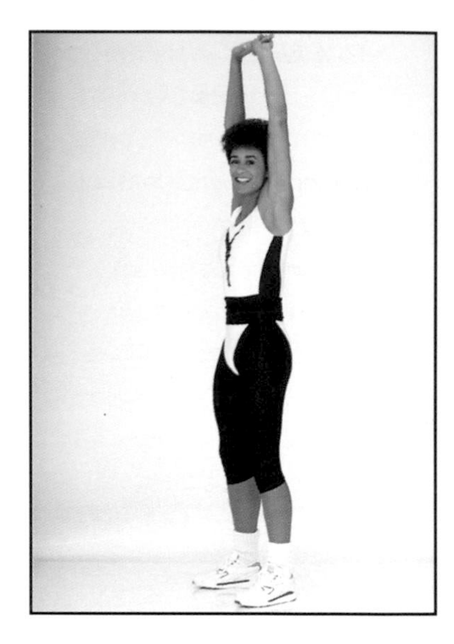

STANDING SHOULDER STRETCH 2 x 4 counts

EXERCISE 2

CHEST STRETCH

PURPOSE:
To stretch the pectorals (chest)

- Standing with your feet hip-width apart, clasp your hands together behind your back.

- Pulling in your tummy muscles to prevent your lower back from arching, extend your arms out to the back and raise them slightly until you feel a stretch across the front of your chest.

- Hold for a count of 4, rest and repeat.

Take a deep breath in as you ease into the stretch then breathe out as you hold it

To assist stretch, try to rotate the shoulders backwards

Check that you maintain a correct pelvic tilt throughout

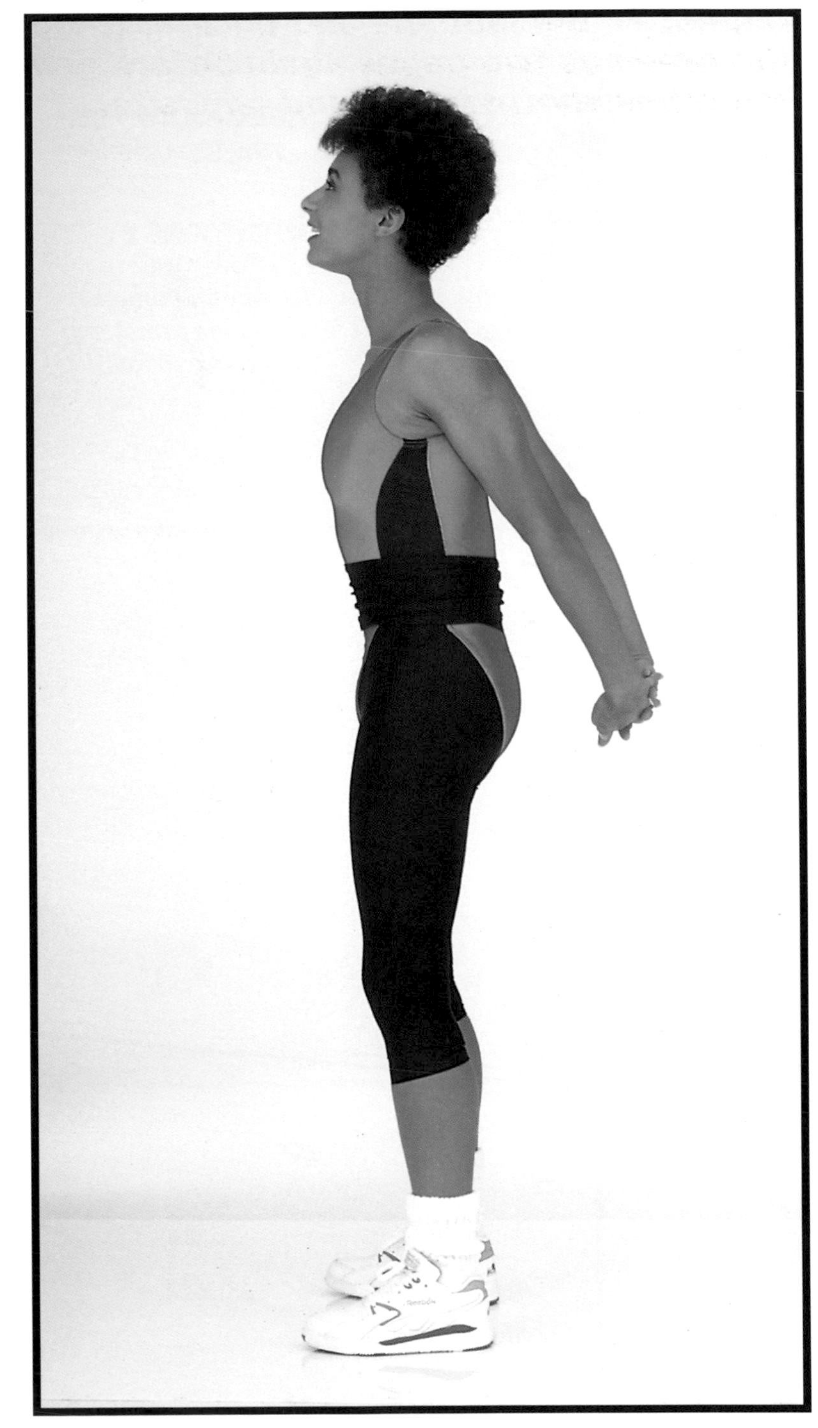

Repeat all these warm-up stretches before going on to the toning exercises.

The number of sets and repetitions of each exercise has increased since Level 1 and the exercises themselves in many cases have become harder. Keep referring to the check points to ensure that you are doing each exercise correctly, remember the muscles should feel a little tired but not exhausted after each set if the exercise is to be safe and effective. (The tummy muscles will now be referred to as abdominals.)

EXERCISE 1

THREE-QUARTER PRESS-UPS

REPETITIONS *2 x 4*
PURPOSE:
To tone the triceps (back of the arms) and pectorals (chest)

- With your hands and knees on the floor, place your shoulders over your hands and your knees far enough back for your body to be in a straight line from knees to shoulders.

- Bend your arms to lower the body, so that thighs, hips, chest and nose touch the floor simultaneously, then return to the start.

- Do this 4 times, rest then repeat it 4 more times.

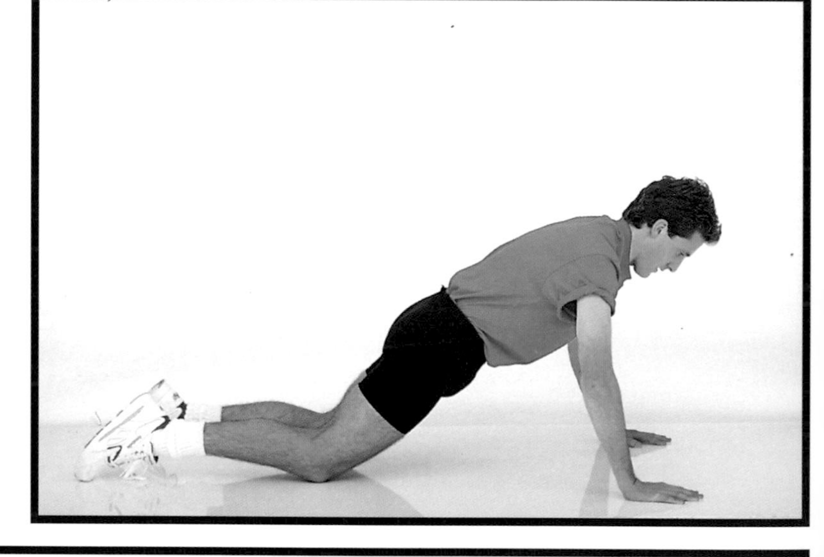

Feel the chest and upper arm muscles working

Tilt your pelvis, using your abdominal muscles to prevent a dip in the lower back and keep your shoulders over your hands

Breathe out as you push up each time

If this is too uncomfortable or too much of a strain, go back to the Box Press-ups (page 84) and do 12 repetitions, rest, then repeat.

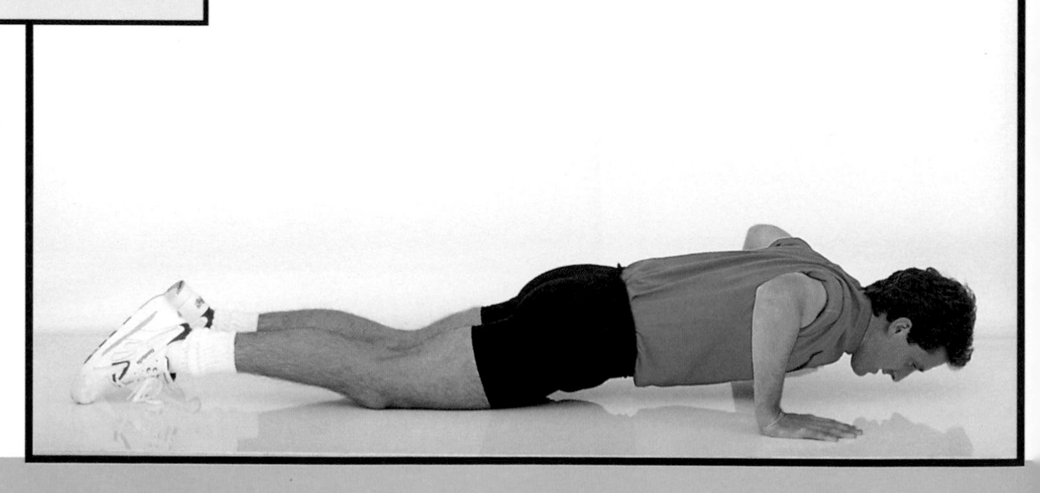

EXERCISE 2

LYING REAR LEG RAISES

REPETITIONS
12 Right 12 Left
PURPOSE:
To tone the gluteals (bum)

- Lie flat on your front with your hands on the floor under your face.
- Keeping both hips down on the floor, raise then lower one leg.
- Do this 12 times, then repeat with the other leg.

If your back hurts try doing the same exercise on all-fours. You must, however, ensure that your back is flat and held firmly throughout the exercise in this position.

Feel the buttock muscles working

Try to relax the rest of the body

The leg will not go very high

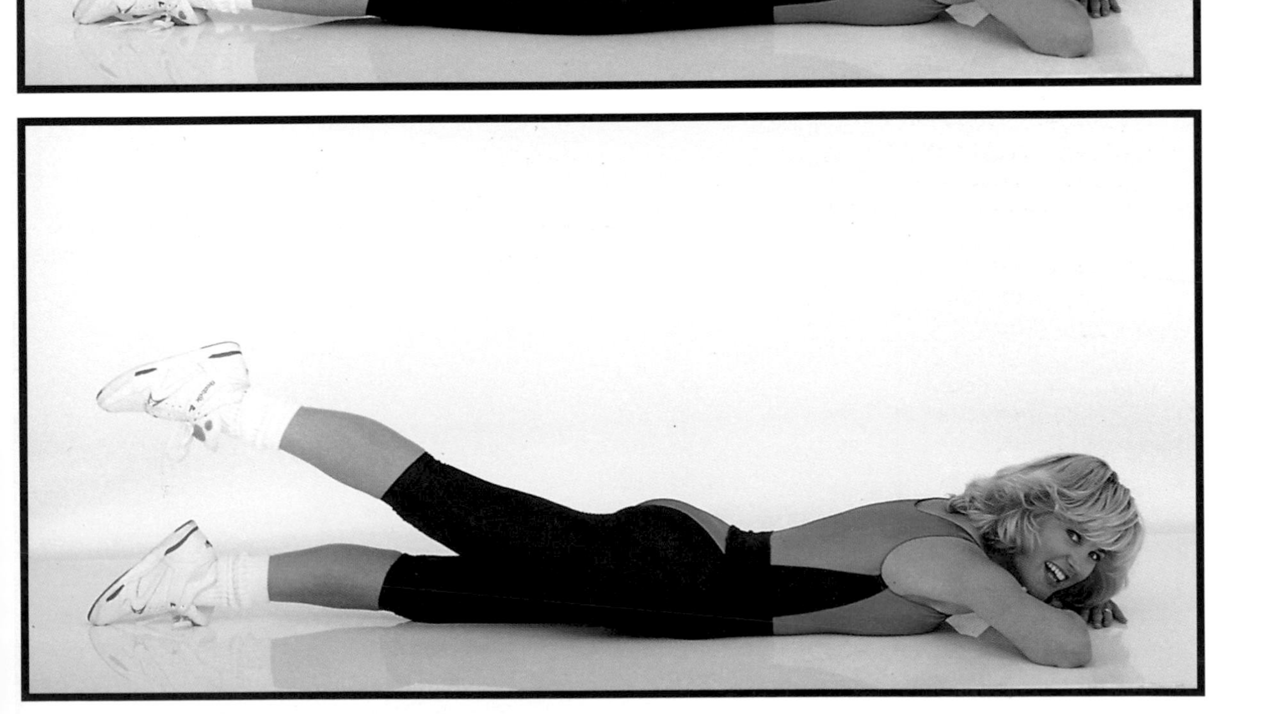

EXERCISE 3

REPEAT THE THREE-QUARTER PRESS-UPS. REPETITIONS 2 x 4

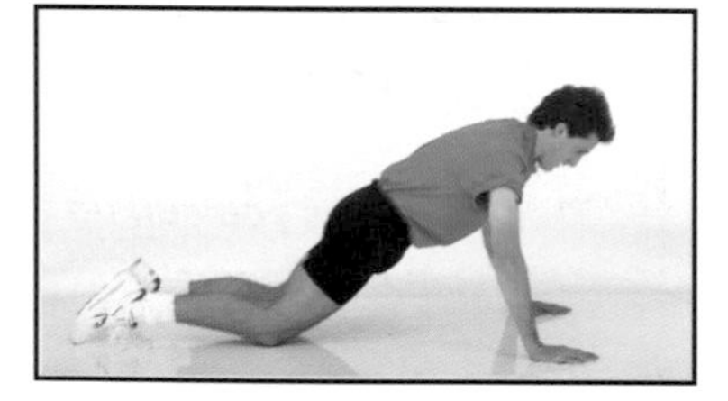

EXERCISE 4

REAR ARM RAISES

REPETITIONS 8
PURPOSE:
To tone the triceps (back of the arms)

- Lying flat on your front, with your face towards the floor, place your arms down by your sides with your palms to the floor.
- Keeping your arms straight, slowly raise them up off the floor as high as possible, then, breathing out, slightly raise your shoulders off the floor rotating them backwards (your thumbs will point up to the ceiling) and squeezing the shoulder blades together. Look forwards. Relax.
- Do this 8 times.

If your back feels uncomfortable, keep your chest on the floor.

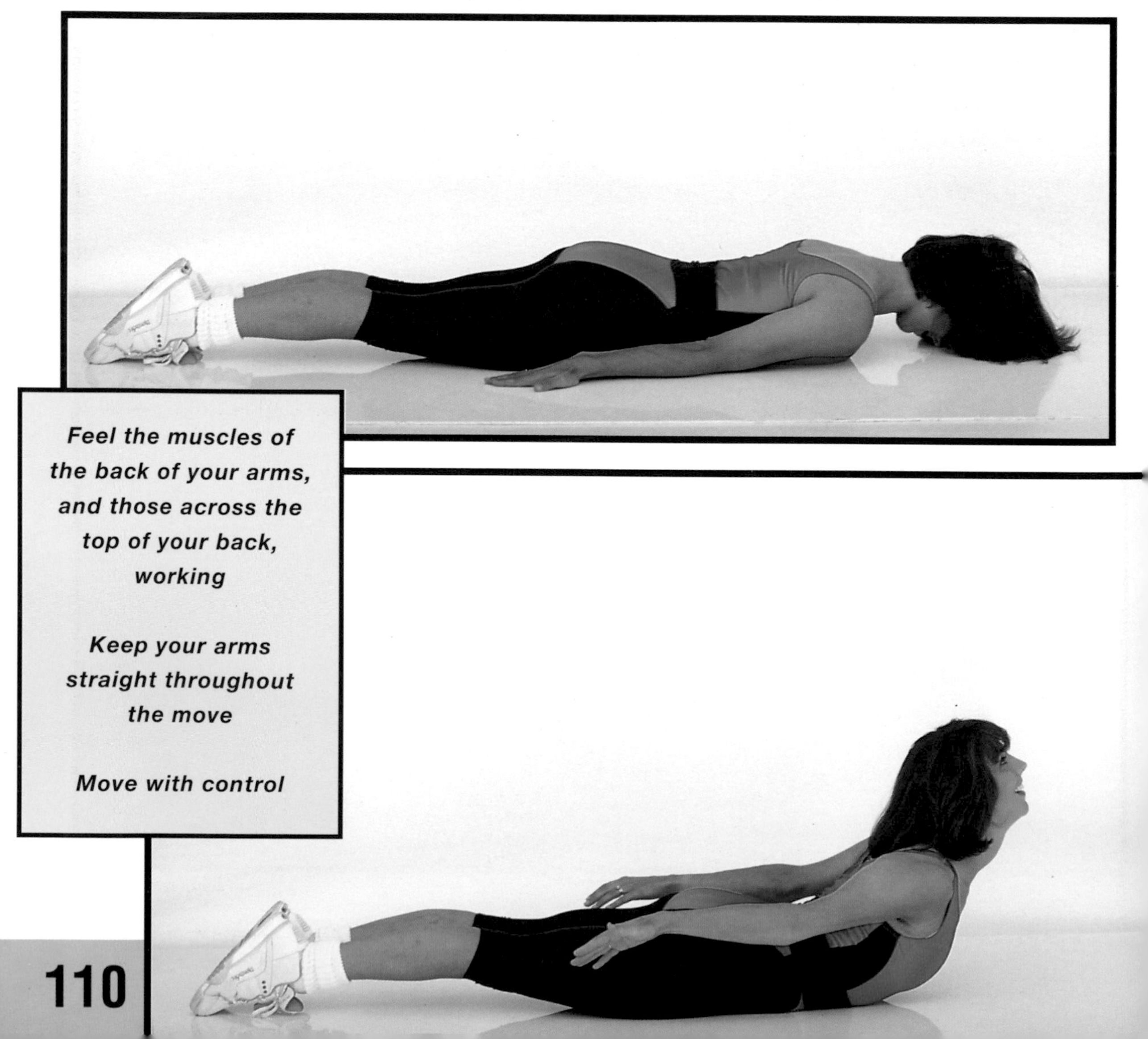

Feel the muscles of the back of your arms, and those across the top of your back, working

Keep your arms straight throughout the move

Move with control

Exercise 5

CURL-UPS

REPETITIONS *2 x 8*
PURPOSE:
To tone the abdominals (tum)

- Lie on your back, legs bent and feet flat on the floor. Rest your head in your fingertips and keep your elbows back.

- Tightening your abdominals to pull in your tummy, slowly curl your head and shoulders up off the floor, supporting your head by your fingertips. Relax.

- Do 8 times. Repeat.

Feel your abdominals working

Check that you don't pull on your head with your hands

Breathe out as you curl up
To make the exercise harder, try to curl up a little bit more and hold it for a split second at the top

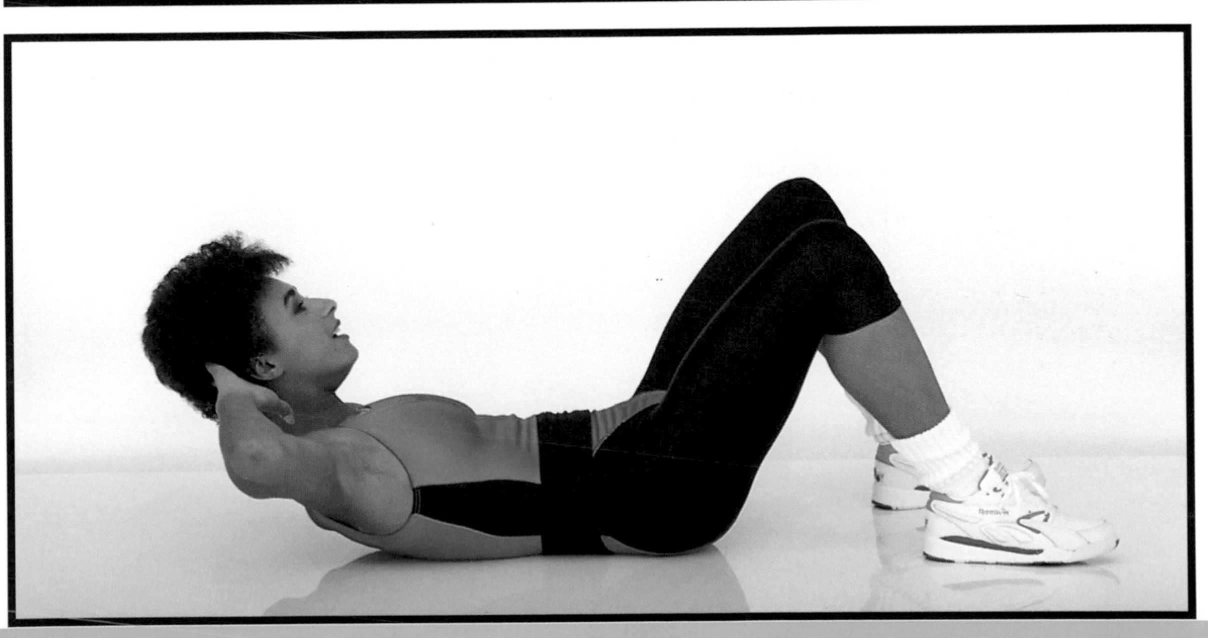

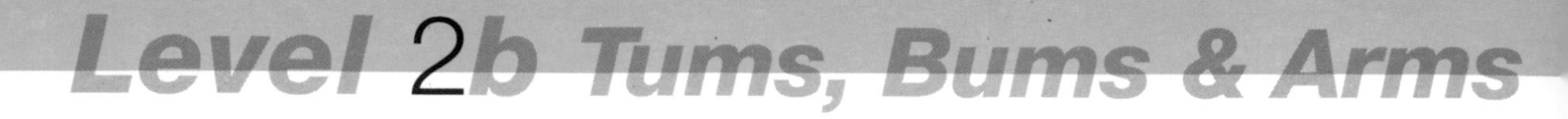

EXERCISE 6

BUTTOCKS AND THIGH SQUEEZES

REPETITIONS *12*
PURPOSE:
To tone the gluteals (bum) and adductors (inner thighs)

- Lie on your back with your legs together and knees bent; tilt your pelvis to flatten your stomach.

- Raise your hips off the floor to make a straight line from your knees to your chest.

- Keeping the lower back still, tighten your buttocks and squeeze your knees together, relax.

- Do this 12 times.

Feel the buttocks and the inner thigh muscles working

Take care to keep the upper back (shoulder blades) in contact with the floor

Ensure you do not arch your back

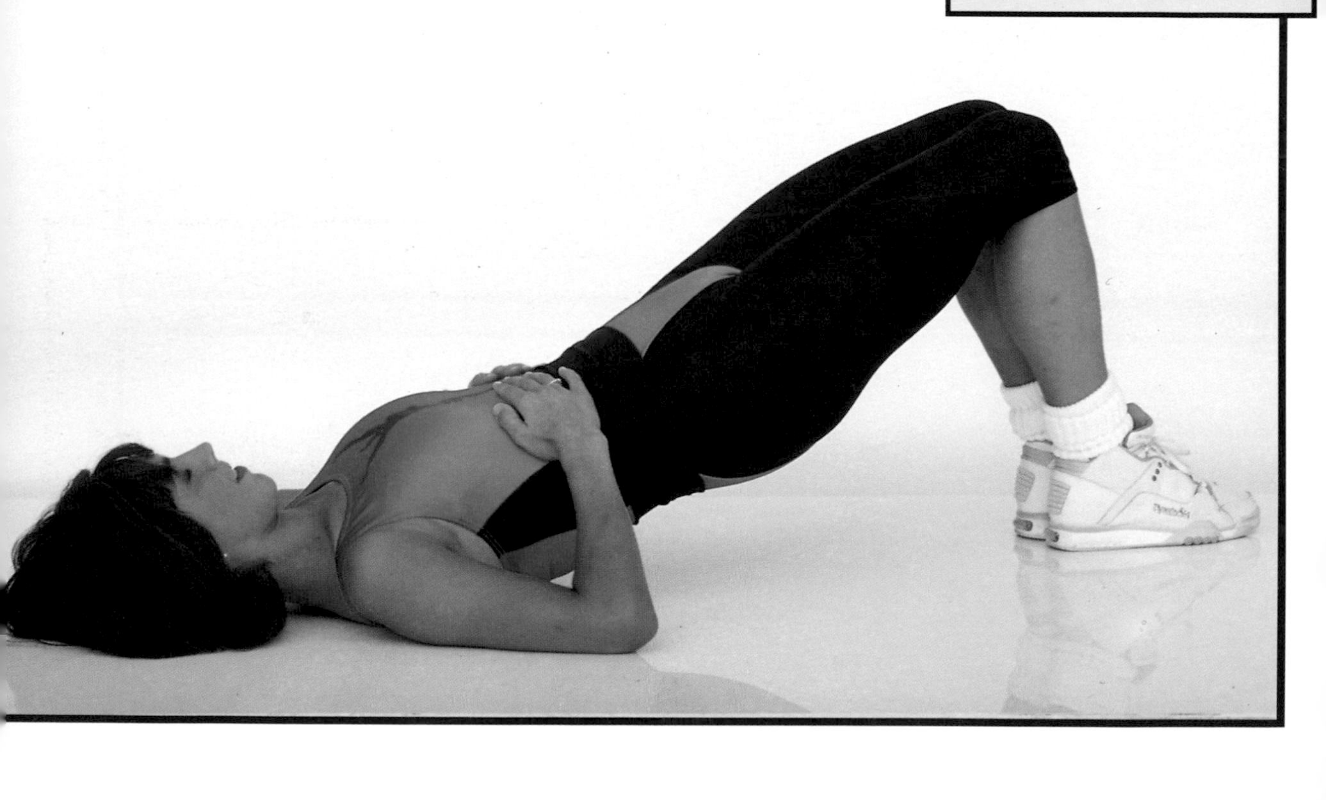

EXERCISE 7

TWISTING CURL-UPS

REPETITIONS
6 Right 6 Left
PURPOSE:
To tone the abdominals (tum)

- Lie on your back with your legs bent and your head resting in your fingertips.

- Place your right ankle over your left knee and keep your right knee pushed away from you.

- Holding your tummy in flat, curl your head and shoulders off the floor, twisting to the right to lean on your right elbow and taking your left elbow across to touch the right knee. Relax.

- Do this 6 times then change the legs over and repeat the exercise twisting to the other side.

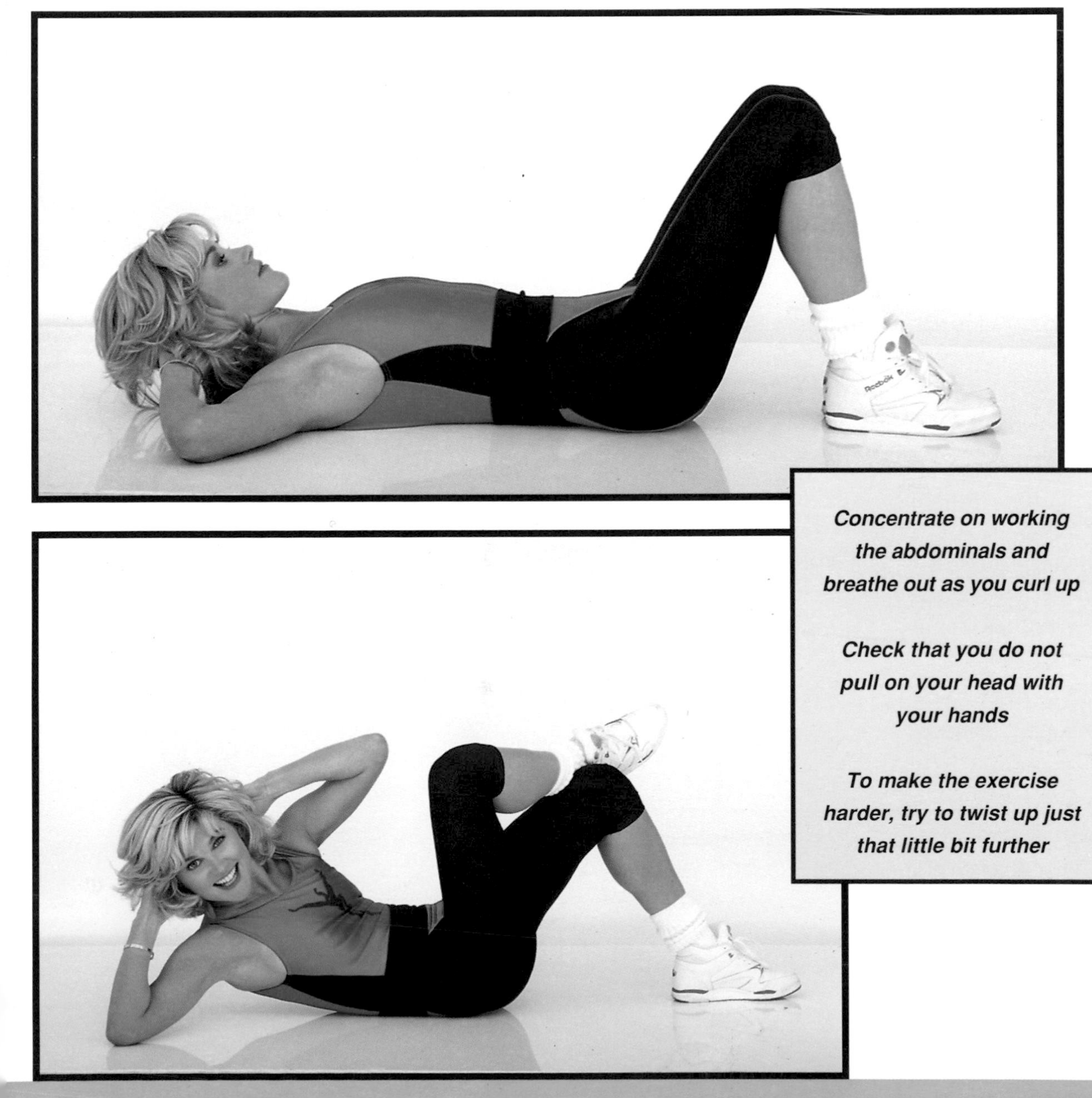

Concentrate on working the abdominals and breathe out as you curl up

Check that you do not pull on your head with your hands

To make the exercise harder, try to twist up just that little bit further

Exercise 8

REPEAT BUTTOCK AND THIGH SQUEEZES x 12

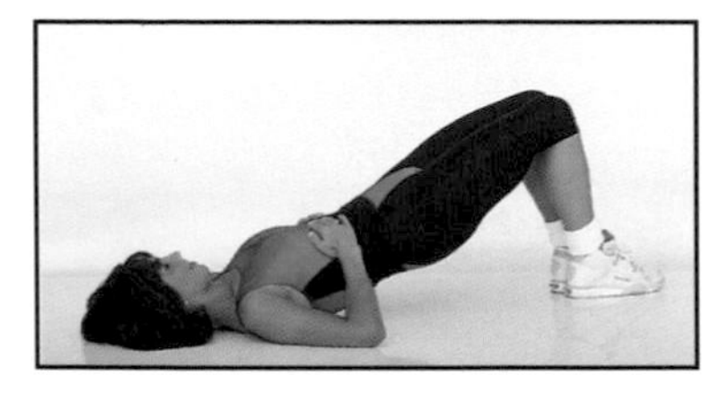

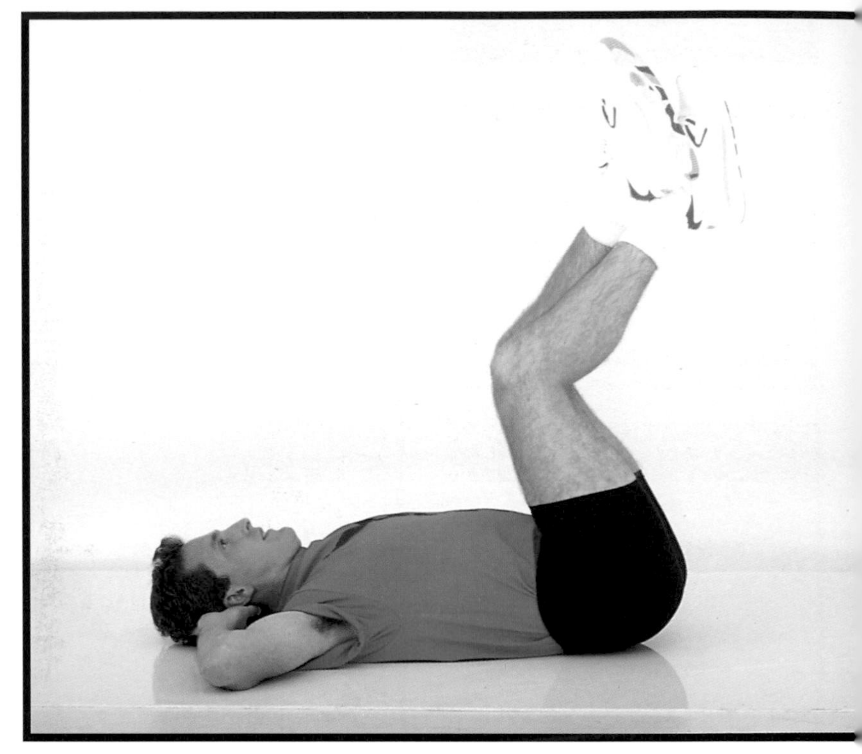

Exercise 9

CRUNCHIES

REPETITIONS *2 x 6*
PURPOSE:
To tone the abdominals (tum)

- Lie on your back with your legs bent up over your chest and your head resting in your fingertips.
- Keeping your knees still and your tummy held in flat, curl your head and shoulders up towards your knees. Relax.
- Do this 6 times, rest then repeat a further 6 times.

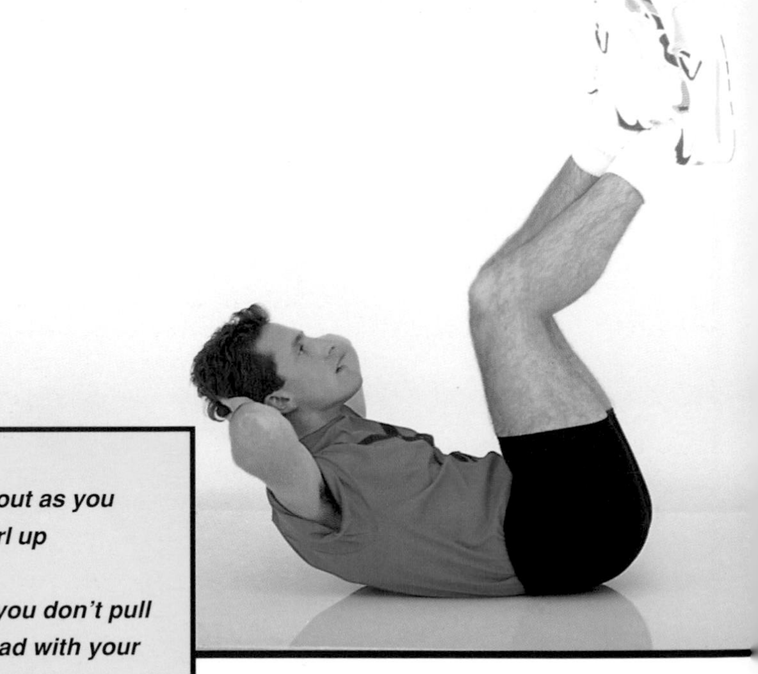

Feel your abdominals working

Breathe out as you curl up

Check that you keep your knees over your tummy throughout

Check that you don't pull on your head with your arms

EXERCISE 10

REPEAT BUTTOCK AND THIGH SQUEEZES x 12

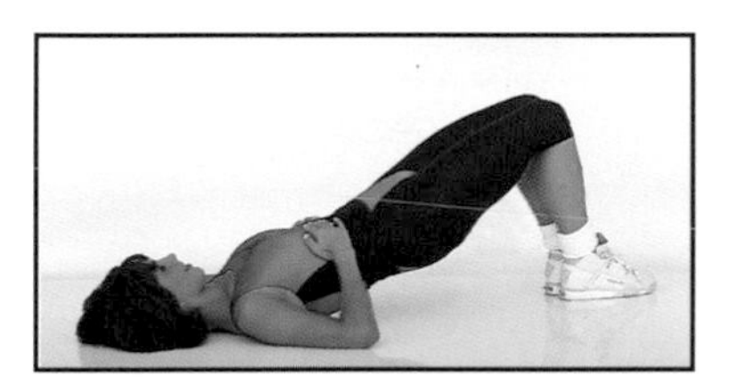

EXERCISE 11

SEATED DIPS

REPETITIONS *12*
PURPOSE:
To tone the triceps (back of the arm)

- Sit on the floor with your legs bent and your feet flat on the floor in front of you.
- Place your hands on the floor as far behind you as you can with your fingers pointing back towards you.
- Bend, then gently straighten your arms.
- Do this 12 times.

If you find this exercise uncomfortable, do 12 Rear Arm Raises instead (see page 110).

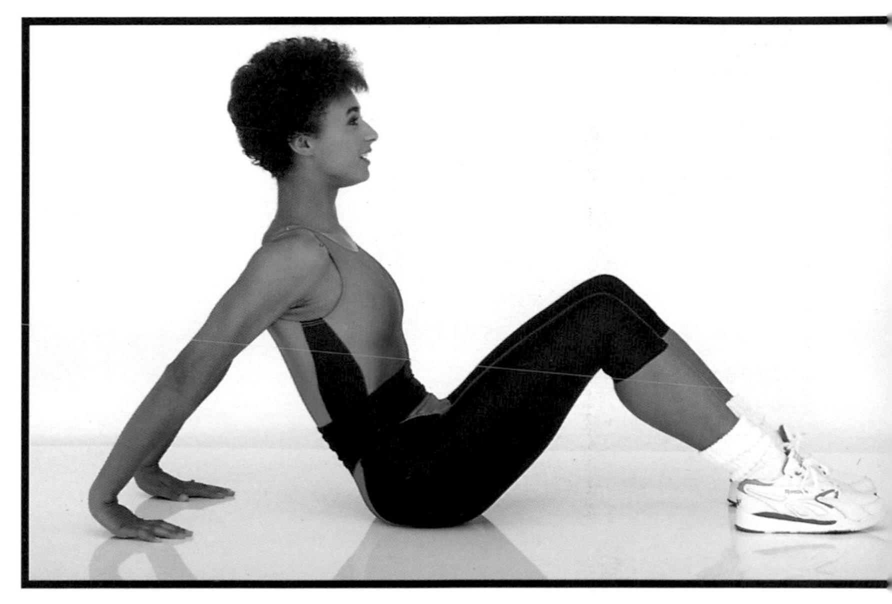

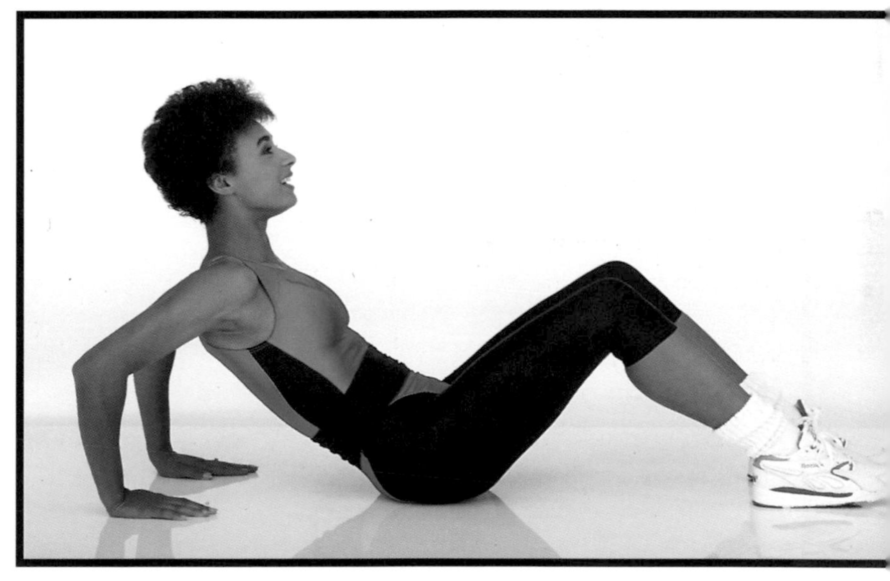

Feel the muscles around the back of your arms working

You will probably also feel a stretch across the front of the shoulder. Don't expect to go too low - it's the flexibility of your shoulder that is limiting you

Check your hands are in the correct position and do not lock out the elbows as you straighten your arms

Try to keep your back as straight as possible

The time allocated to the cool-down has been slightly reduced from that in Level 1 but this is a minimum and is only meant as a guide. Ensure that the exercises are all performed correctly and held for long enough, so that the muscles do not stiffen up and feel uncomfortable the next day. Repeat the cool-down exercises from Level 1b and add the two new ones to your regime.

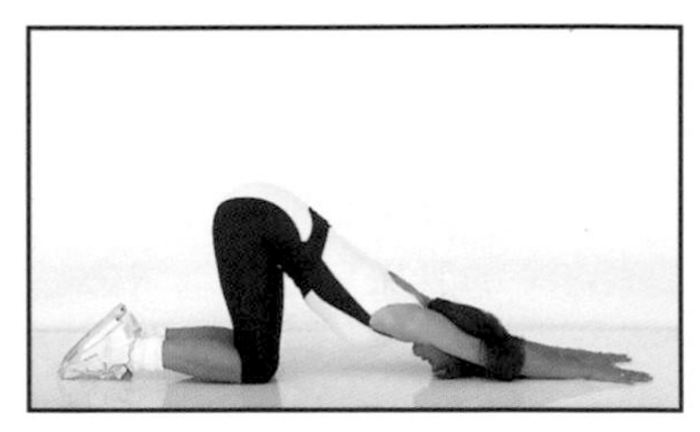

KNEELING SHOULDER STRETCH
8 counts

EXERCISE 1

SEATED SHOULDER STRETCH

PURPOSE:
To stretch the anterior deltoids (front of the shoulder)

- Sitting on the floor with your legs bent and your feet flat on the floor in front of you, place your hands close together on the floor behind you with your fingers pointing away from you.
- Keeping your elbows very slightly bent to protect the elbow joint, slide your bottom forwards away from your hands until you feel the stretch across the front of your shoulders.
- Hold for a count of 8, rest and repeat.

Check that your fingers point away from you

Ease into the stretch very gently and don't expect to get very far at first

Ensure that you keep your elbows slightly bent throughout

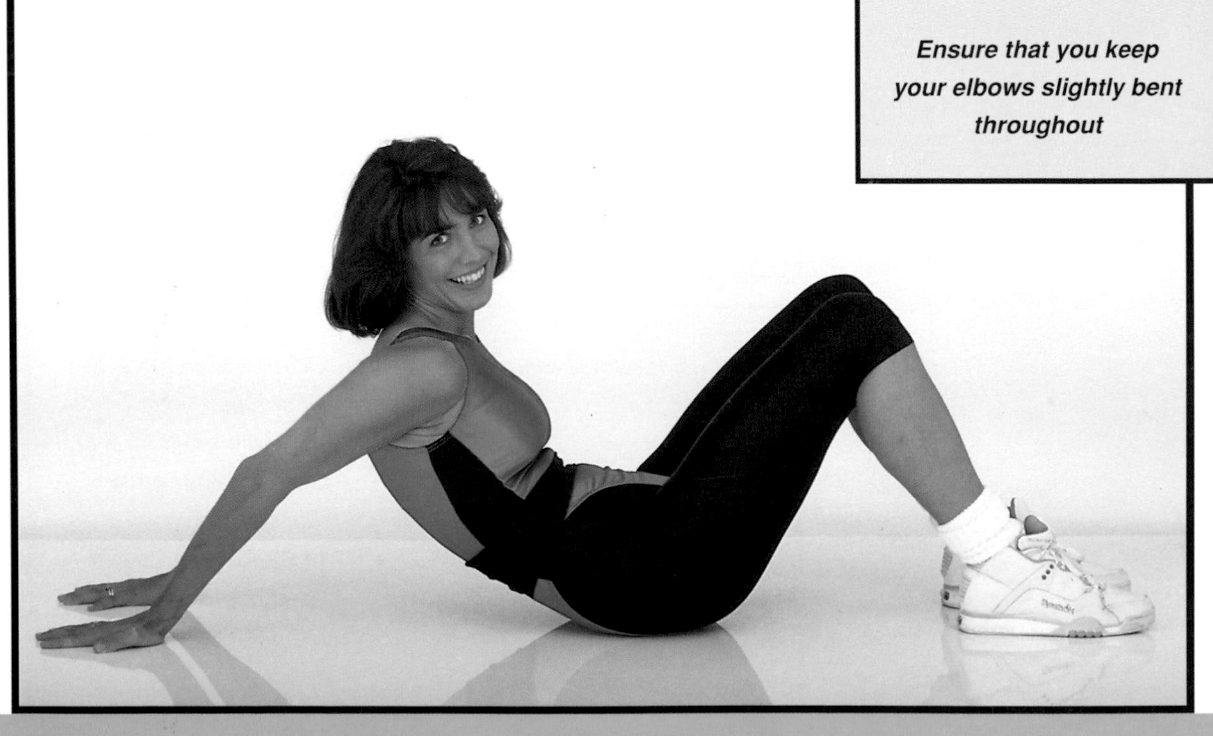

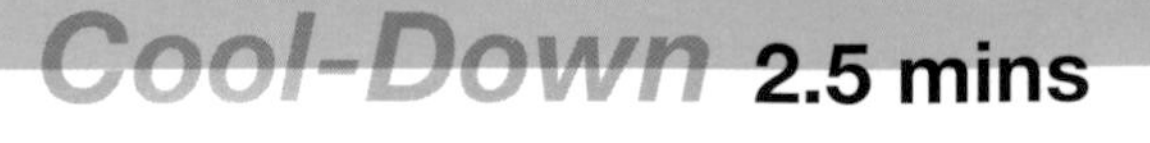

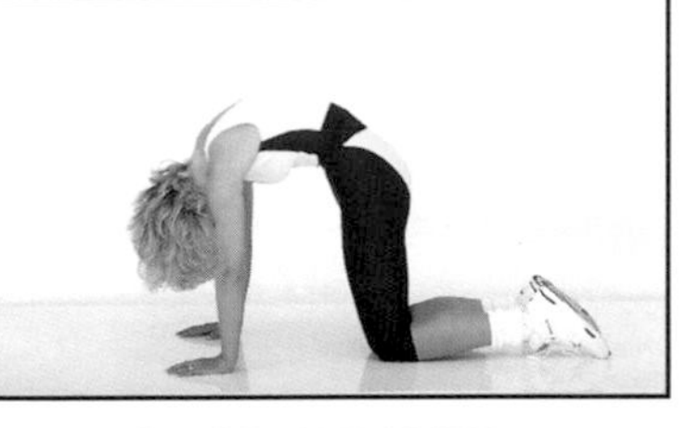

HOLLOW AND HUMP x 4

SEATED TRICEP STRETCH
8 counts each arm

SEATED HAMSTRING STRETCH
16 counts each leg

EXERCISE 2

TUM STRETCH

PURPOSE:
To stretch the abdominals (tum) and mobilize the spine

- Lie on your front, your legs straight out behind you and your hands on the floor in front of your head (arms slightly bent).

- Gently lift your head and shoulders off the floor by pushing on your hands and straightening your arms, then, keeping your hips on the floor and your arms straight, shuffle your hands in slightly towards you until you feel a stretch down the front of your tummy.

- Hold for a count of 4, rest, then repeat.

Check that your hips are supported on the floor throughout

Think of lengthening your spine rather than curling it backwards

Don't try to push up too far

Breathe naturally

Level 3a Hips and Thighs

You may find by now that you can compile your own set of warm-up exercises by choosing previously relevant ones. That is fine as long as they provide a balance of mobility and pulse-raising (warming) exercises and an adequate set of stretches relevant to the muscles to be worked.

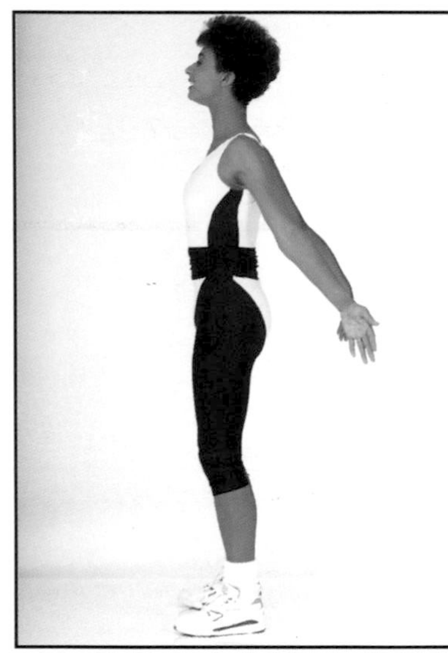

SHOULDER SQUEEZES x 4

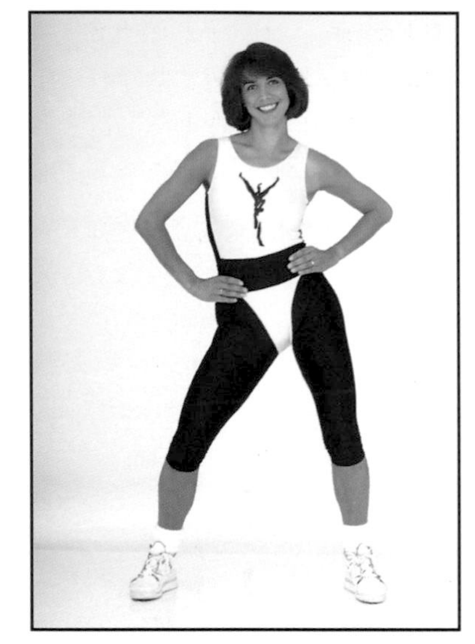

HIP CIRCLES x 2 Right 2 Left

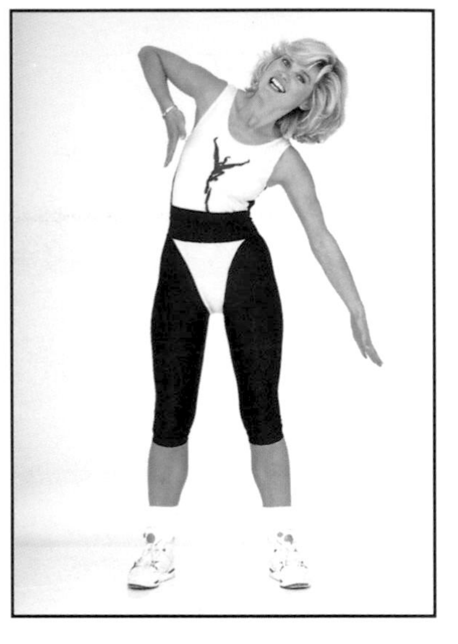

SIDE BENDS x 4

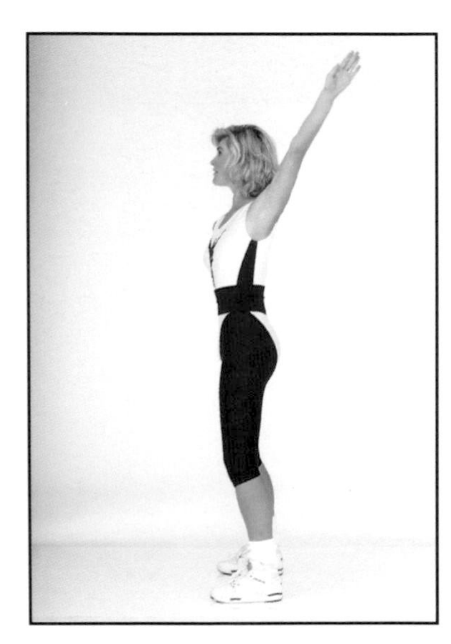

FORWARD ARM CIRCLES x 2 Right 2 Left

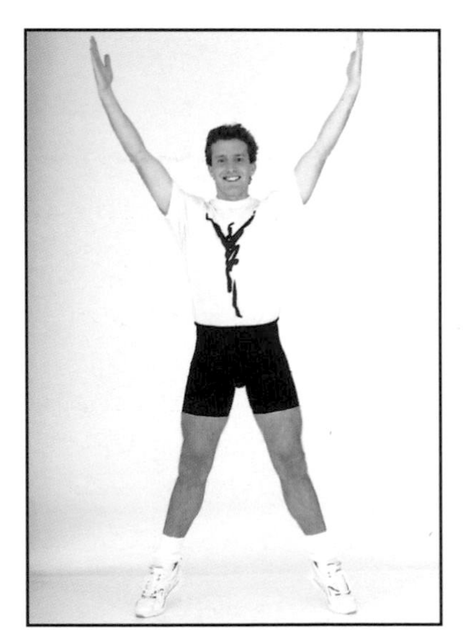

SQUAT AND REACH WITH HEEL RAISES x 4

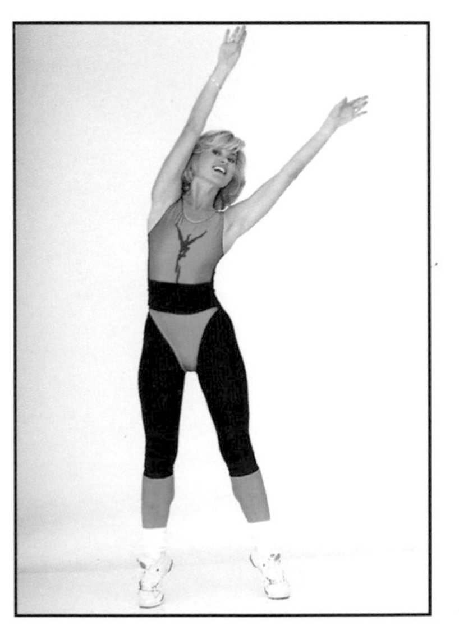

FULL CIRCLE SWINGS x 8

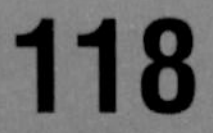

EXERCISE 1

WAIST TWISTS WITH ARM PUSHES

REPETITIONS *8*
PURPOSE:
To mobilize the spine

- Stand with good posture, your feet shoulder width apart, knees slightly bent and your fingertips resting on your shoulders.

- Keeping your hips still and facing the front with elbows pointing out, slowly twist your head, shoulders and arms to the right as far as you can, return to the front then extend your arms forwards at shoulder height and replace the hands on your shoulders.

- Repeat to the left and continue alternate sides until you have done it 8 times.

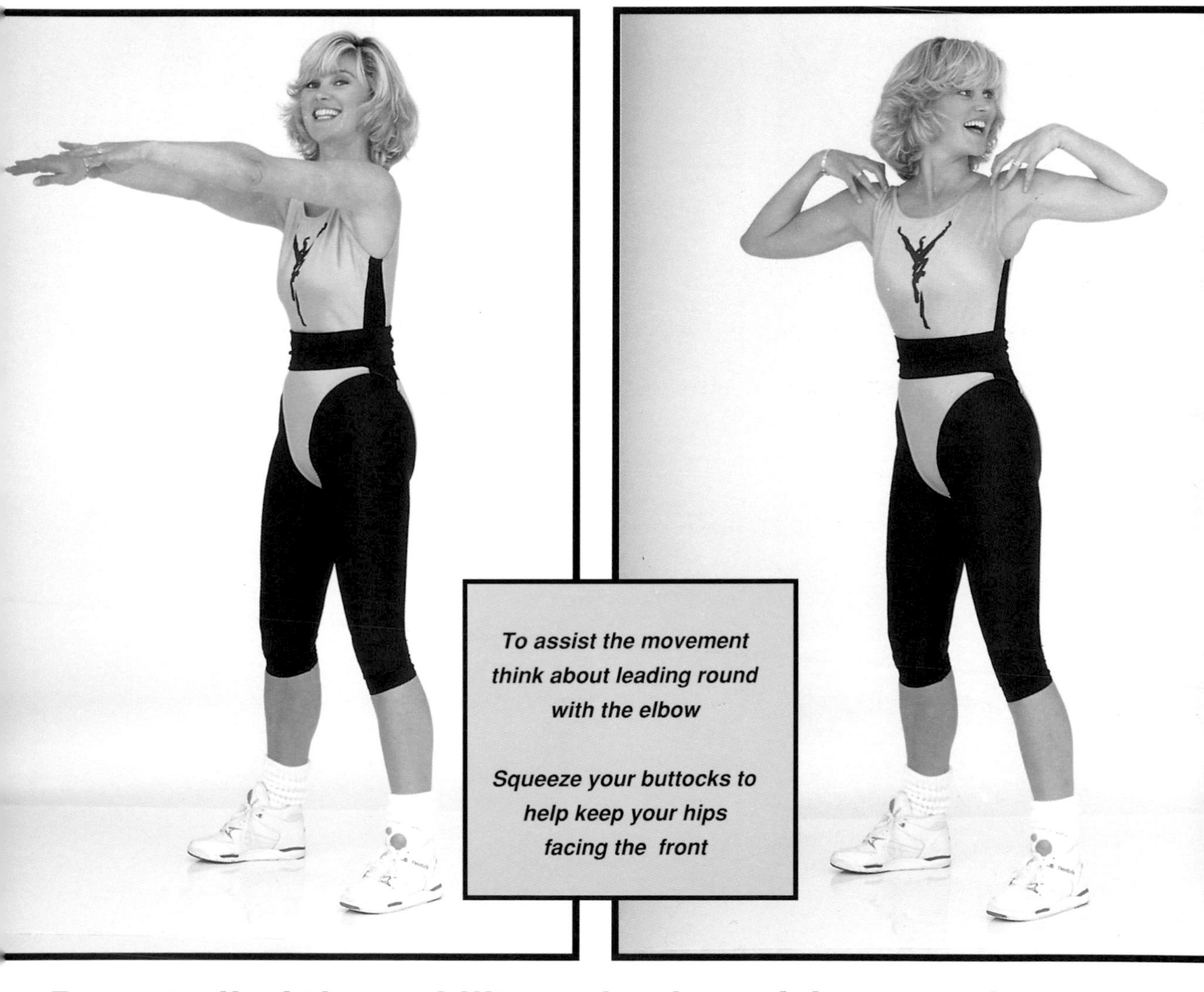

To assist the movement think about leading round with the elbow

Squeeze your buttocks to help keep your hips facing the front

Repeat all of the mobility and pulse-raising exercises before moving on to the warm-up stretches.

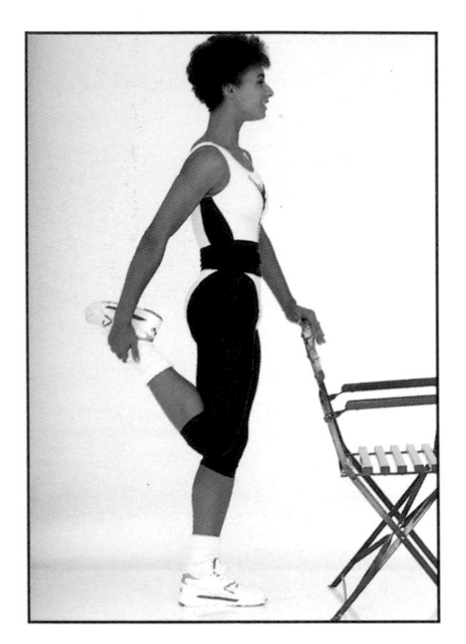

STANDING QUAD STRETCH
8 counts for each leg

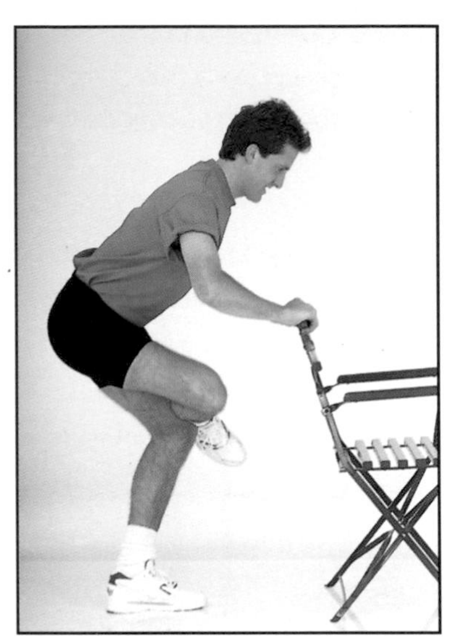

STANDING BUTTOCK STRETCH
8 counts for each side

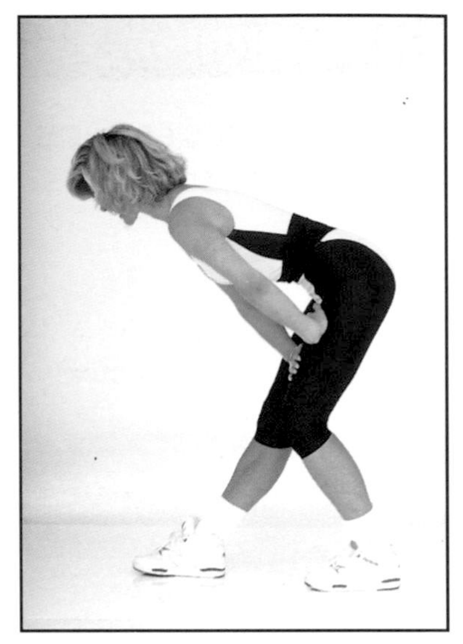

STANDING HAMSTRING STRETCH 8 counts for each leg

EXERCISE 2

LOW FORWARD LUNGE STRETCH

PURPOSE:
To stretch the gluteals (buttocks) and adductors (inner thigh)

- Step forward, bend the front knee and place your hands on the floor either side of your front foot.

- Keeping the knee of the front leg in line with its heel and sliding the back foot backwards, lower your hips until you feel a stretch in the inner thigh and/or buttocks.

- Hold for a count of 8, then repeat with the other leg in front.

Try to keep your back leg straight

Do not bounce - it is quite tempting in this position

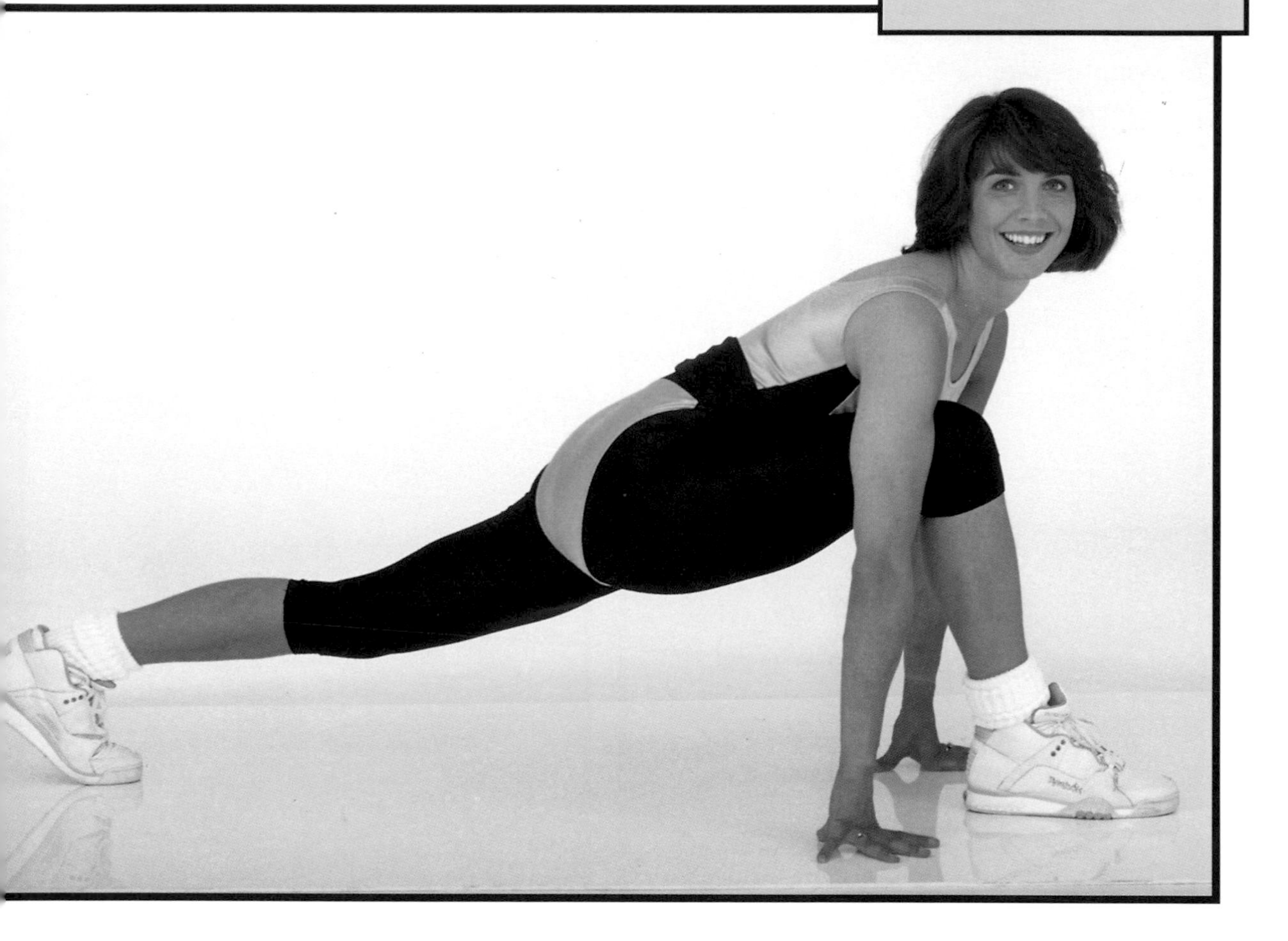

Some exercises now require you to alternate sets of different exercises so that instead of resting between sets, you do the next exercise then return to the first one for the repeat. This allows the muscles to recover between sets but it reduces the actual time for which you are resting. Overall this will enable you to do more exercise in the same amount of time.

EXERCISE 1

ADVANCED FRONT LEG RAISES

REPETITIONS
2 (8 Right 8 Left)
PURPOSE:
To tone the quadriceps (front of thigh) and the gluteals (buttocks)

- Stand left side on to a chair, hold onto it for support and. extend the right leg in front of you.

- Keeping your back still, bend the supporting leg and slowly raise the right leg as high as you can. Lower the right leg and straighten the supporting leg to recover.

- Do this 8 times, turn round then repeat 8 times using the other leg.

- Repeat the whole exercise again.

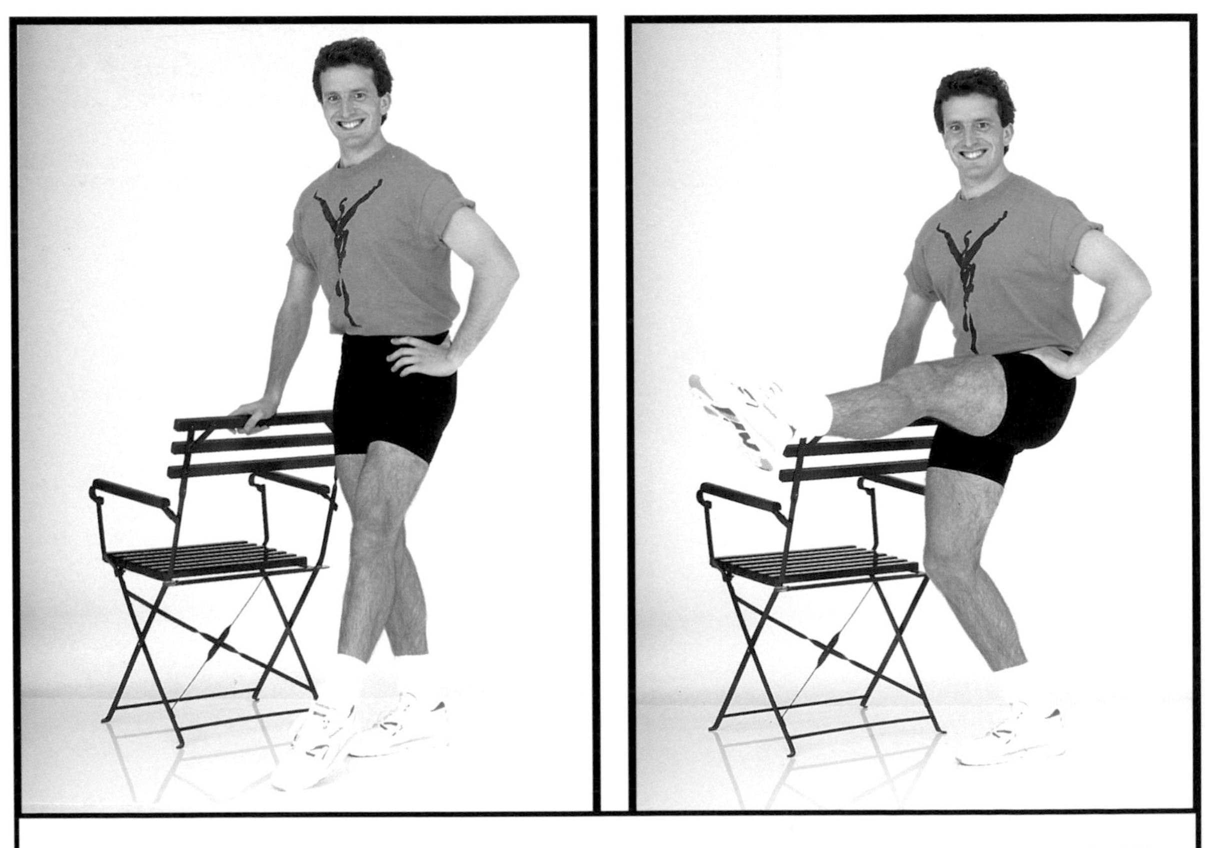

Squeeze your buttocks to work them and to support your hips

Feel the thigh muscles working

Keep the working leg straight throughout the exercise

Keep your abdominals held in tightly to support your back

EXERCISE 2

ADVANCED REAR LEG CURLS

REPETITIONS
2 x 8 Left 2 x 8 Right
PURPOSE:
To tone the hamstrings (back of the thigh), gluteals (buttocks) and quadriceps (front of the thigh)

- Standing left side on to the chair and holding on for balance, bend forwards from the hips, and extend the left leg (inside leg) slightly off the floor behind you.

- Keeping the left thigh back, curl the left heel in towards your buttocks, bending the supporting leg at the same time.

- Gently straighten both legs to recover.

- Do this 8 times, turn round then repeat 8 times using the right leg.

- Repeat the whole exercise again.

Feel the muscles at the back of your thigh and your buttocks working

Squeeze your buttocks to support your hips

Keep your hips level and your abdominals tight and keep your pelvis correctly tilted to support your back

There should be a straight line from the back of your head to the knee of the back leg

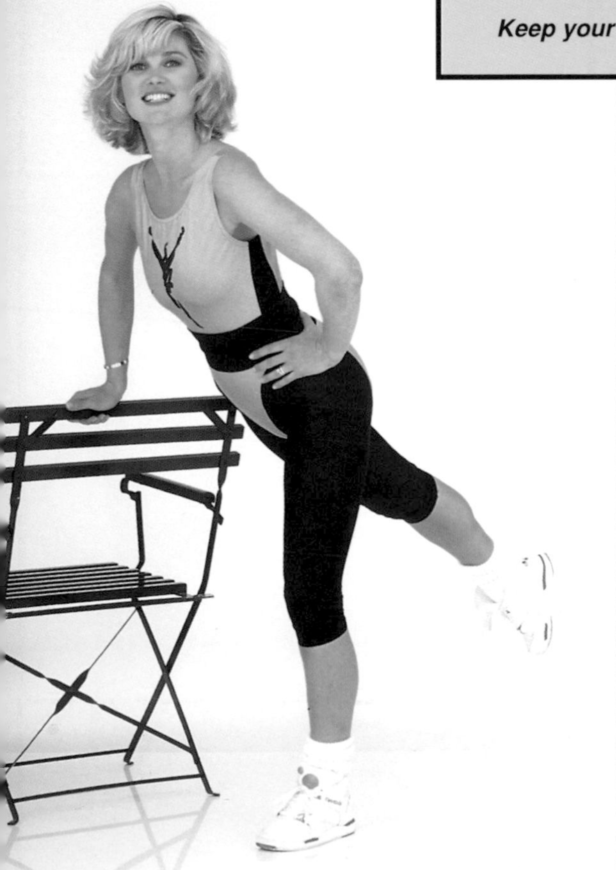

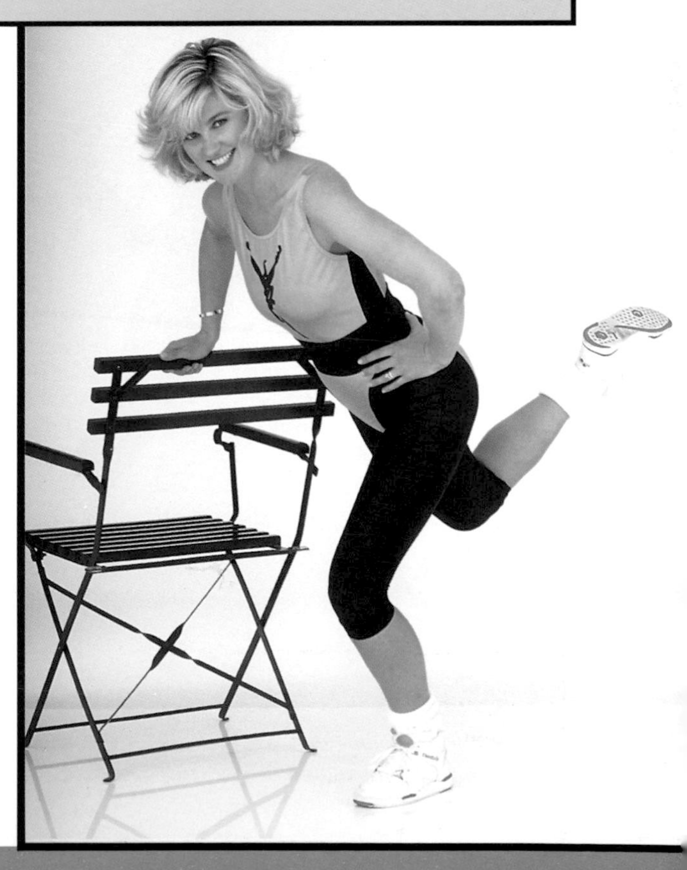

Exercise 3

FORWARD SQUATS

REPETITIONS
8 Right 8 Left
PURPOSE:
To tone the quadriceps (front of thigh) and gluteals (buttocks)

- Stand side on to a chair, holding on for support, one leg forwards and the other back (feet quite a way apart), your legs straight and the heel of your back foot off the floor. Your weight should be evenly balanced between your feet.

- Keeping your back upright and abdominals tight, bend both legs at the same time, taking the knee of the back leg down towards the floor, to end up just behind the heel of the front foot. Straighten them again.

- Do this 8 times, rest, change legs and repeat with the other leg in front.

Feel your thigh and buttock muscles working

Make the bend shallow at first and progress to the deeper bend as your muscles get stronger

The thigh of your back leg should be vertical when your knees are bent

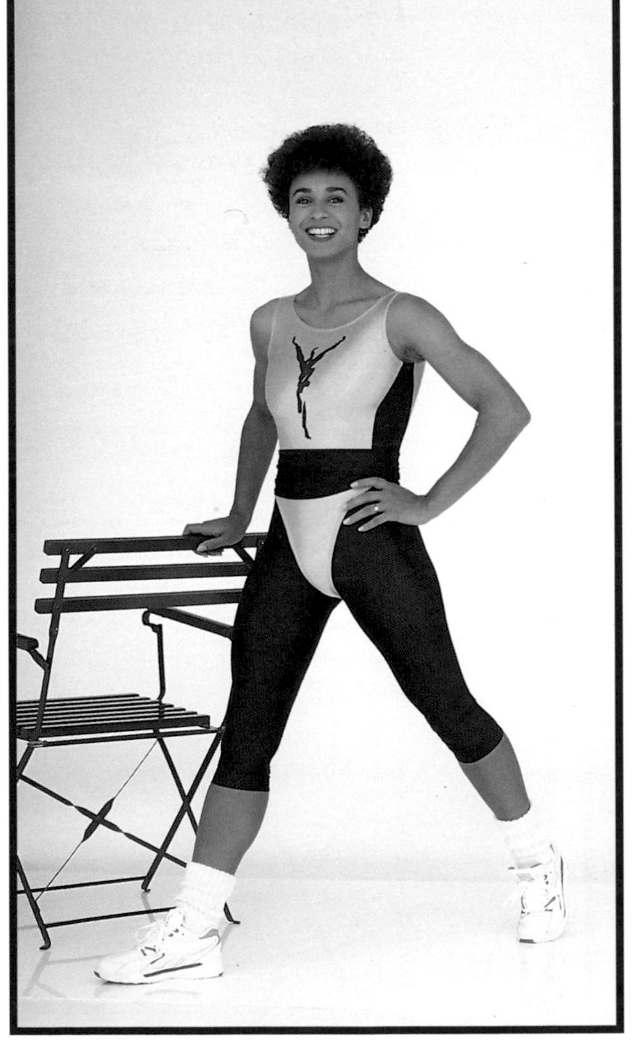

If your knees feel uncomfortable do another set of the Front Leg Raises as in Exercise 1 (see page 122).

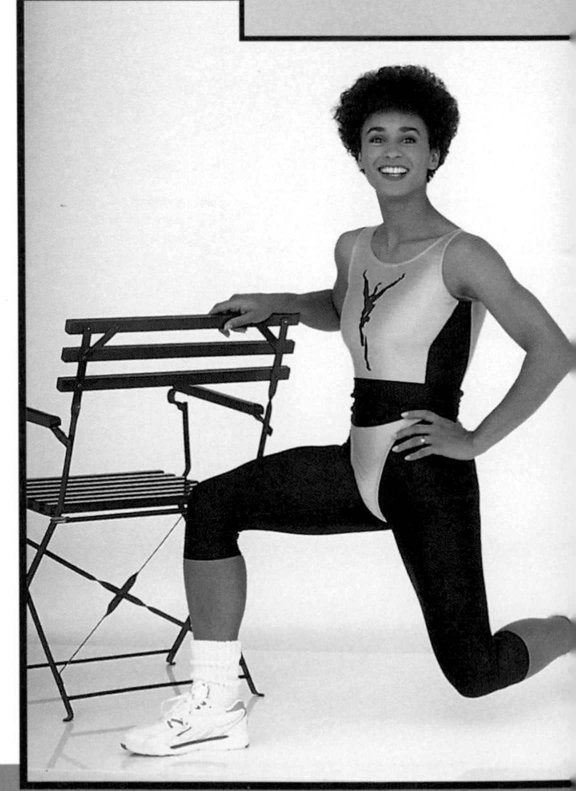

EXERCISE 4

LUNGE AND SQUAT COMBINATION

REPETITIONS
2 x 4
PURPOSE:
To tone the quadriceps (front of thigh)

- Stand with your feet wide apart, toes pointing slightly out and your hands on your hips.

- Keeping both feet flat on the floor, bend and straighten your right leg (as in a lunge), bend and straighten both knees, bend and straighten your left leg, bend and straighten both knees.

- Repeat this combination until you have done it 4 times, rest then repeat it another 4 times.

If your knees feel uncomfortable check that your feet are wide enough apart, or try performing just the squats and miss out the lunges.

Feel your thigh muscles working

During the lunge, keep the thigh muscles of the straight leg really tight and its foot flat on the floor

Check that your hips face the front and your pelvis remains correctly tilted

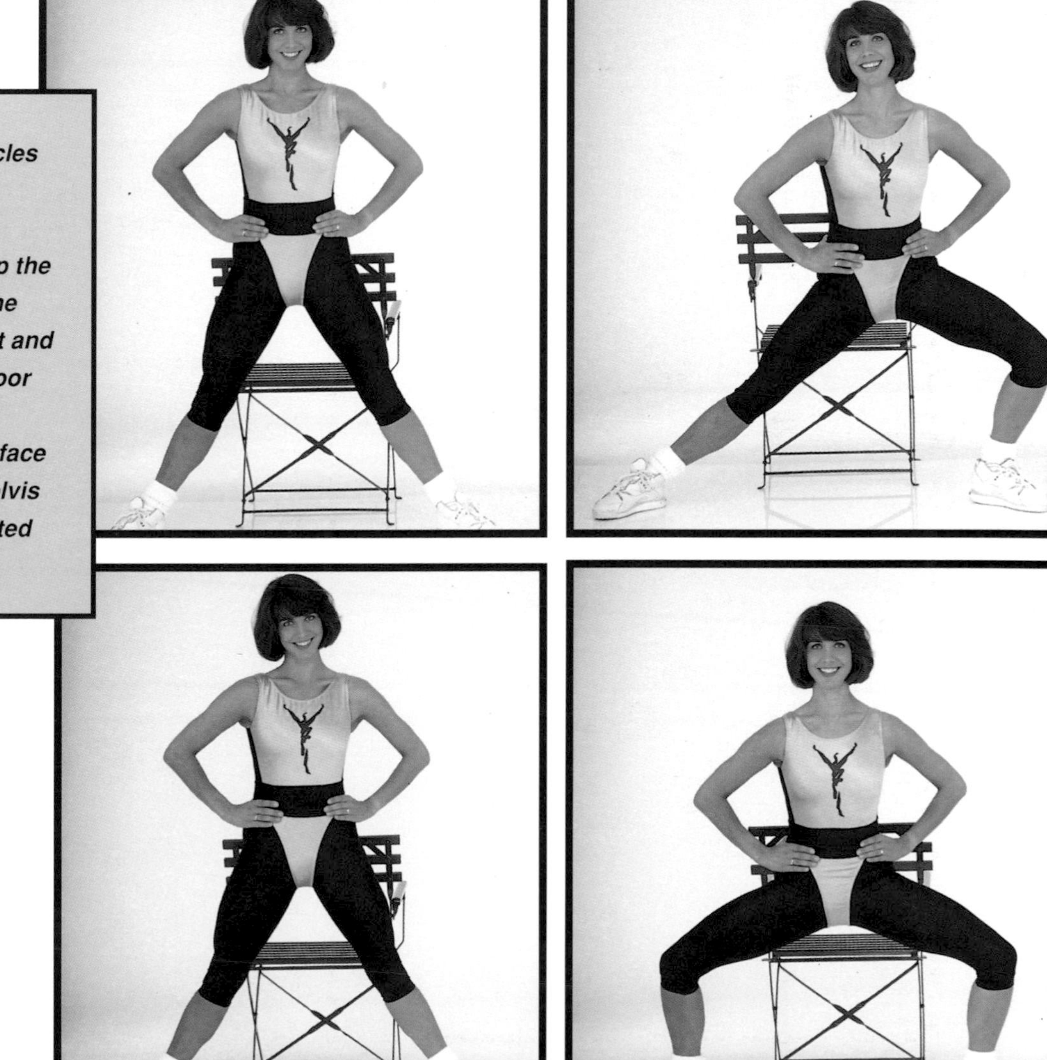

Exercise 5

OUTER AND INNER THIGH COMBINATION

(EXERCISE A + EXERCISE B)

REPETITIONS
16 + 8 Right, 32 + 16 Left, 16 + 8 Left, 32 + 16 Right

Feel the muscles around the hip working

Check that your hips stay still; the leg will not go very high

Keep the working leg straight

A) LYING SIDE LEG RAISES

REPETITIONS *16 + 8 Right*
PURPOSE:
To tone the abductors (outer hip and thigh)

- Lie on your left side, resting your head in your hand, the bottom leg bent backwards for stability and the top leg straight out in line with your body, thighs parallel. Place the spare hand on the floor in front of you for balance.

- Making sure your hips and tummy face forwards and keeping the hips completely still, slowly raise and lower the top leg.

- Do this 16 times, have a short rest and then repeat it another 8 times with the same leg. Now move on to the next part of this combination on the next page.

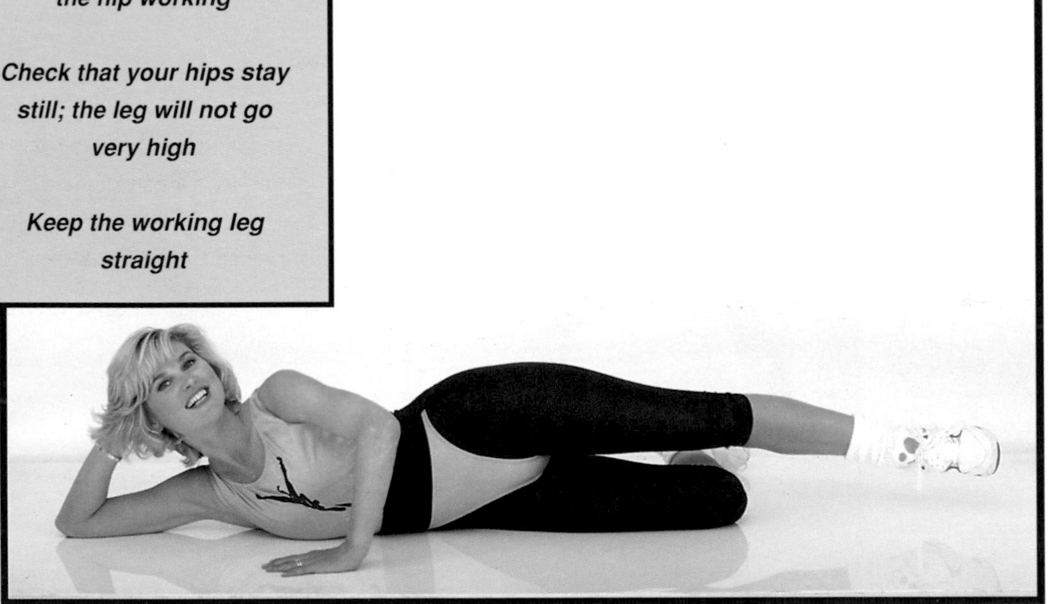

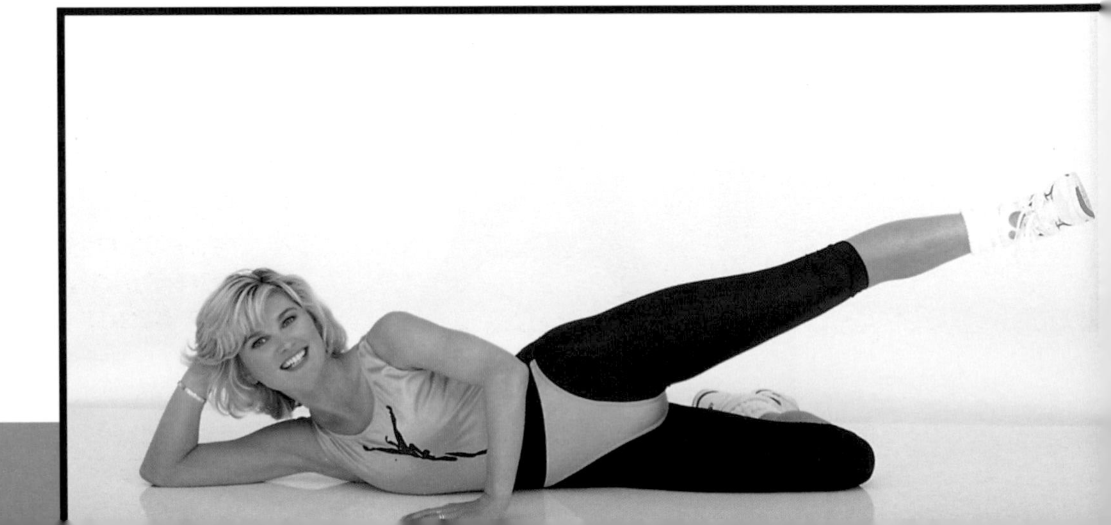

B) LYING INNER THIGH RAISES

REPETITIONS *32 + 16 Left*
PURPOSE:
To tone the adductors (inner thigh)

- Stay on your left side, resting your head in your hand (as opposite). Straighten the lower leg, bend the top leg, rest the knee on the floor and the ankle on top of the knee of the lower leg. Place your spare hand on the floor in front of you for balance.

- Keeping your hips facing forwards and the hips and trunk still, think of squeezing the inner thighs together as you raise and lower the bottom leg.

- Do this 32 times, rest and repeat 16 more times with the same leg.

Feel the inner thigh muscles working

The ankle resting on the knee makes it harder work for the inner thigh muscles

Relax the rest of your body

Don't expect to lift your leg very high - the exercise only requires a small range of movement

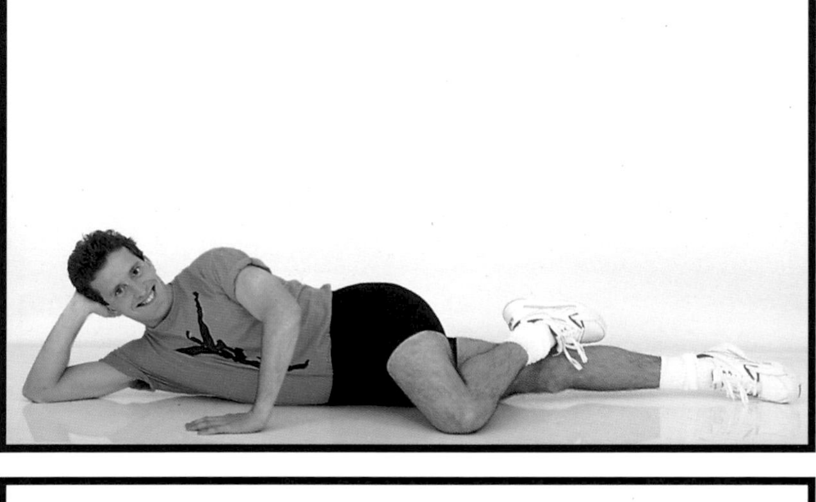

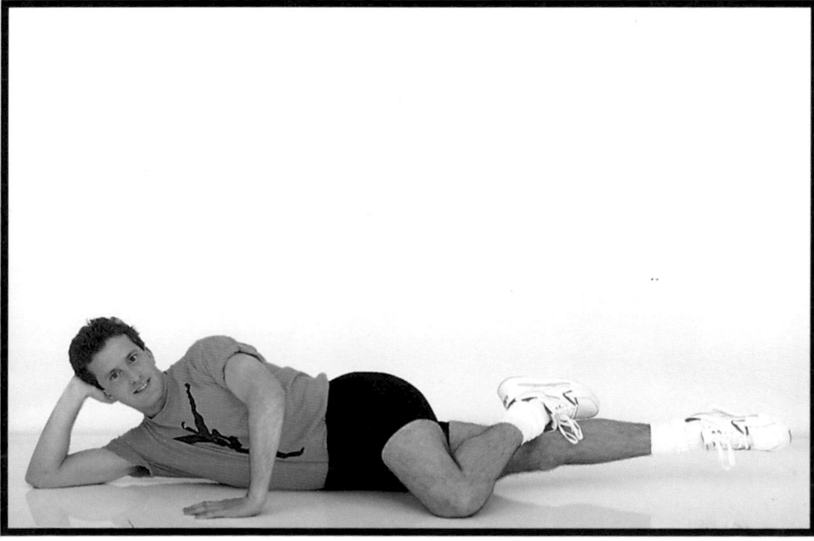

Roll over and repeat the combination on the other side.

Although the time indicated for the cool-down is only two minutes, whenever possible extend this to allow you to perform a comprehensive developmental stretch section. You may find that you have a preference for alternative stretches to those included in this section. As long as the stretch is for the same muscle group and feels comfortable for you, feel free to choose any alternative from other stretch sections.

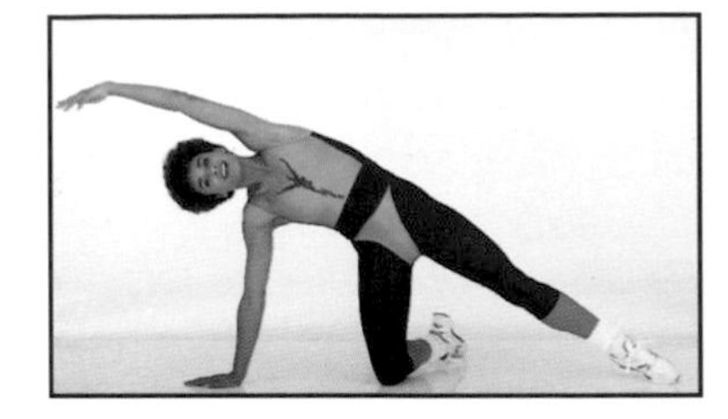

KNEELING SIDE STRETCH
8 counts for each side

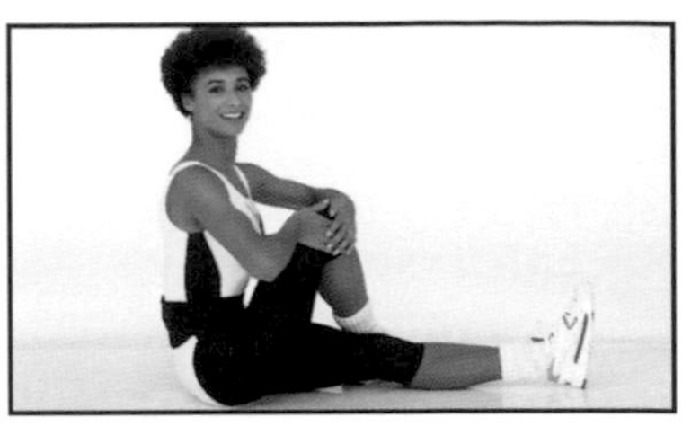

SEATED BUTTOCK TWIST
8 counts for each side

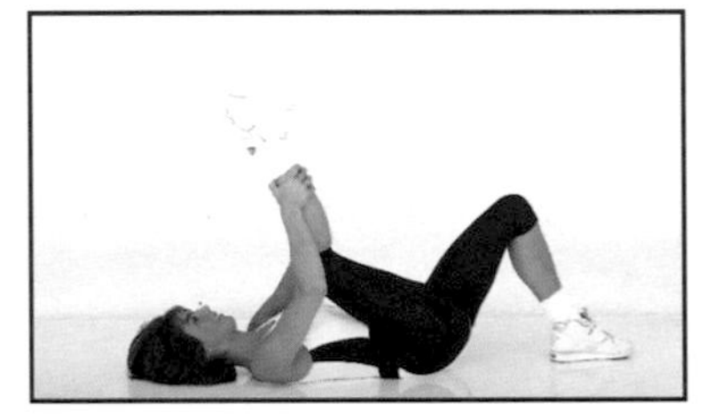

LYING HAMSTRING STRETCH
16 counts for each leg

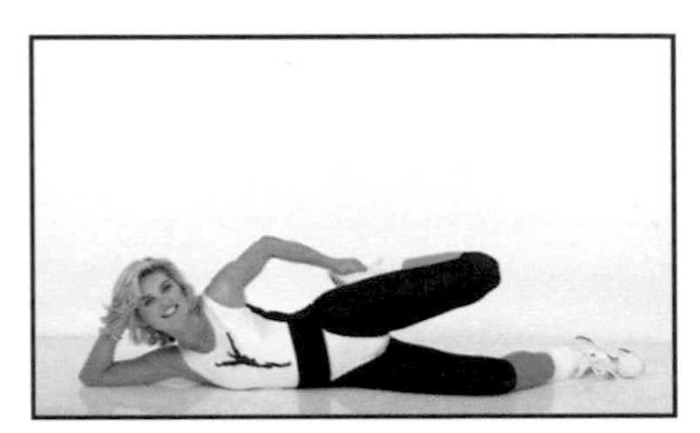

SIDE LYING QUAD STRETCH
8 counts for each side

EXERCISE 1

STRADDLE STRETCH

PURPOSE:
To improve the suppleness of the hip joint by stretching the adductors (inner thigh) and hamstrings (back of the thigh)

- Sit up tall with your legs extended as wide apart as possible and your hands on the floor in front of you.
- Keeping your knees pointing towards the ceiling, lean forwards from the hips until you feel a stretch along the inside and back of your thighs.
- Hold for a count of 16 trying to relax and develop the stretch further.

If you feel at all uncomfortable, use a hamstring stretch from any of the previous levels instead.

Try to keep your back straight as you lean forwards and use your hands on the floor for support

Don't expect to get very far at first

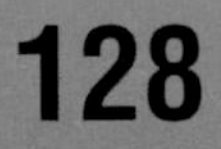

Exercise 2

SEATED ARM CIRCLES

REPETITIONS
2 Right 2 Left
PURPOSE:
To relax the muscles around the shoulder

- Sit up tall with one hand resting on the floor beside you and your legs in any position that's comfortable.
- Keeping your shoulders facing forwards, circle the other arm forwards and up, brushing your ear as you take the arm past your head, back and down to return to the start position.
- Do this twice with one arm then repeat with the other.

Feel the movement in your shoulder

Try to make as large a circle as possible with your hand

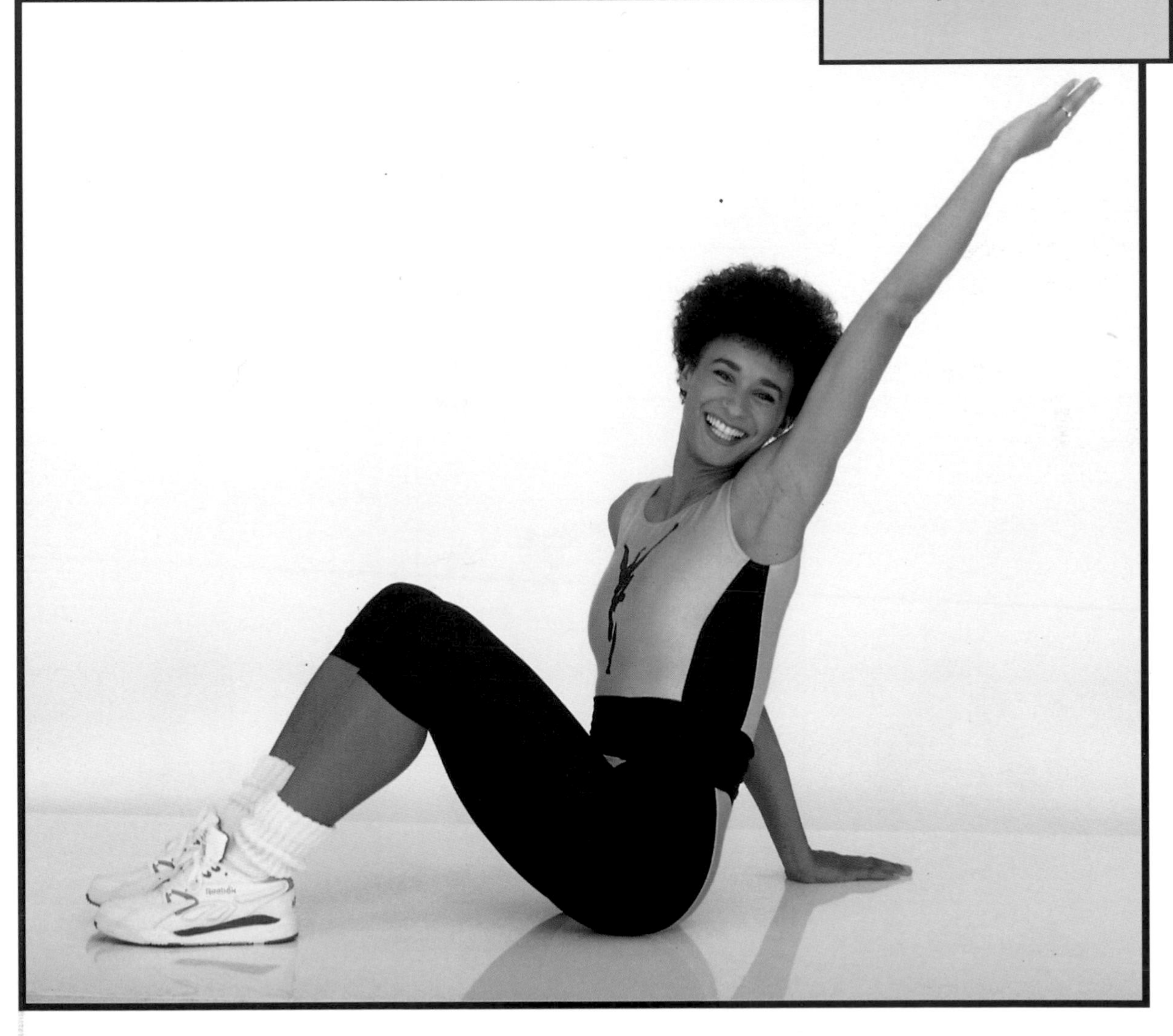

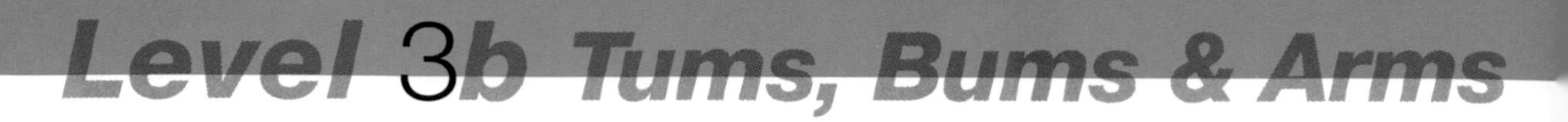

Level 3b Tums, Bums & Arms

You should be able to develop quite a neat routine from these exercises if you perform them with continuity. You may even want to play a piece of music with a steady beat at the same time - but take care that the speed of it does not make you rush.

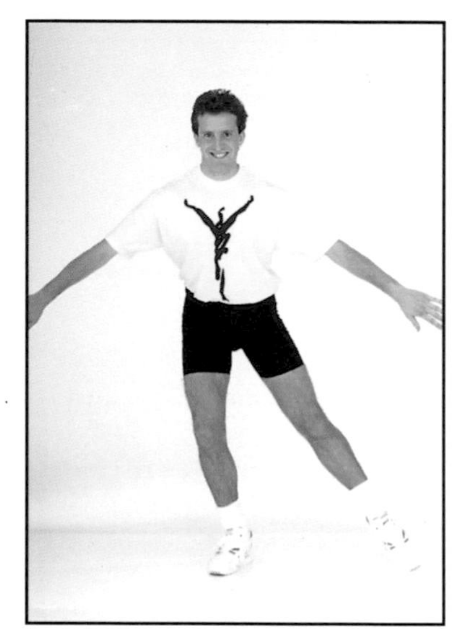

TAP LEG OUT
x 4 Right 4 Left

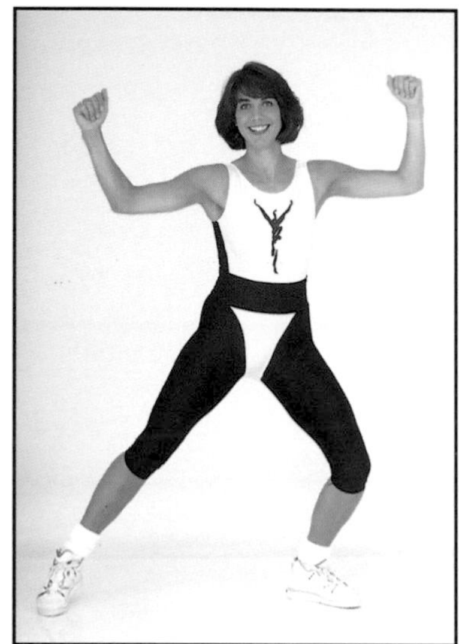

SIDE SPRINGS x 8

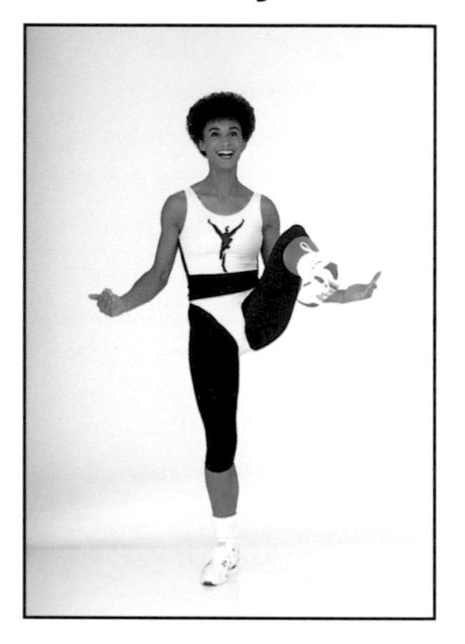

KNEE LIFTS WITH ARM PULL DOWNS x 8

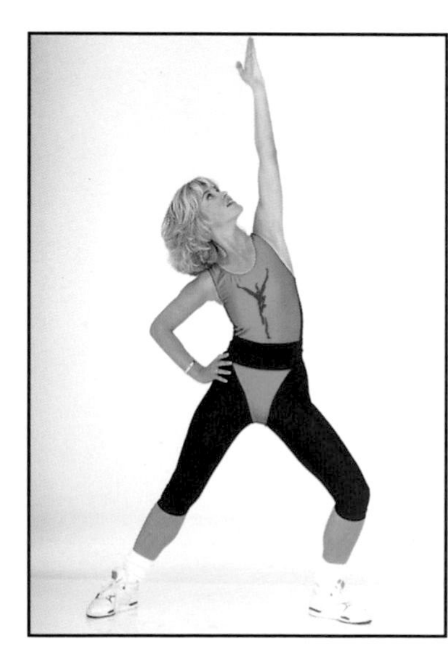

REACHES WITH KNEE BENDS x 8

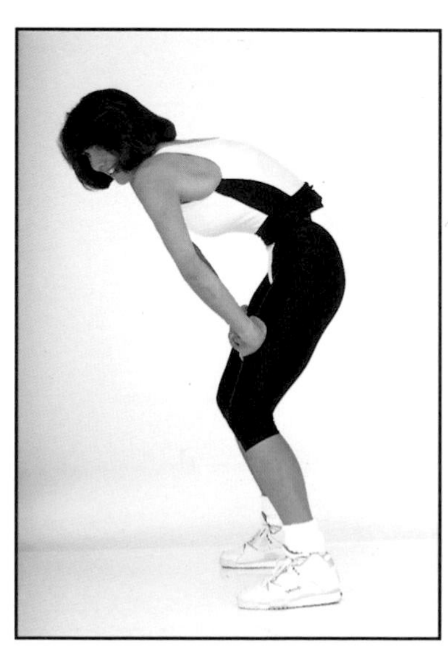

HOLLOW AND HUMP x 4

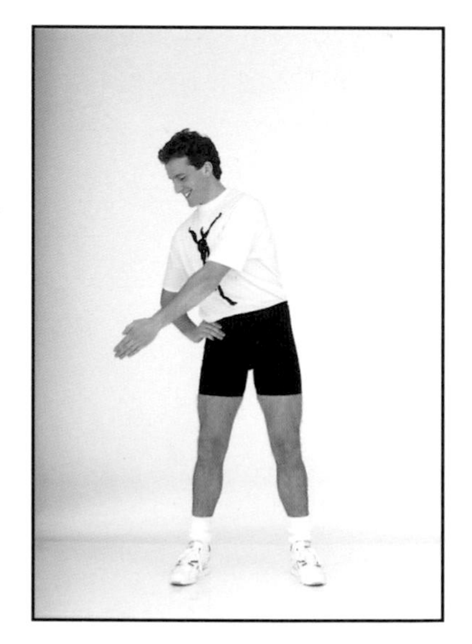

ARM CIRCLES ACROSS BODY
x 2 Right 2 Left

EXERCISE 1

LUNGES WITH ARMS

REPETITIONS *8*
PURPOSE:
To warm the muscles

- Start with feet wide apart, the right leg bent and left leg straight as for a lunge, left arm up and the other extended out to the side at shoulder height.
- Change over to the other side, touching your shoulders with your hands on route.
- Repeat this 4 times.

Keep your hips facing forwards and your pelvis correctly tilted

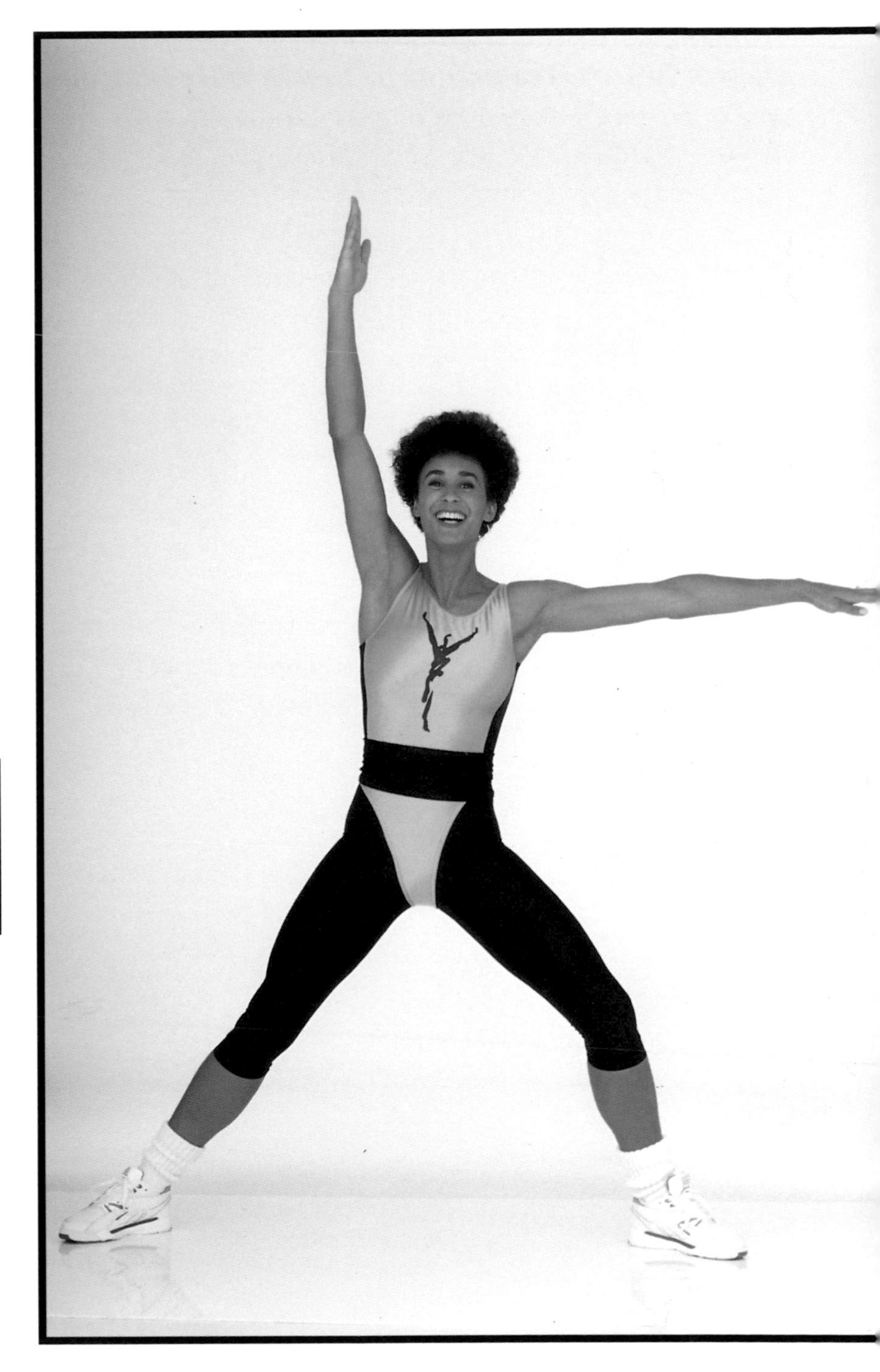

Repeat all of the mobility and pulse-raising exercises on the previous pages before moving onto these warm-up stretches.

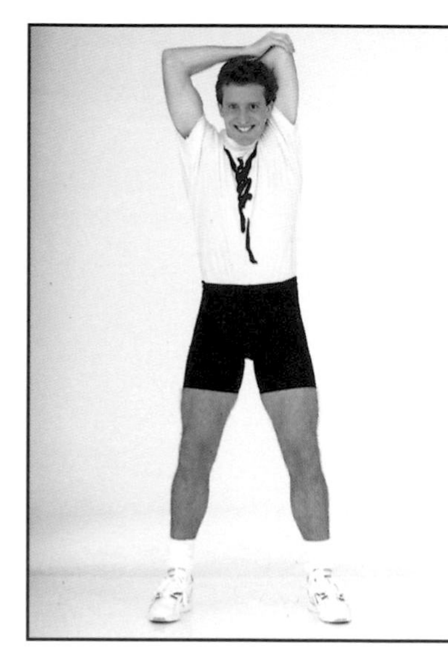

STANDING TRICEPS STRETCH
4 counts on each arm

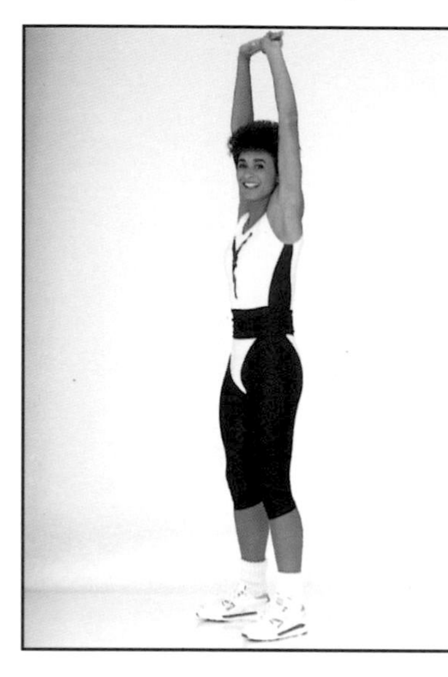

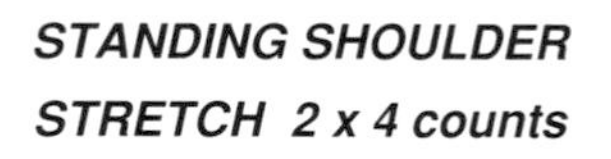

STANDING SHOULDER STRETCH 2 x 4 counts

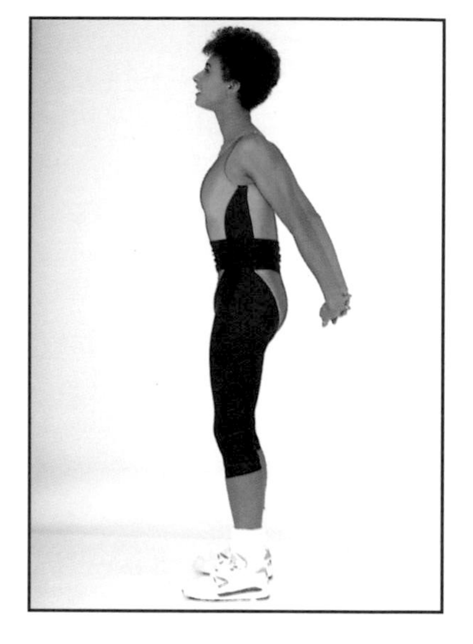

CHEST STRETCH
2 x 4 counts

EXERCISE 2

INNER THIGH AND SIDE STRETCH

PURPOSE:
To stretch the adductors (inner thigh) and obliques (waist)

- Stand with your feet wide apart, toes pointing slightly out and your left hand on your left hip.

- Bend your right leg until you feel a stretch in the inner thigh (if you do not feel a stretch, slide your left leg further to the side). Keeping your hips still and holding the inner thigh stretch, take your right arm up above your ahead and bend sideways to the left until you feel an additional stretch down your right side.

- Hold for a count of 8, then repeat on the other side, bending the left leg and stretching the left side.

Breathe out as you go into the side stretch

Check that your hips, chest and shoulders face the front throughout

Check that your feet are wide enough apart for the lunge to be comfortable and effective

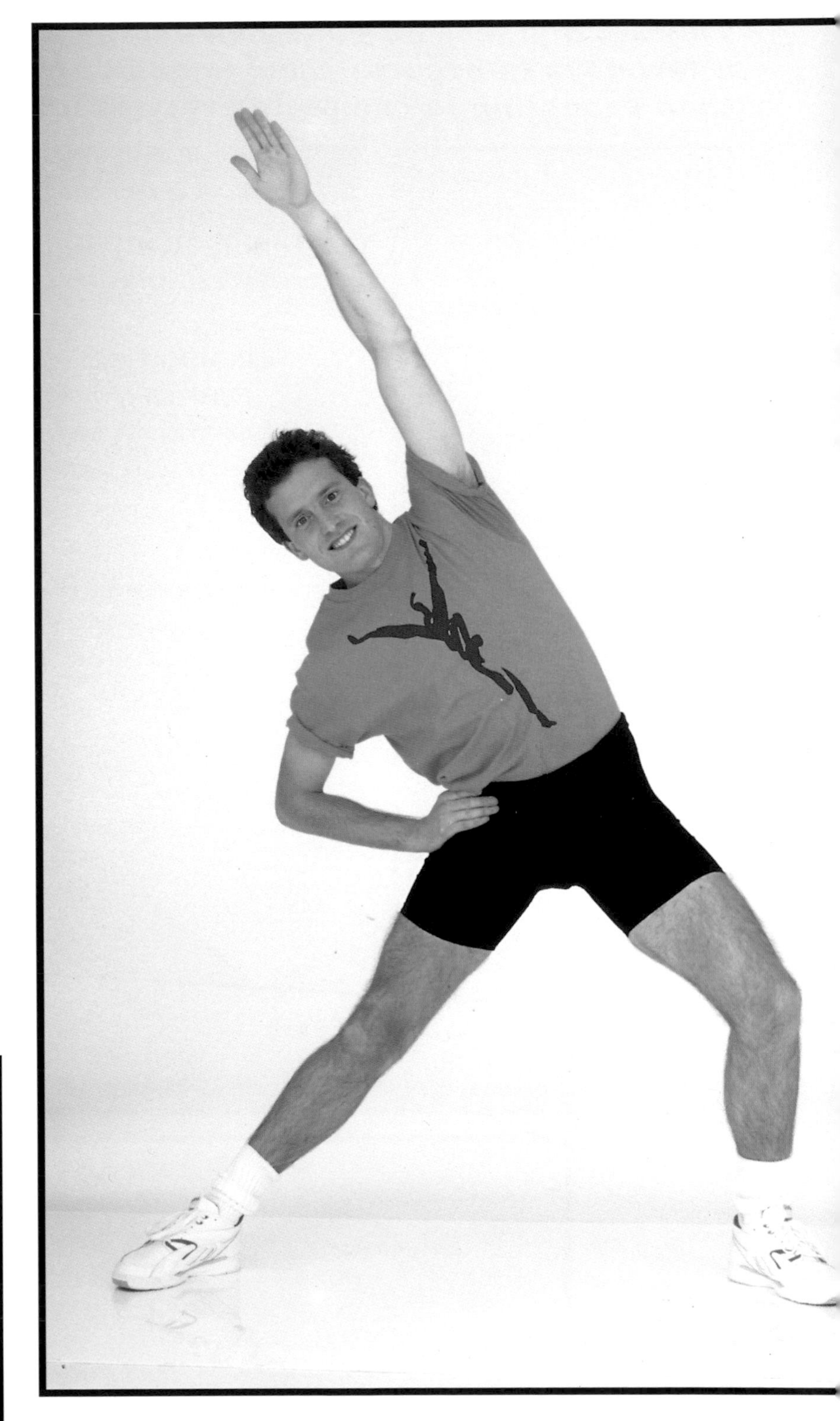

This section may be quite demanding at first. Give yourself a few days to become accustomed to the exercises rather than expecting to complete every exercise fully first time.

Feel the chest and upper arm muscles working

Tilt your pelvis and use your abdominals to prevent a dip in the lower back

Breathe out and keep your shoulders over your hands as you push up each time. Straighten the arms carefully

If this exercise is uncomfortable, go back to the box press-ups (see page 84) and do 16 repetitions. Rest then repeat

EXERCISE 1

THREE-QUARTER PRESS-UPS

REPETITIONS *12*
PURPOSE:
To tone the triceps (backs of the arms) and pectorals (chest)

- With your hands and knees on the floor, place your shoulders over your hands and your knees far enough back for your body to be in a straight line from knees to shoulders.
- Bend your arms to lower the body, so that thighs, hips, chest and nose touch the floor simult aneously, then return to the start.
- Do this 12 times.

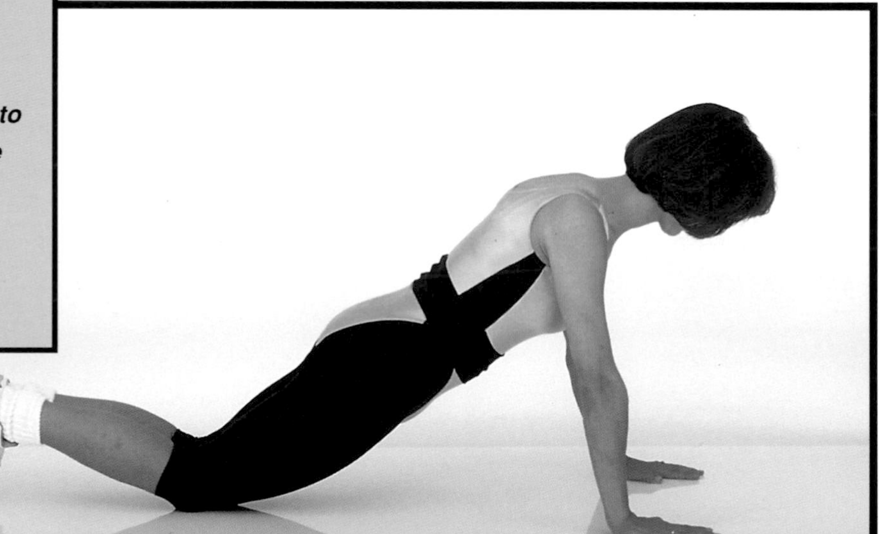

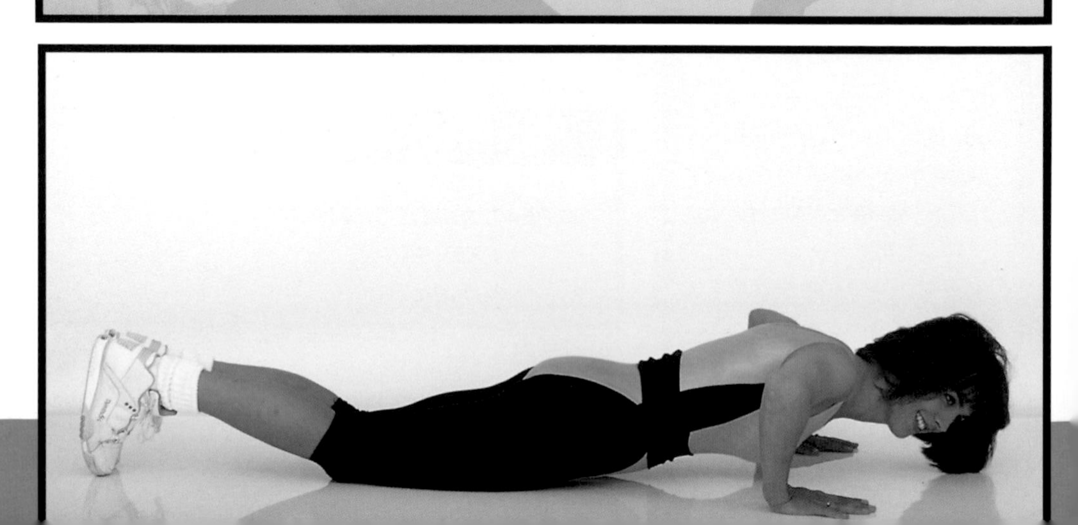

Exercise 2

DOUBLE LEG RAISES WITH CURL

REPETITIONS *16*
PURPOSE:
To tone the gluteals (buttocks)

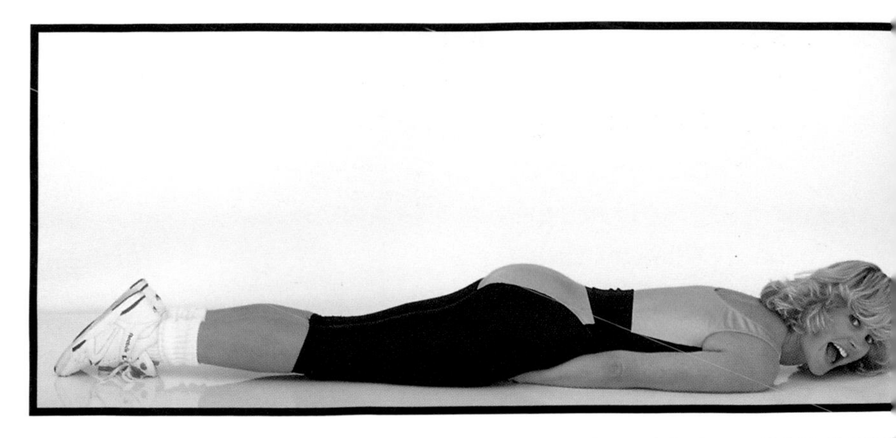

- Lie flat on your front with your face resting on the floor and, for comfort, place your hands, palms up, under your thighs.

- Tighten your buttocks and raise both legs a little way off the floor, then, keeping your thighs still and your knees off the floor, curl your heels into your buttocks, straighten your legs again and then lower them to the floor, breathing out as you relax.

- Do this exercise 16 times.

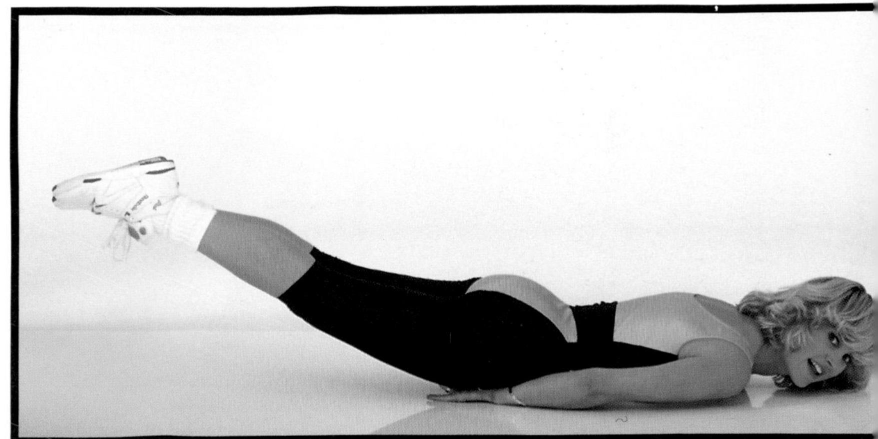

Feel your buttocks muscles working. Keep your face and chest resting on the floor

To make the exercise harder, hold your knees as far as you can off the floor as you really squeeze your heels in towards your buttocks

If your back feels uncomfortable or hurts in any way, find an alternative exercise for the gluteals on all fours that works one leg at a time.

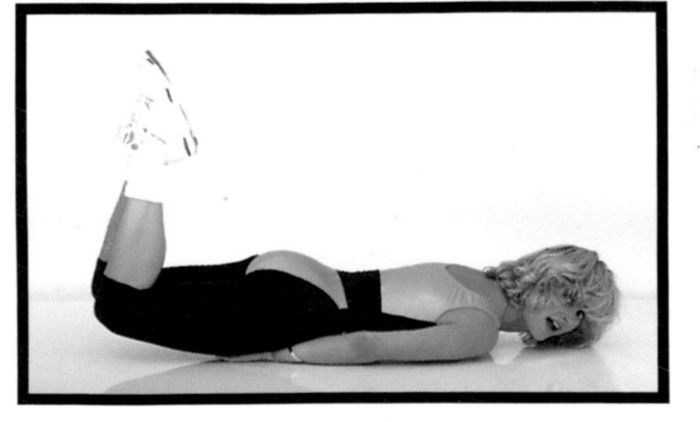

Exercise 3

REPEAT THREE-QUARTER PRESS-UPS
See opposite

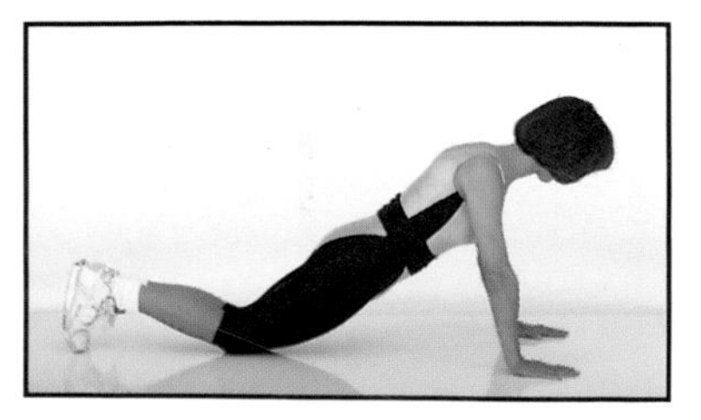

EXERCISE 4

CURL-UPS COMBINATION

REPETITIONS *4*
PURPOSE:
To tone the abdominals (tum)

- Lie on your back with your knees bent, feet flat on the floor and your head resting on your fingertips.

- Curl your head and shoulders off the floor and recover, curl up again, this time twisting to the left, reaching your left hand to touch the outside of your right knee, recover, repeat the first curl-up, then repeat the twisting curl-up, this time twisting to the other side (reach your right hand to the outside of your left knee.

- Repeat this combination until you have done it 4 times in total.

Feel your abdominals working

Remember to keep breathing

Keep your chin down towards your chest

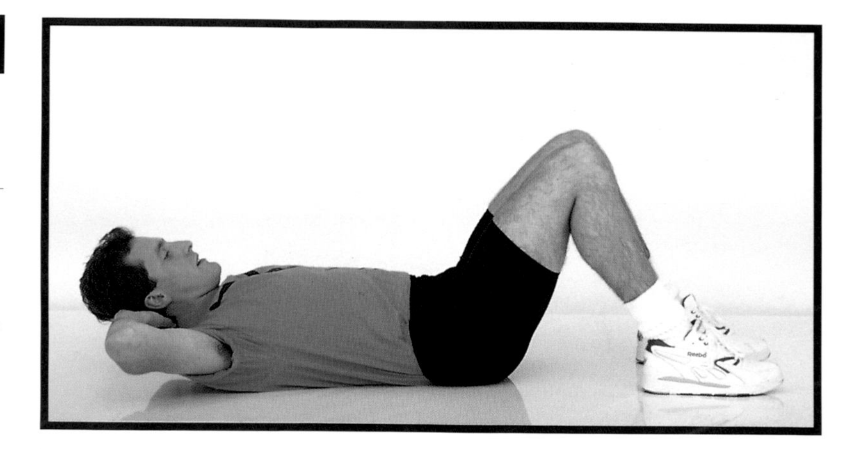

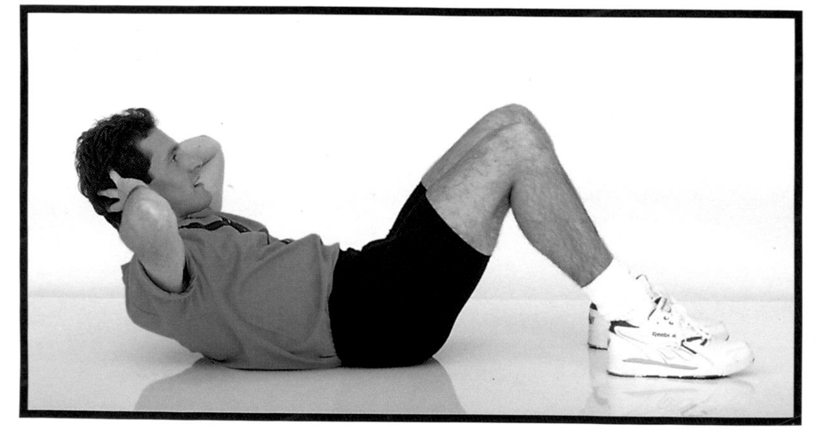

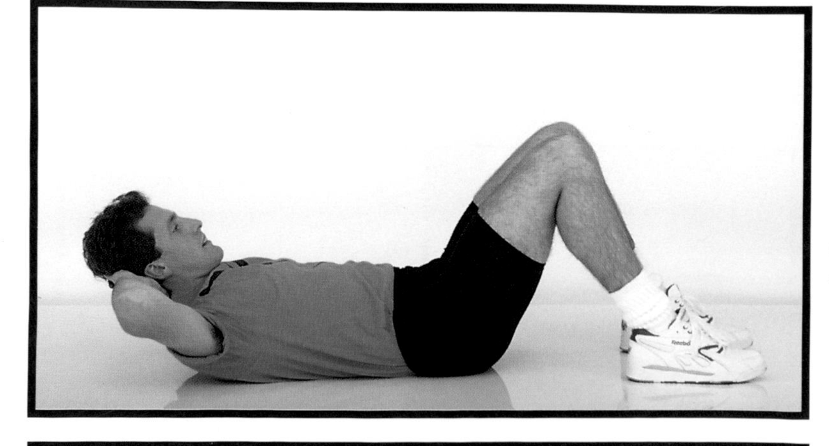

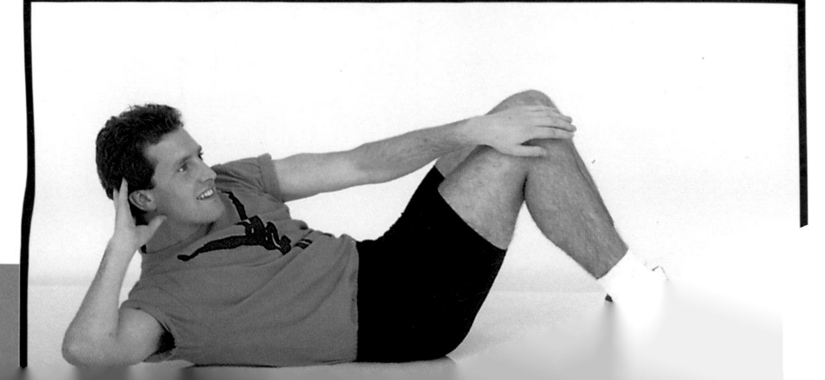

EXERCISE 5

CRUNCH COMBINATION

REPETITIONS *4*
PURPOSE:
To tone the abdominals (tum)

● Lie on your back with your legs bent up over your chest and your head resting in your fingertips.

● Keeping your knees still and your tummy flat, curl your head and shoulders towards your knees, recover, then curl up with a twist, taking your left elbow to your right knee. Recover, repeat the first crunchie, then repeat the twisting crunchie, this time twisting to the other side (right elbow to left knee).

● Repeat this combination until you have done it 4 times in total.

Feel your abdominals working

Breathe out as you curl up

Check that you keep your knees over your tummy throughout

Check that you do not allow your abdominals to bunch up, especially as they get tired

Check that you don't pull on your head with your arms

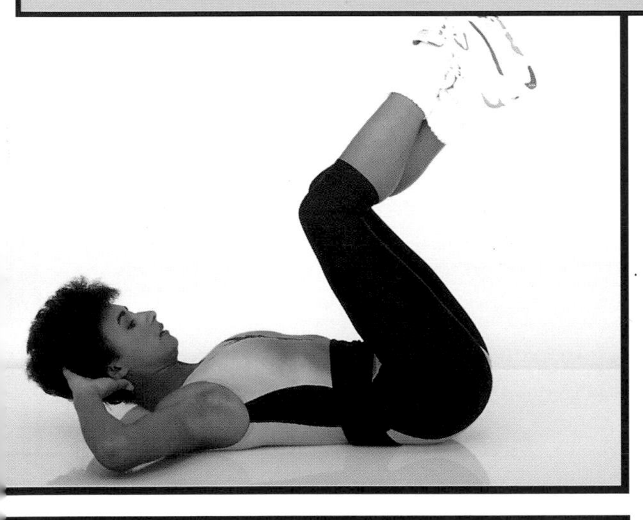

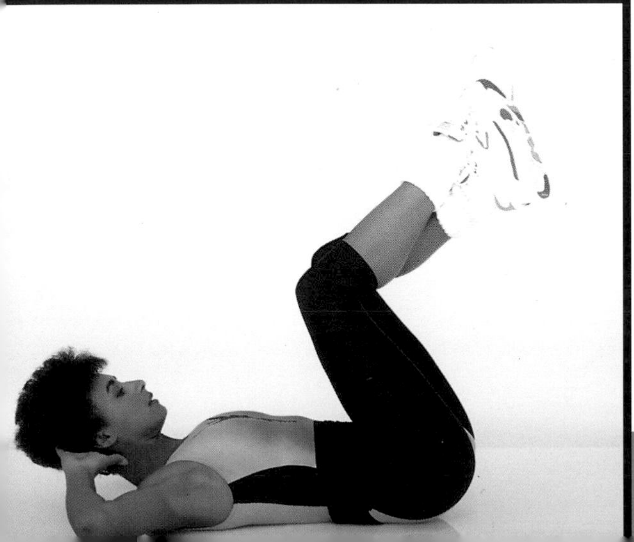

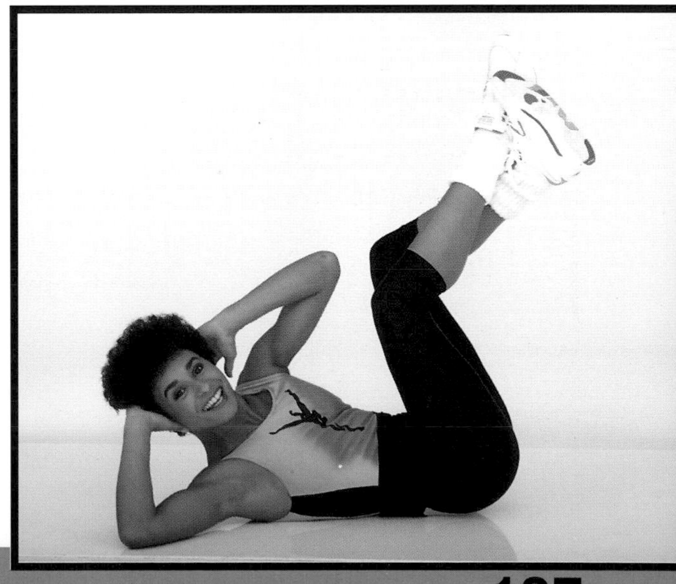

EXERCISE 6

ADVANCED BUTTOCK SQUEEZES

REPETITIONS
16 Right 16 Left
PURPOSE:
To tone the gluteals (buttocks)

- Lie on your back with one leg bent, foot flat on the floor and the other ankle resting on its knee, knee pushed out away from you.
- Raise your hips off the floor so that they make a straight line from your ribs to your knee.
- Keeping your hips still, tighten your buttocks and hold for a moment, then relax.
- Do this 16 times, change legs and repeat.

Feel the buttocks working

Remember to keep your shoulder blades in contact with the floor and your pelvis tilted the correct way

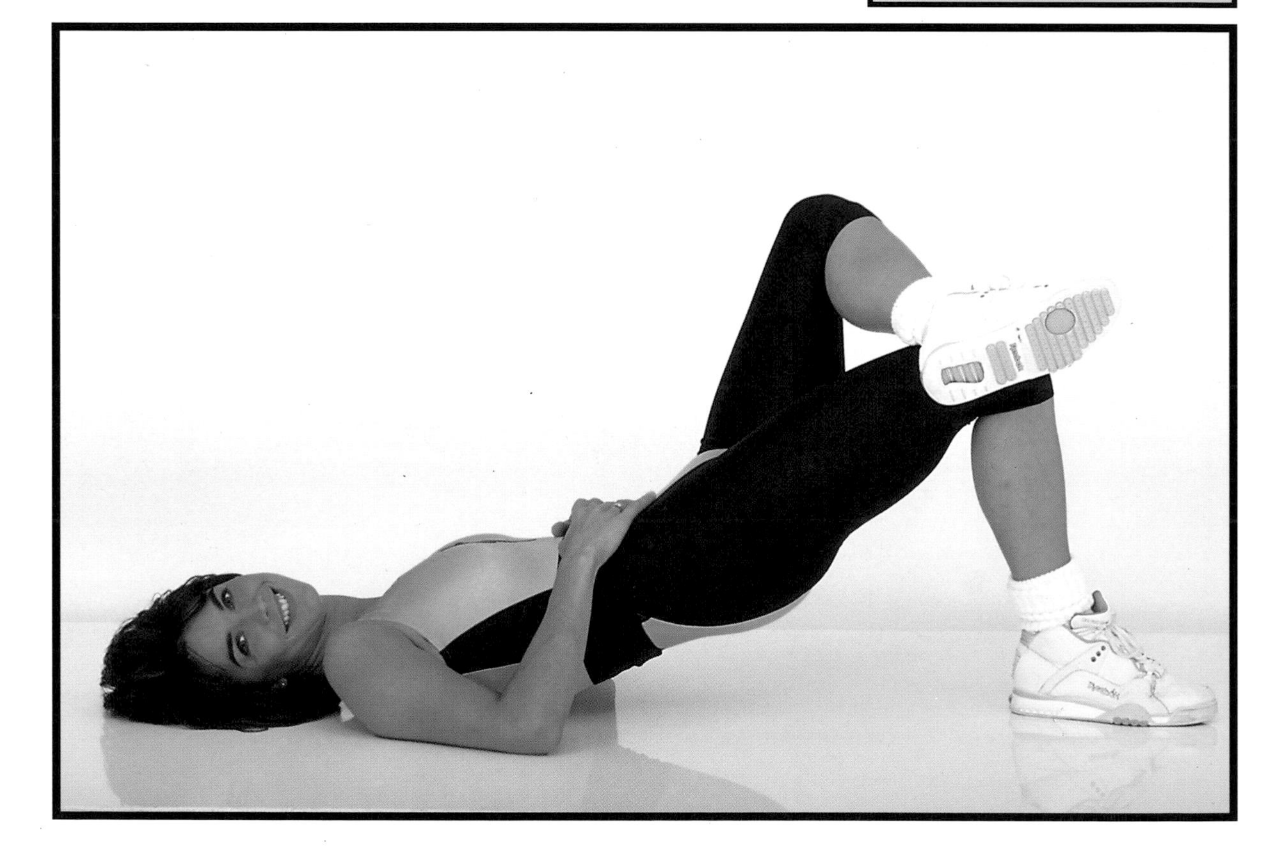

EXERCISE 7

BUTTOCKS AND THIGH SQUEEZES

REPETITIONS *16*
PURPOSE:
To tone the gluteals (buttocks)

- Lie on your back with your legs together and knees bent; tilt your pelvis to flatten the stomach.
- Raise your hips off the floor to make a straight line from your knees to your chest.
- Keeping the lower back still, tighten your buttocks and squeeze your knees together, hold for a moment, relax.
- Do this 16 times.

Feel the buttock and inner thigh muscles working

Take care to keep the upper back (shoulder blades) in contact with the floor

Ensure you do not arch your back

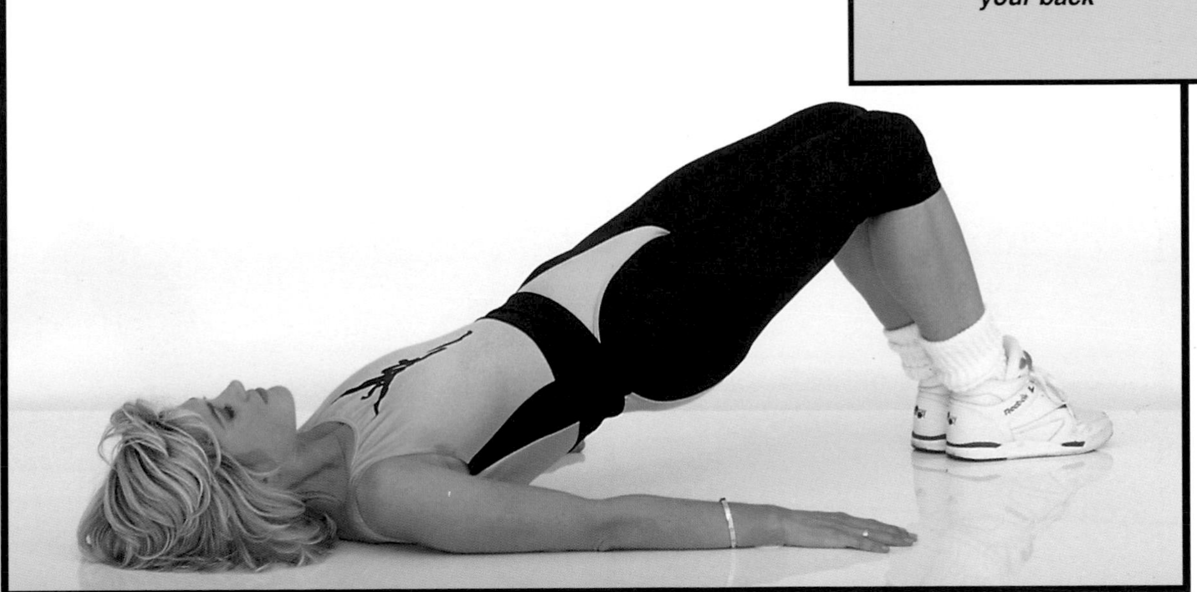

EXERCISE 8

REPEAT CURL-UP COMBINATION
REPETITIONS x 4
See page 136

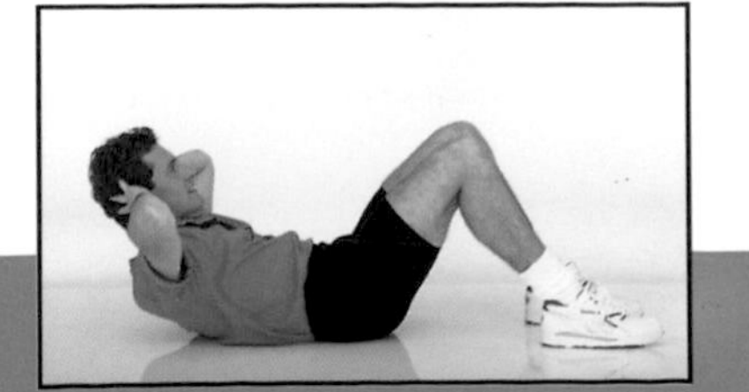

EXERCISE 9

REPEAT CRUNCH COMBINATION
REPETITIONS x 4
See page 137

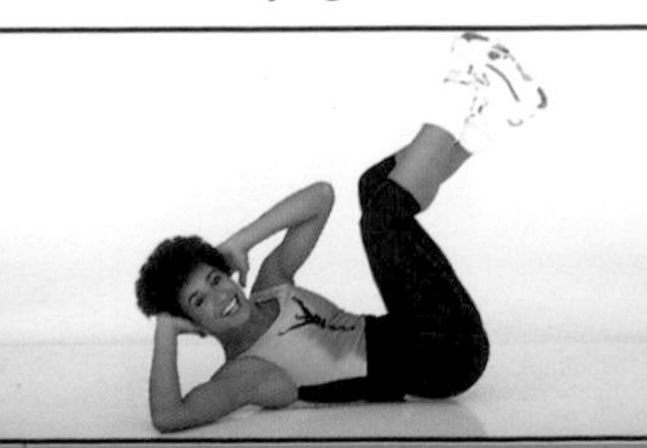

EXERCISE 10

CURL AND ROUND

REPETITIONS *4*
PURPOSE:
To tone the abdominals (tum)

● Lie on your back with both legs bent and feet flat on the floor.

● Do one curl-up to the centre and recover, then curl up to the centre again and bend round to the right to touch your right heel with your right hand, recover, repeat curl-up to the centre then repeat curl-up with bend to the other side (left hand to touch left heel).

● Repeat this combination until you have done it 4 times in total.

Feel your abdominals working, especially around the waist

Check that you bend to the side and don't twist

Keep your feet flat on the floor

To make the exercise harder, keep your shoulder blades off the floor as you bend to the side

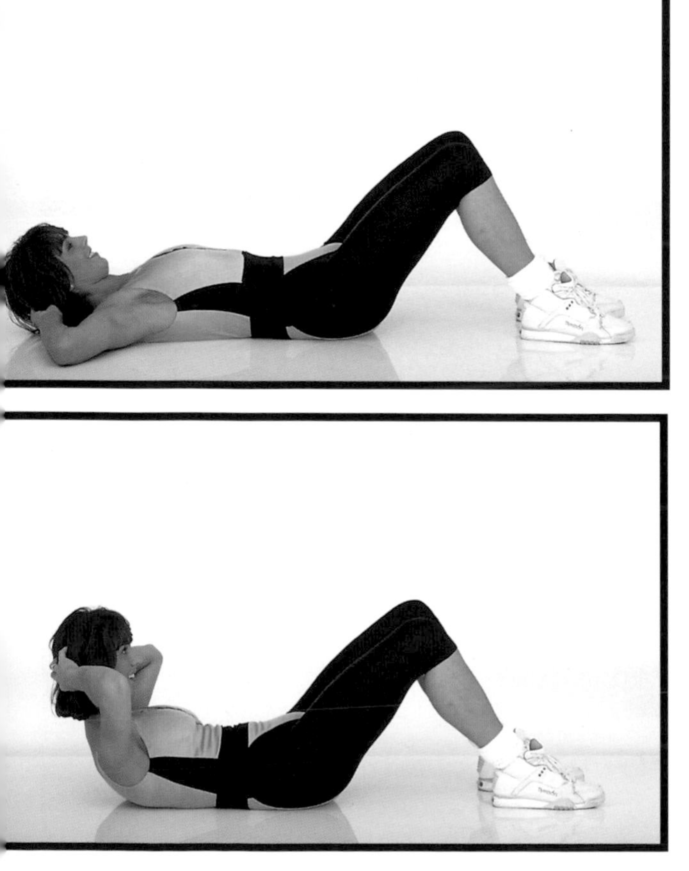

If you find it difficult to balance, try it with your feet a little further away from your buttocks.

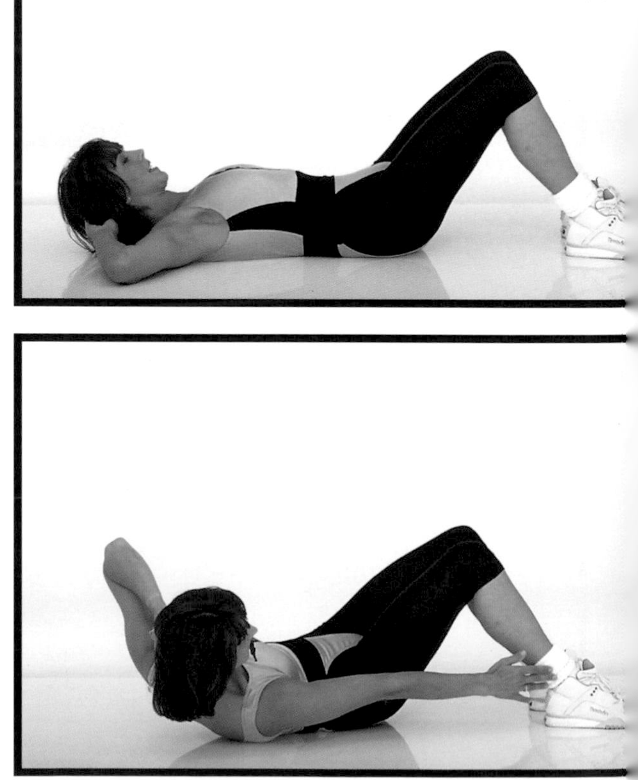

EXERCISE 11

DIPS

REPETITIONS
12 + 12
PURPOSE:
To tone the triceps (back of the arms)

- Sit on the floor with your legs bent and your feet flat on the floor.
- Place your hands on the floor behind you with your fingers pointing in towards you, then lift your hips off the floor and take the weight on your hands and feet.
- Keeping your trunk as still as possible, bend your arms as far as comfortable then straighten them again.
- Do this 12 times, rest and then repeat another 12 times.

If you find this exercise too strenuous to perform correctly, keep your hips on the floor as for Seated Dips (see page 115).

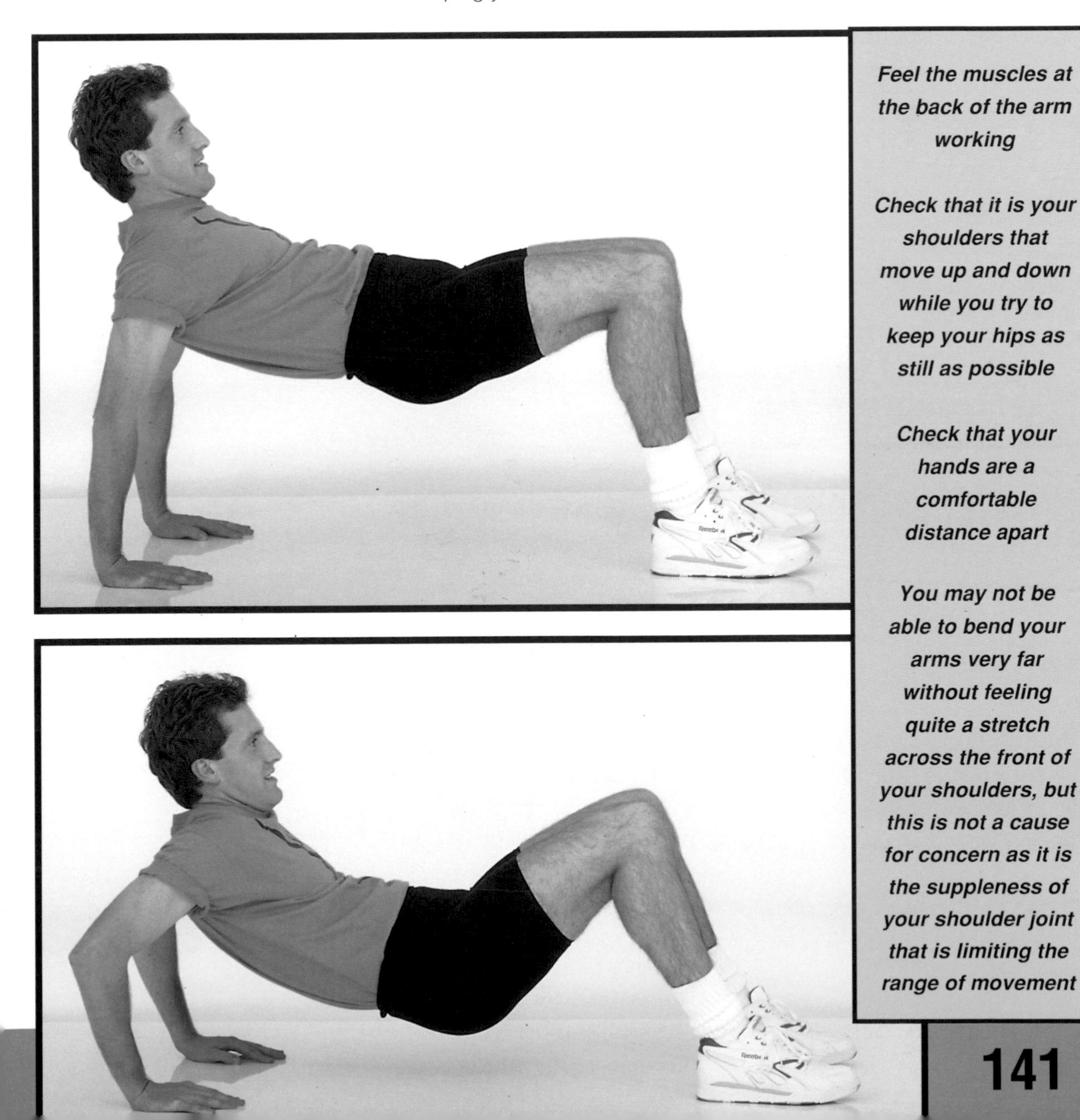

Feel the muscles at the back of the arm working

Check that it is your shoulders that move up and down while you try to keep your hips as still as possible

Check that your hands are a comfortable distance apart

You may not be able to bend your arms very far without feeling quite a stretch across the front of your shoulders, but this is not a cause for concern as it is the suppleness of your shoulder joint that is limiting the range of movement

Level 3b Tums, Bums & Arms

Your muscles deserve a good relaxing stretch now, so allow yourself as much time as you can for this section. Think about what you are aiming to achieve and perhaps play a piece of smooth, relaxing music at the same time. The two new stretches provide alternatives to those previously incorporated into the programme. Choose whichever is more comfortable for you.

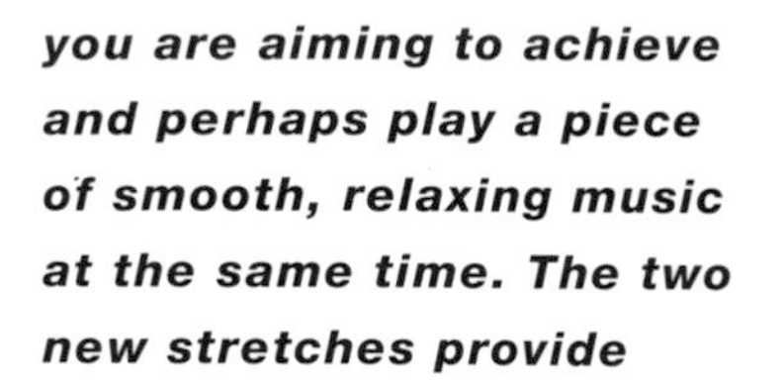

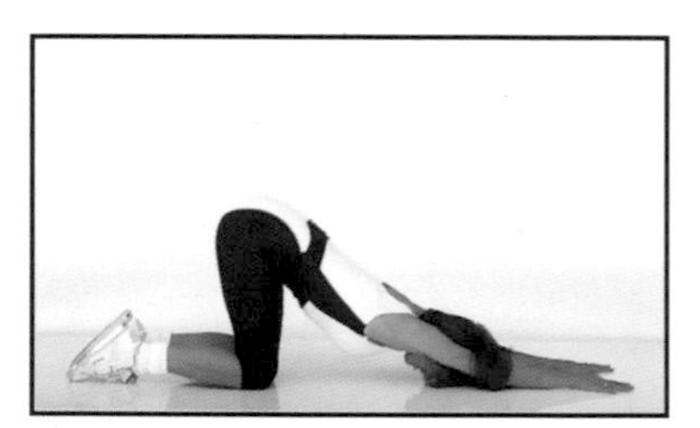

KNEELING SHOULDER STRETCH
8 counts

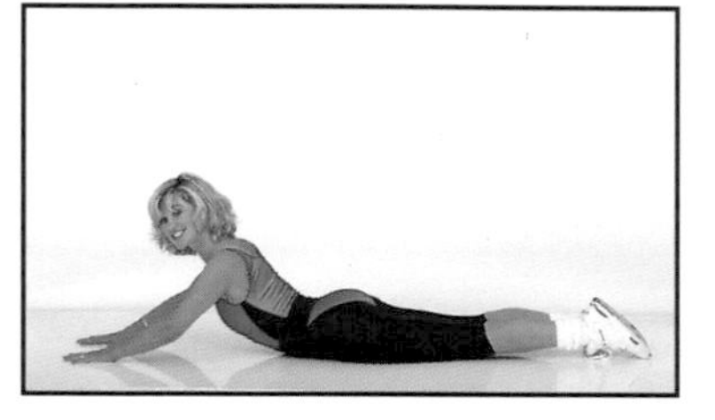

TUM STRETCH
2 x 4 counts

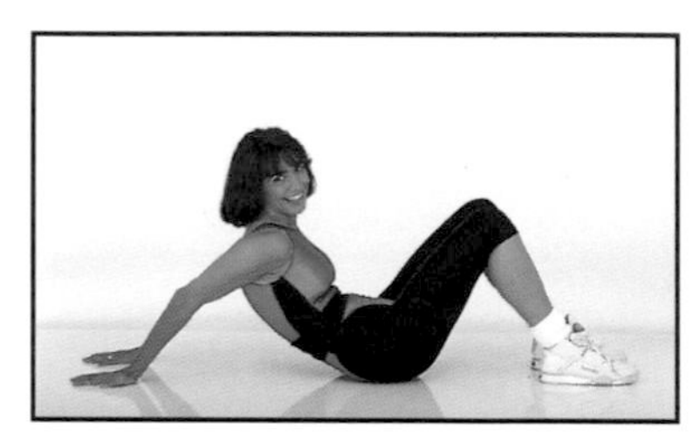

SEATED SHOULDER STRETCH
8 counts

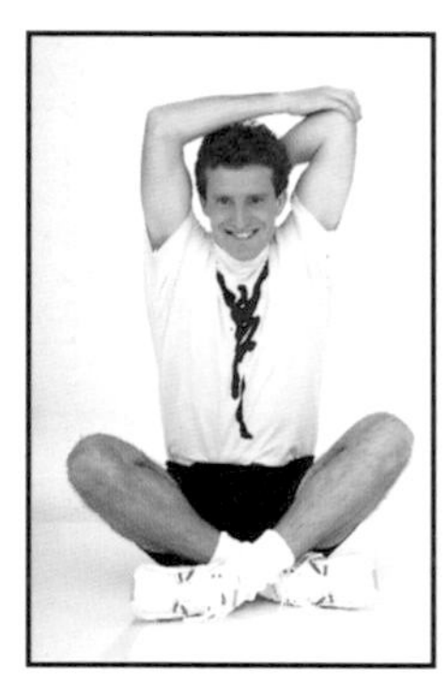

SEATED TRICEP STRETCH
8 counts each arm

EXERCISE 1

FORWARD HAMSTRING STRETCH

PURPOSE:
To stretch the hamstrings (back of the thigh)

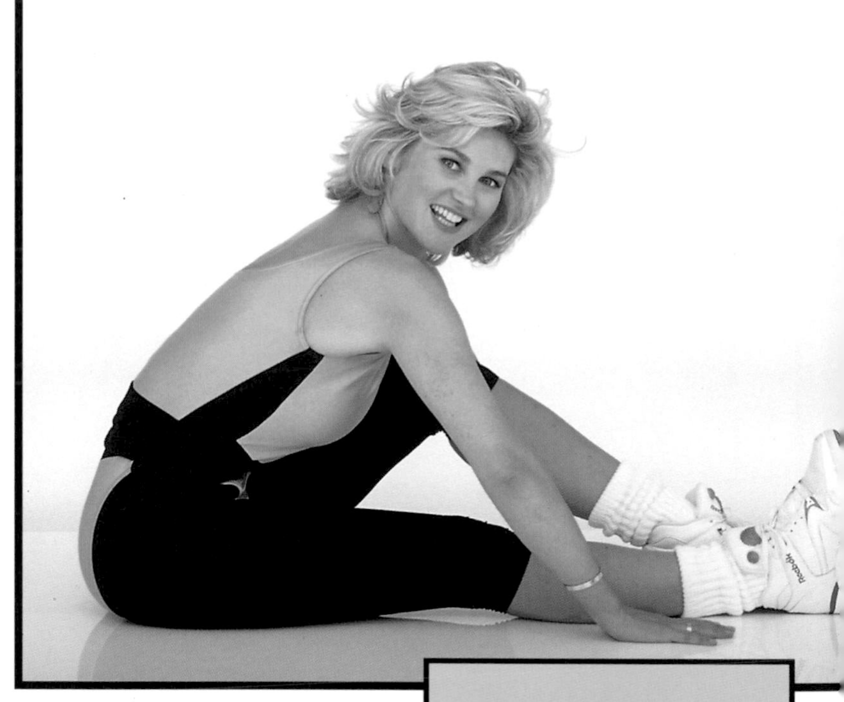

- Sitting with your legs slightly bent in front of you, lean forwards over your thighs and use your hands on the floor as a slight support.

- Keeping your trunk still, gently straighten one leg and flex your foot until you feel the stretch down the back of the thigh.

- Hold for a count of 16, trying to relax and develop the stretch. Repeat for the other leg.

Try to keep your back straight and bend from the hips

If you feel a pull in your lower back, do another hamstring stretch that is more comfortable for you.

EXERCISE 2

SEATED BUTTOCK STRETCH

PURPOSE:
To stretch the gluteals (buttocks)

- Leaning back on your hands for support, sit with your left leg bent, the foot flat on the floor, and the other leg bent with the ankle resting on the left knee.

- Using your arms to assist the movement, sit up so that your take your tummy and chest towards your thighs until you feel a stretch in the buttocks of the right leg.

- Hold for a count of 16, trying to develop the stretch, then repeat for the other leg.

You may find this exercise more comfortable if you do it lying on your back as opposed to sitting up

Keep your back straight and try to fold at the hips as much as possible

Keep your right knee pushed away

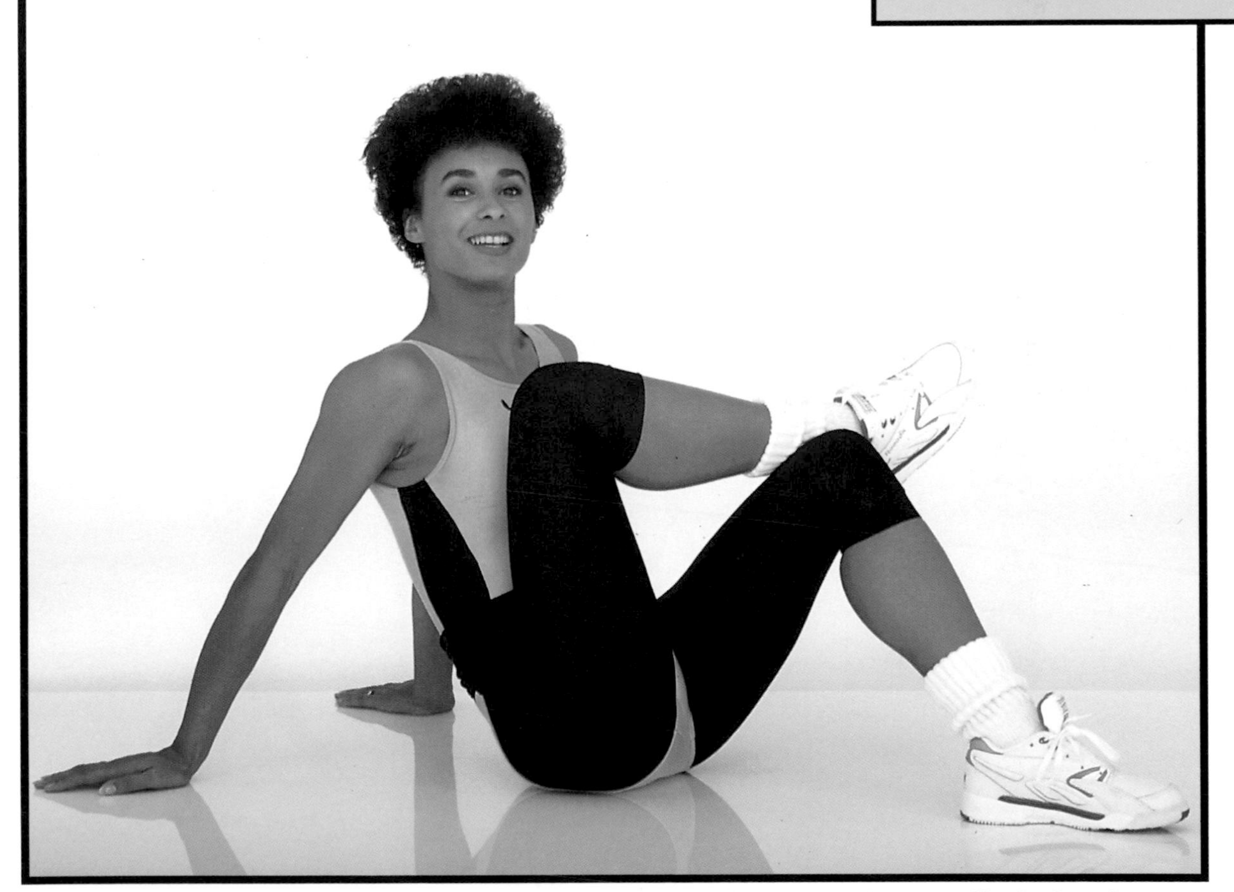

Well done. After two weeks on Level 3 you have finished the Countdown – now maintain your new-found figure with Supertone three times a week.

Now you have completed the 36-day Countdown you should move on to this Supertone block that combines the two different types of workout into one block. You should aim to do this at least three times a week, on alternate days to allow your muscles time between workouts

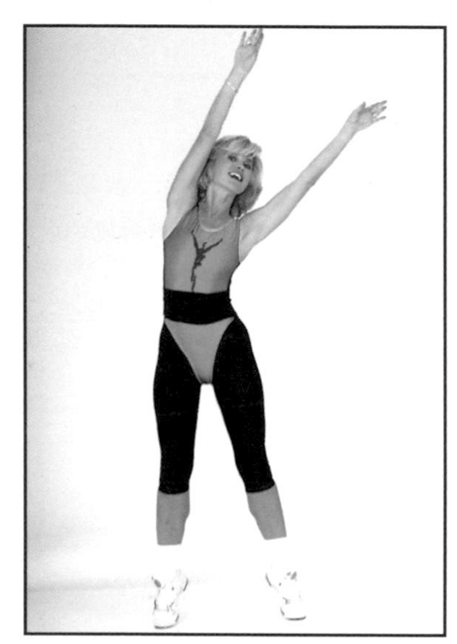

FULL CIRCLE SWINGS x 8

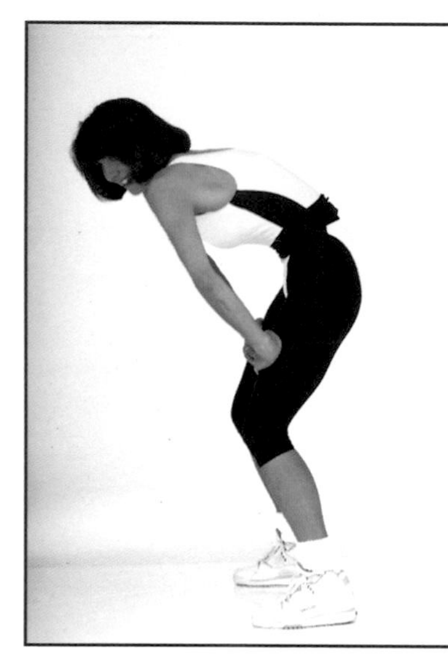

HOLLOW AND HUMP x 4

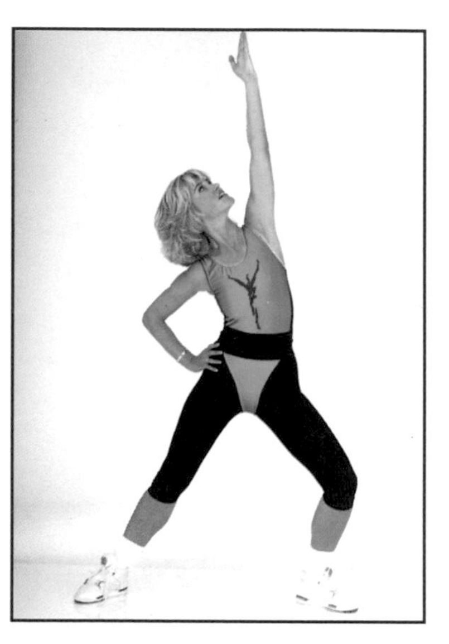

REACHES WITH KNEE BEND x 8

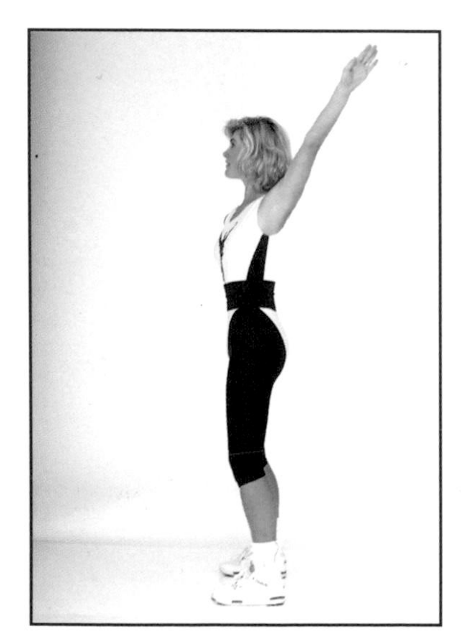

FORWARD ARM CIRCLES x 2 Right 2 Left

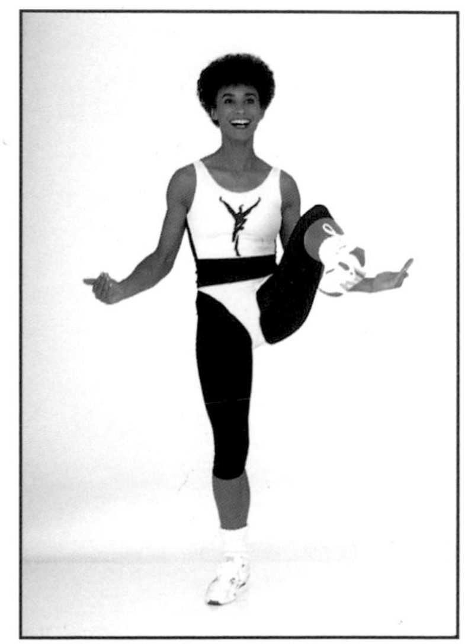

KNEE LIFTS WITH ARM PULL DOWNS x 8

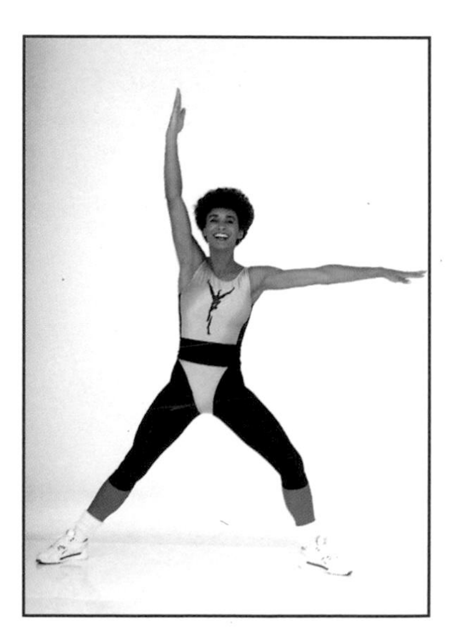

LUNGES WITH ARMS x 8

in which to recuperate. Most of the toning exercises have been taken from Level 3 and are therefore of the same intensity (there are some new ones for variety). This supertone programme is designed to maintain the muscle tone that you have developed through Countdown.

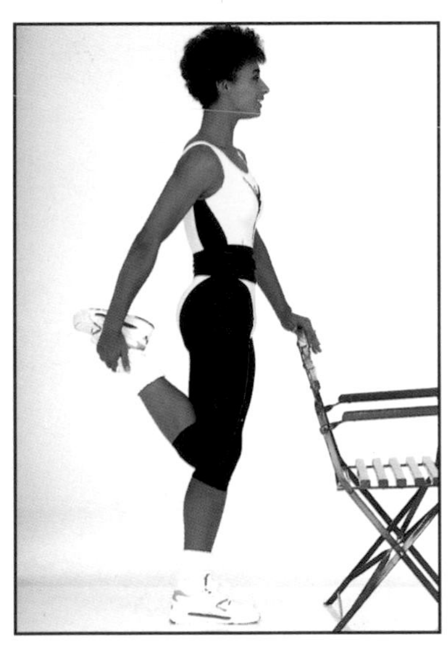

STANDING QUAD STRETCH
x 8 counts each leg

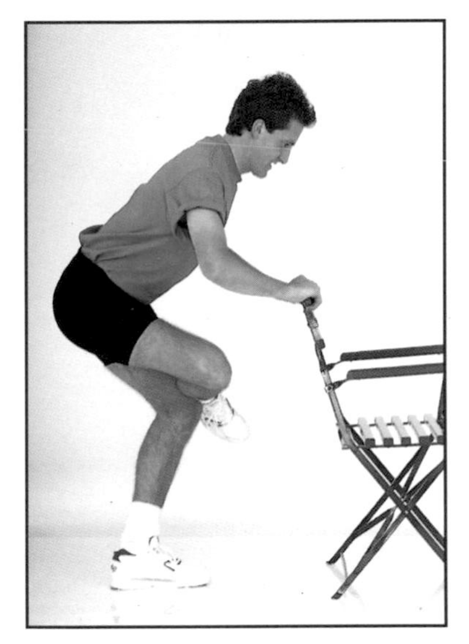

STANDING BUTTOCK STRETCH
x 8 counts each sice

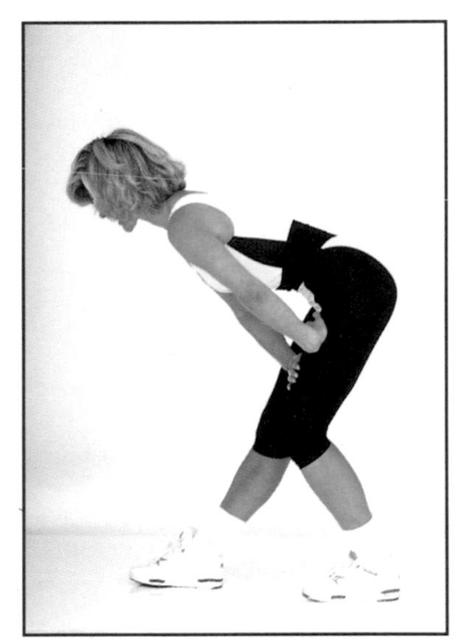

STANDING HAMSTRING STRETCH
x 8 counts for each leg

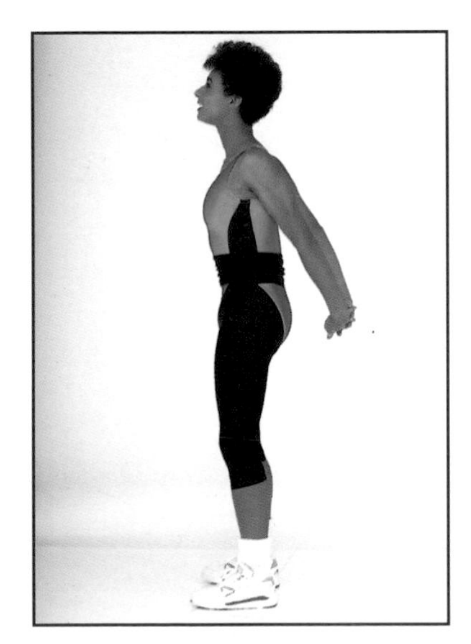

CHEST STRETCH
2 x 4 counts

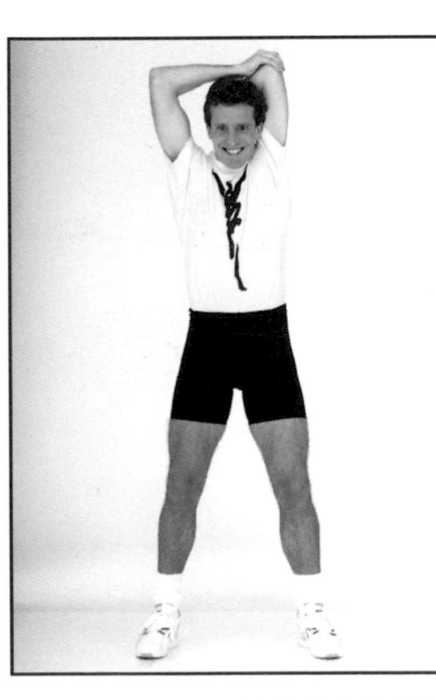

STANDING TRICEP STRETCH
2 x 4 counts each arm

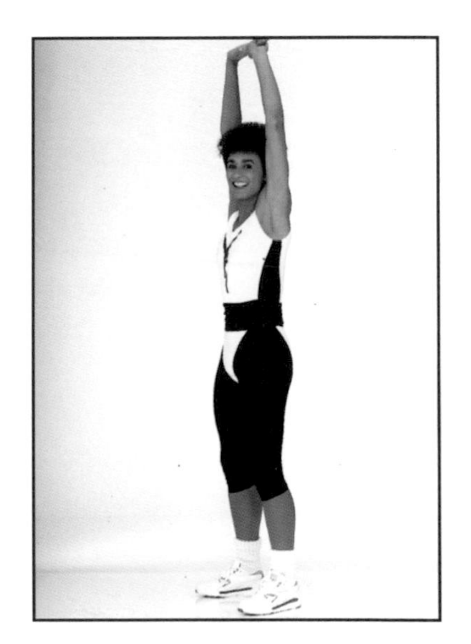

STANDING SHOULDER STRETCH 2 x 4 counts

EXERCISE 1

STANDING LEG RAISER COMBINATION

(EXERCISE A
+ EXERCISE B)

REPETITIONS
16 Right, 16 Left,
16 Left, 16 Right

A) ADVANCED FRONT LEG RAISES WITH BICEPS CURL

REPETITIONS
16 Right
PURPOSE:
To tone the quadriceps (front of the thigh) and biceps (front of the upper arm).

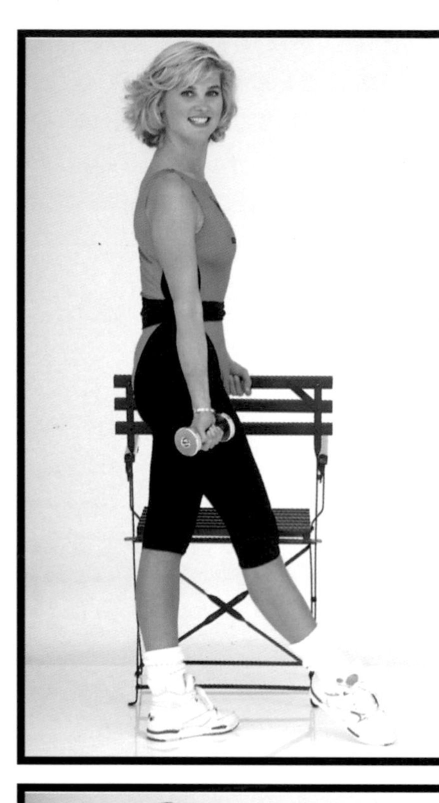

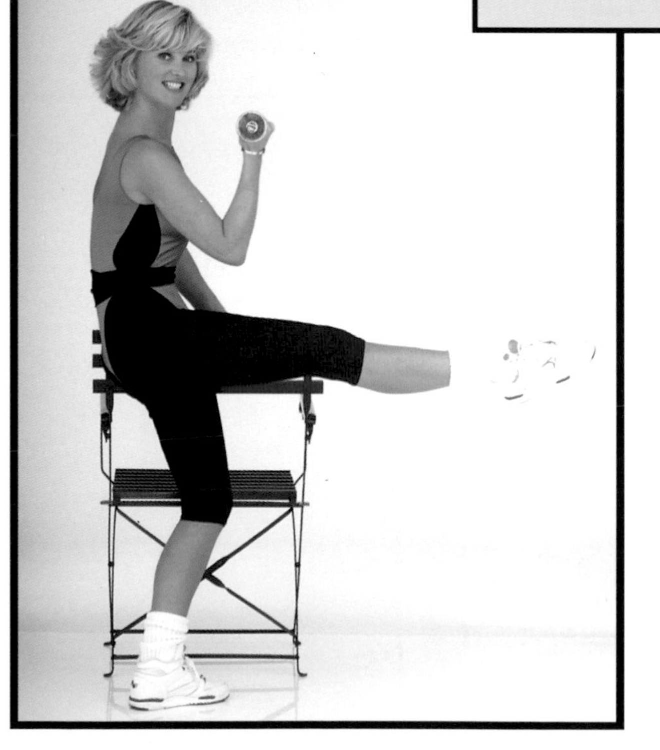

- Stand with your left side on to a chair and hold on for support. Follow the instructions for the front leg raises in Level 3a (see page 122) but this time hold an object that weighs about 0.5-1kg (1-2lb) in your right hand (the same side as the working leg) with your arm straight down by your side.

- As you move your legs, bend your arm, lifting the object up towards your right shoulder, then lower it again.

- Do this 16 times with the right leg and right arm, then move on to the next exercise (rear leg raises with lateral arm raises).

The abductors (hip muscles) of the supporting leg will work hard to stabilize the leg.

Feel your biceps working as well as your quadriceps

Keep your upper body still and keep firm centre control

B) REAR LEG RAISES WITH LATERAL ARM RAISES

REPETITIONS
16 Left
PURPOSE:
To tone the quadriceps (thigh), gluteals (buttocks), hamstrings (back of the thigh) and deltoids (shoulder muscles).

- Stand on your right leg and work the left leg behind you, as for the rear leg curls in Level 3A (see page 123). To work the shoulder muscles as well, hold an object that weighs 0.5-1kg (1-2lb) in your right hand.

- Lift and lower the right arm out to the sides to shoulder height as you bend and straighten the legs.

- Do this 16 times for the left leg and right arm.

The abductors (hip muscles) of the supporting leg will work hard to stabilize the hip.

Turn round, use the other hand for support and repeat Exercises A and B on the other side.

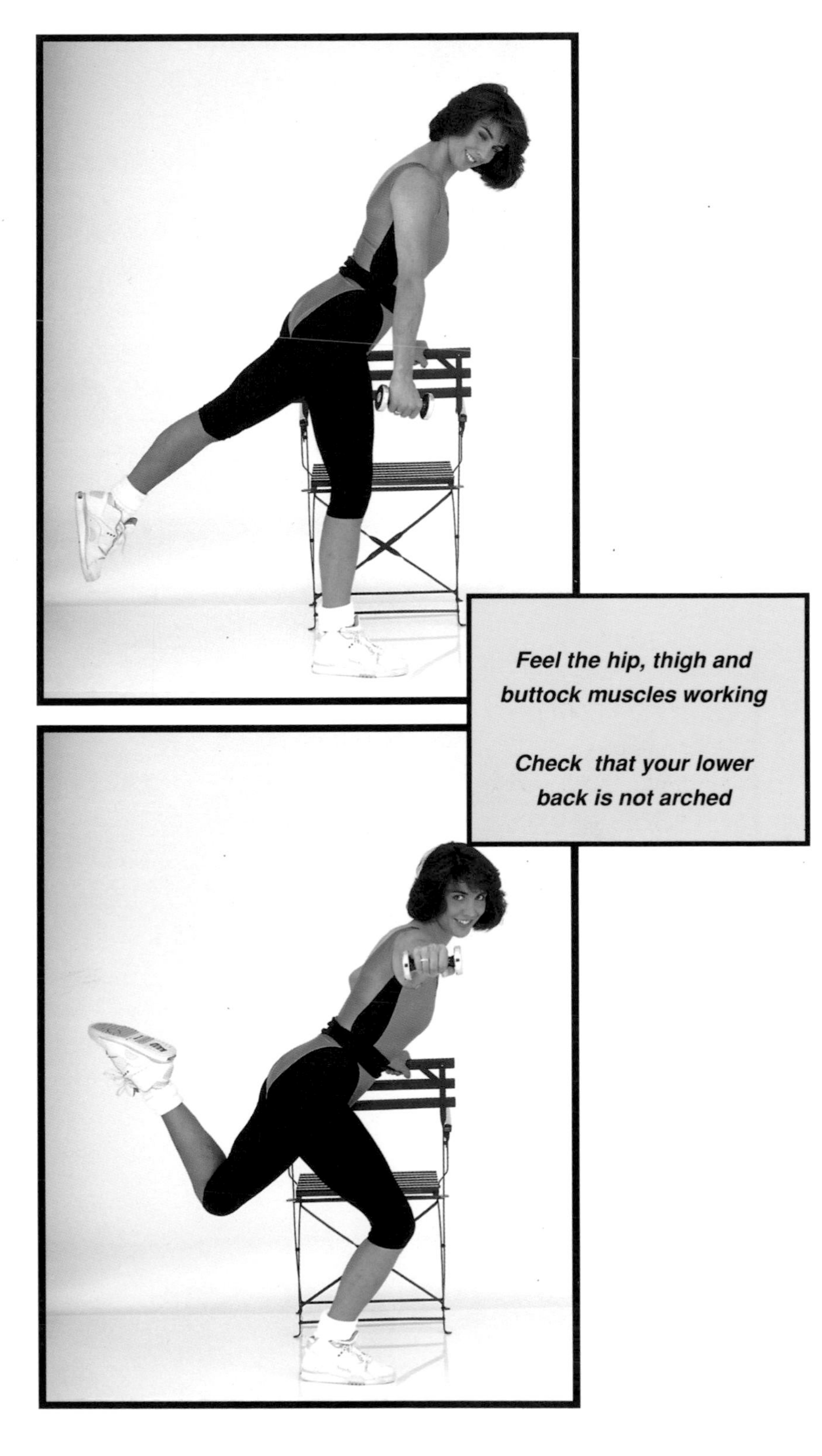

Feel the hip, thigh and buttock muscles working

Check that your lower back is not arched

EXERCISE 2

OUTER AND INNER THIGH COMBINATION

(EXERCISE C + EXERCISE D)

REPETITIONS
16 + 8 Right, 32 + 16 Left, 16 + 8 Left, 32 + 16 Right

C) LYING SIDE LEG RAISES

REPETITIONS *16 + 8 Right*
PURPOSE:
To tone the abductors (outer hip and thigh)

- Lie on your left side, resting your head in your hand, the bottom leg bent backwards for stability and the top leg straight out in line with your body, thighs parallel. Place your spare hand on the floor in front of you for balance.

- Making sure your hips and tummy face forwards and keeping the hips completely still, slowly raise and lower the top leg.

- Do this 16 times, rest for a count of 2 and then do 8 more for the same leg. Now move on to Exercise D.

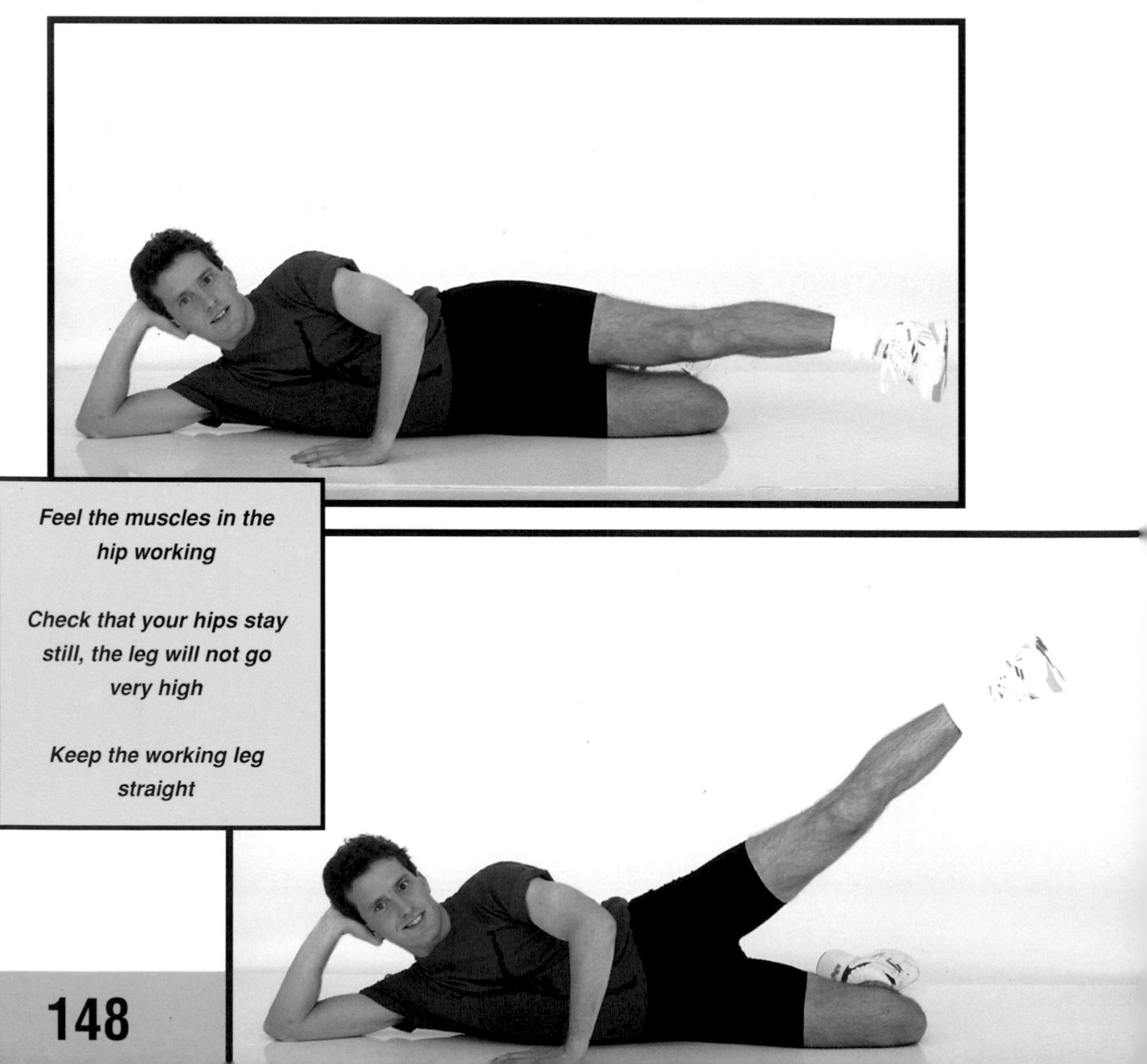

Feel the muscles in the hip working

Check that your hips stay still, the leg will not go very high

Keep the working leg straight

D)'LYING LOWER LEG RAISES

REPETITIONS
32 + 16 Left
PURPOSE:
To tone the adductors (inner thigh)

- Lie on your side resting your head in your hand as above.

Straighten the lower leg, bend the top leg, rest the knee on the floor and the ankle on top of the knee of the lower leg. Place your spare hand on the floor in front for balance.

- Keeping your hips facing forwards and the hips and trunk still, think of squeezing the inner thighs together as you raise and lower the bottom leg.

- Do this 32 times, rest for a couple of counts, then do 16 more.

Roll over and repeat Exercises C and D on the other side.

Feel the inner thigh muscles working

The ankle resting on the knee makes it harder work for the inner thigh muscles. Relax the rest of your body

Don't expect to lift your leg very high; the exercise only requires a small range of movement

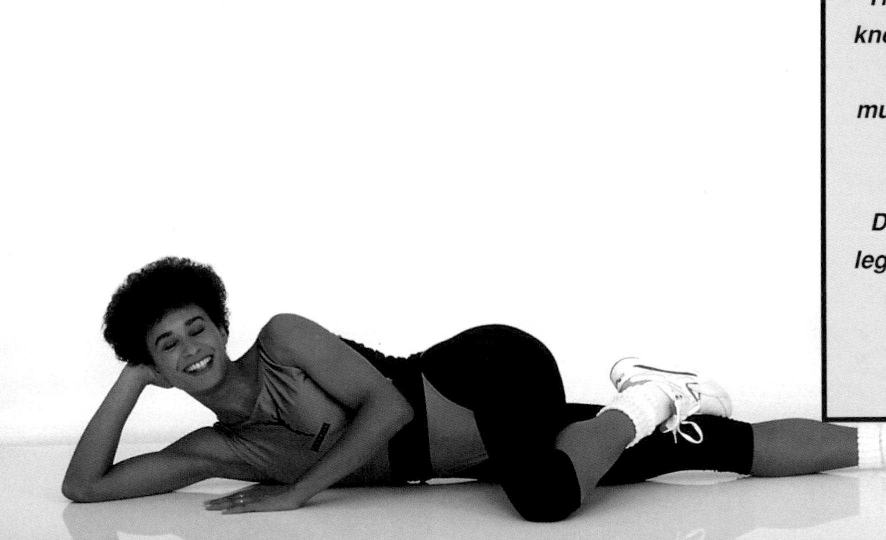

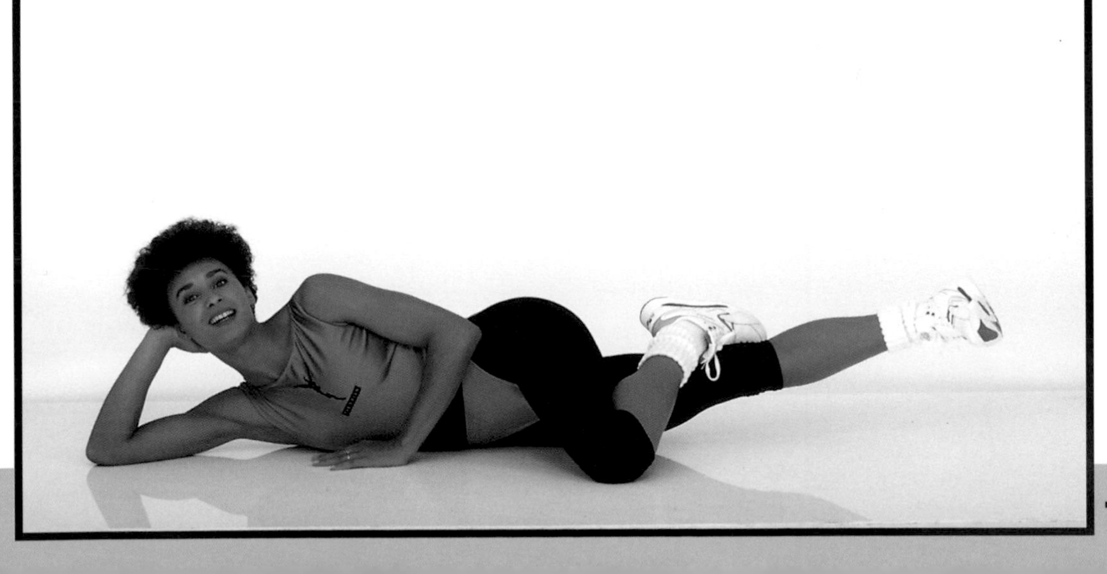

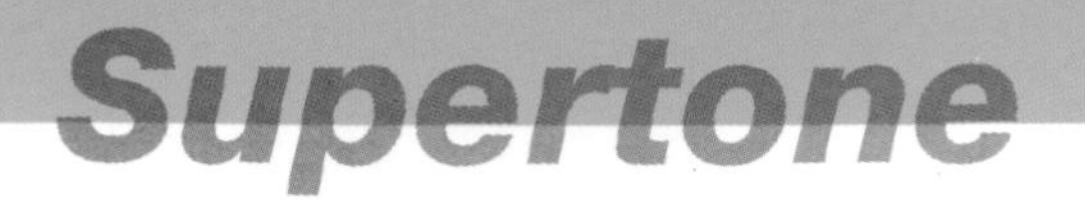

EXERCISE 3

PRESS-UP AND LEG CURL COMBINATION

(EXERCISE E AND EXERCISE F)
REPETITIONS
2 (12 + 12)

E) THREE-QUARTER PRESS-UPS

REPETITIONS *12*
PURPOSE:
To tone the triceps (back of the arms) and pectorals (chest)

- With your hands and knees on the floor, place your shoulders over your hands and your knees far enough back for your body to be in a straight line from knees to hips to shoulders.

- Bend your arms to lower the body, so that thighs, hips, chest and nose touch the floor simultaneously, then return to the start.

- Do this 12 times.

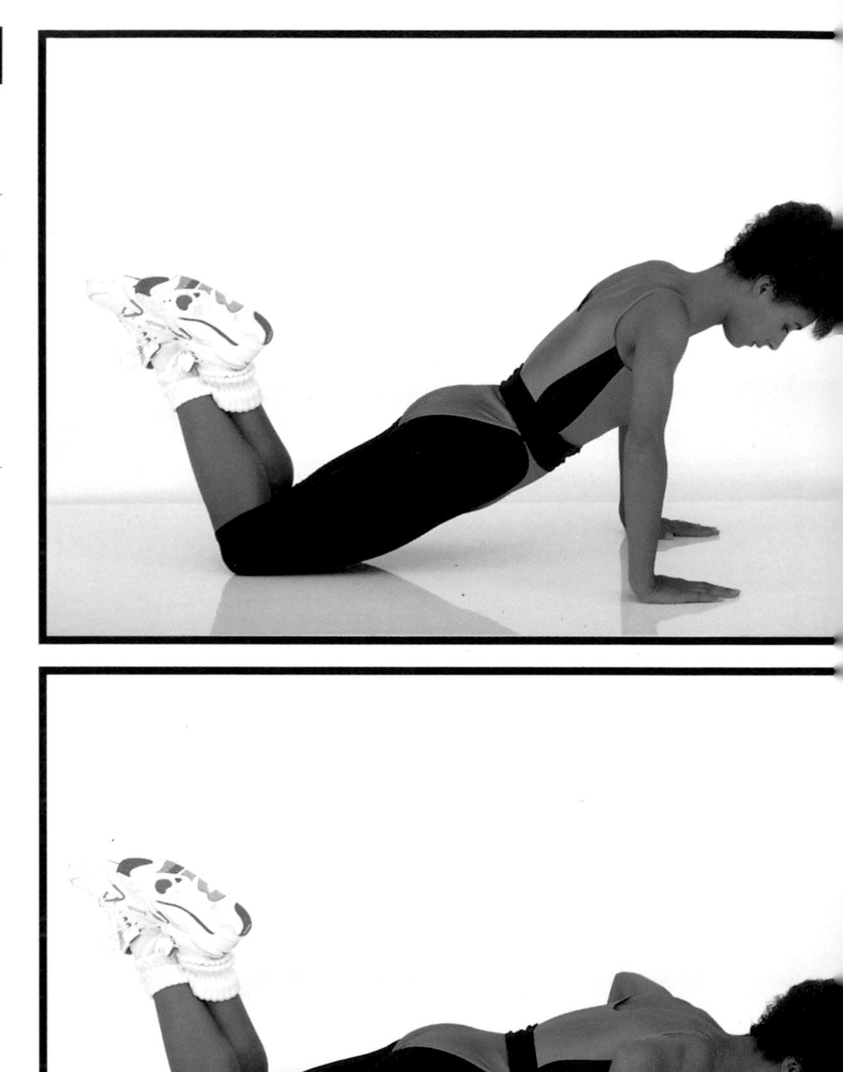

Feel the chest and upper arm muscles working

Tilt your pelvis and use your abdominals to prevent a dip in the lower back and keep your shoulders over your hands

Breathe out and remember, straighten your arms carefully as you push up each time

If this is too uncomfortable or too much of a strain, do 16 box press-ups (see page 84), rest, then repeat

F) DOUBLE LEG RAISES WITH CURL

REPETITIONS *12*
PURPOSE*:*
To tone the gluteals (buttocks)

- Lie flat on your front with your face resting on the floor and, for comfort, place your hands, palms up, under your thighs.

- Tighten your buttocks and raise both legs a little way off the floor. Keeping your knees off the floor, curl your heels into your buttocks, straighten your legs again and lower them to the floor, breathing out as you relax.

- Do this exercise 12 times.

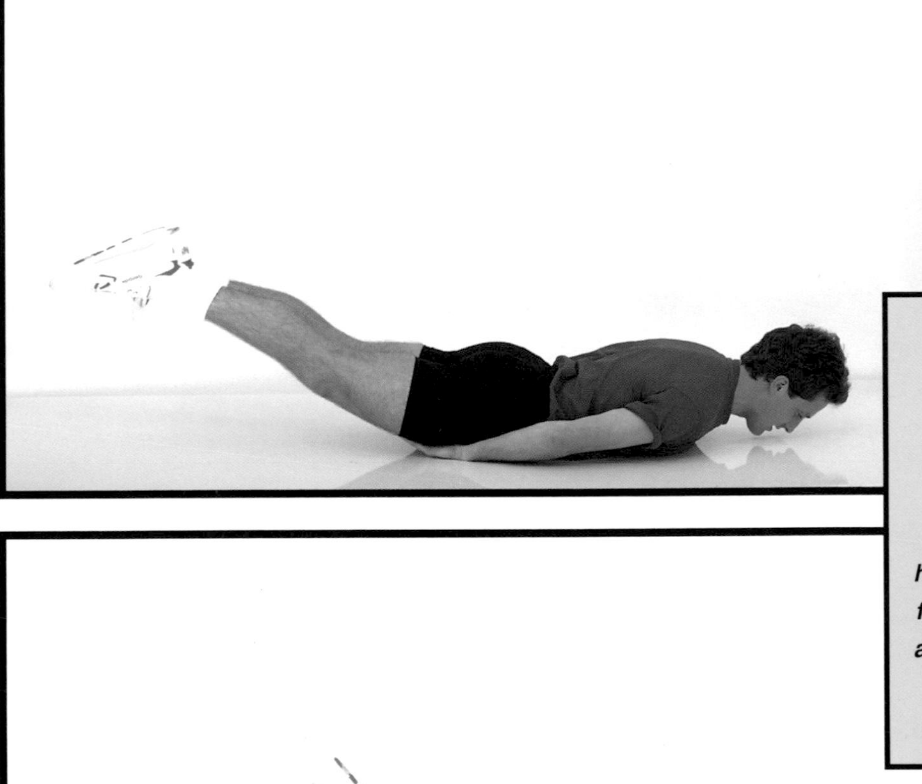

If your back feels uncomfortable or hurts in any way, find an alternative exercise (for the gluteals) on all fours that works one leg at a time.

Feel your buttocks working. Keep your face and chest resting on the floor

To make the exercise harder, hold your knees as far as you can off the floor as you really squeeze your heels in towards your buttocks

Repeat Exercises E and F again.

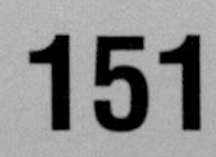

EXERCISE 4

DIPS

REPETITIONS *2 x 12*
PURPOSE:
To tone the triceps (back of the arms)

- Sit on the floor with your legs bent and your feet flat on the floor.

- Place your hands on the floor behind you with your fingers pointing in towards your bottom, then lift your hips off the floor and take the weight on your hands and feet.

- Keeping your trunk as still as possible, bend your arms as far as comfortable then straighten them again.

- Do this 12 times, rest and then repeat another 12 times.

Feel the muscles at the back of the arm working

Check that it is your shoulders that move up and down while you try to keep your hips as still as possible

Check that your hands are a comfortable distance apart

You may not be able to bend your arms very far without feeling quite a stretch across the front of your shoulders, but this is not a cause for concern as it is the suppleness of your shoulder joint that is limiting the range of movement

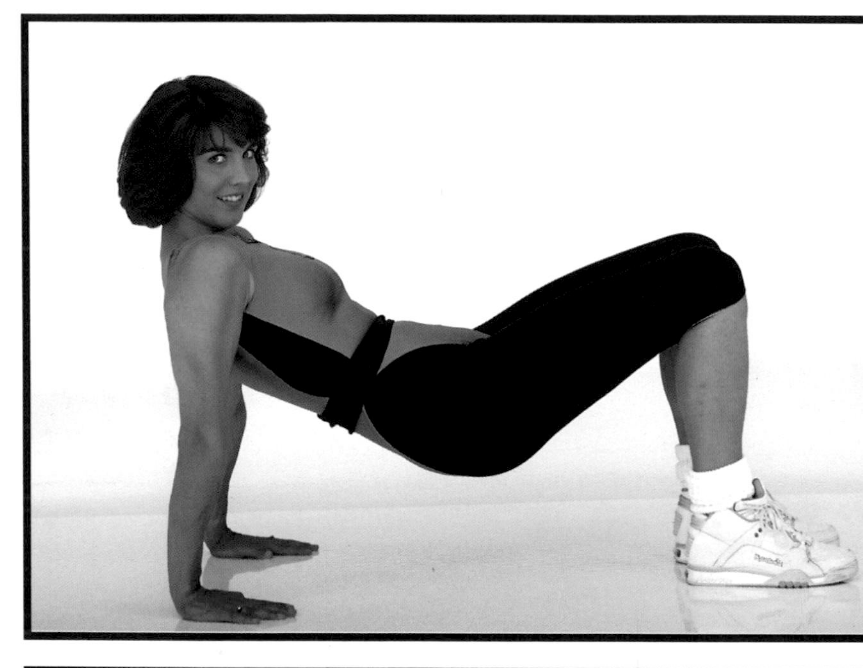

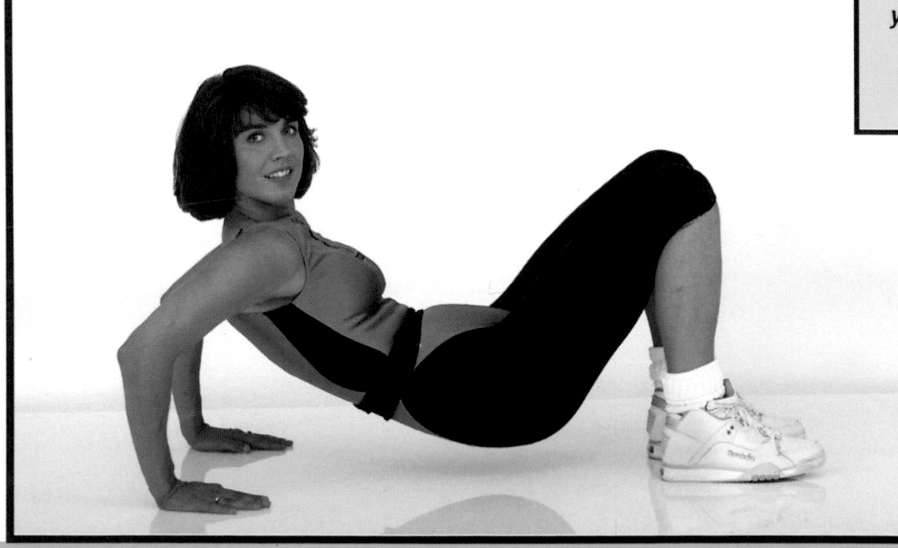

If you find this exercise too strenuous to perform correctly, keep your hips on the floor as for Seated Dips (page 115)

EXERCISE 5

CURL-UPS WITH KNEE IN

REPETITIONS
4 Right 4 Left
PURPOSE:
To tone the abdominals (tum)

- Lie on your back with one leg bent and the foot flat on the floor, the other leg extended off the floor so that the thigh is parallel with that of the bent leg. Tilt your pelvis to protect your back and rest your head on your fingertips with your elbows back.

- Holding your tummy in flat and curling your head and shoulders off the floor, bend the extended leg to bring the knee in to meet the face. Recover, ensuring that your lower back stays on the floor as the leg extends.

- Do this 4 times then change legs and repeat 4 more times.

Feel your abdominals working

Breathe out as you curl up and bring the knee in

As your muscles get tired, make the exercise easier by extending the leg higher than the bent knee

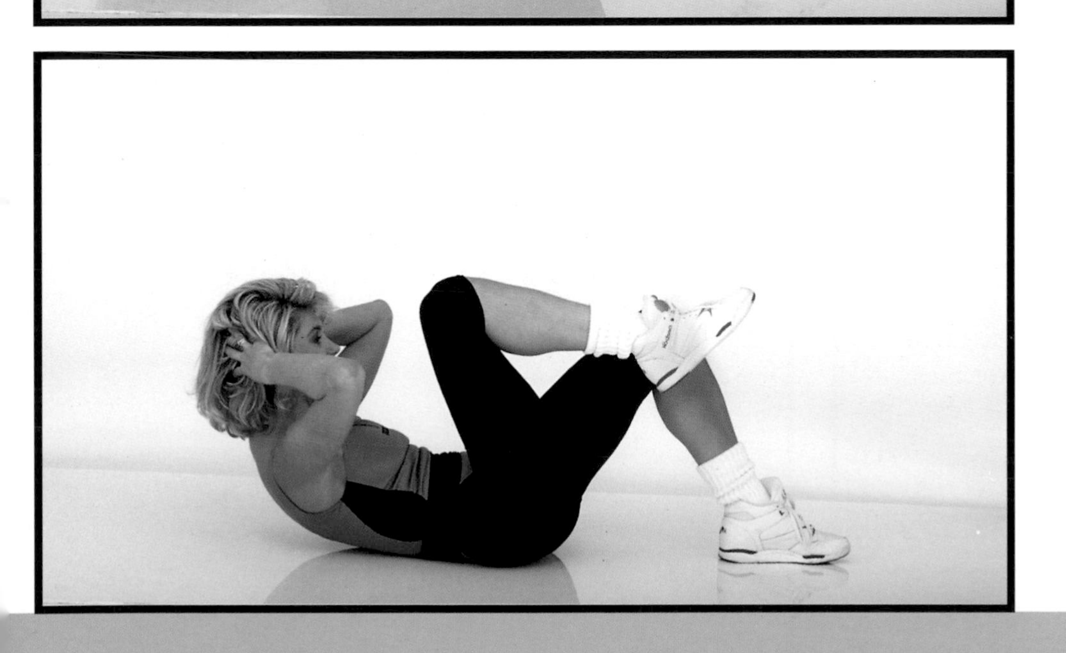

Exercise 6

CRUNCH COMBINATION

PURPOSE:
To tone the abdominals (tum)

- Lie on your back with your legs bent up over your chest and your head resting in your fingertips.

- Keeping your knees still and your tummy flat, curl your head and shoulders towards your knees, recover, then curl up with a twist taking your right elbow to your left knee, recover, repeat the first crunchie, then repeat the twisting crunchie this time twisting to the other side (left elbow to right knee).

- Repeat this combination until you have done it 4 times in total (see Level 3B on page 137).

Feel your abdominals working

Breathe out as you curl up. Check that you keep your knees over your tummy throughout

Check that you do not allow your abdominals to bunch up, especially as they get tired

Check that you don't pull on your head with your arms

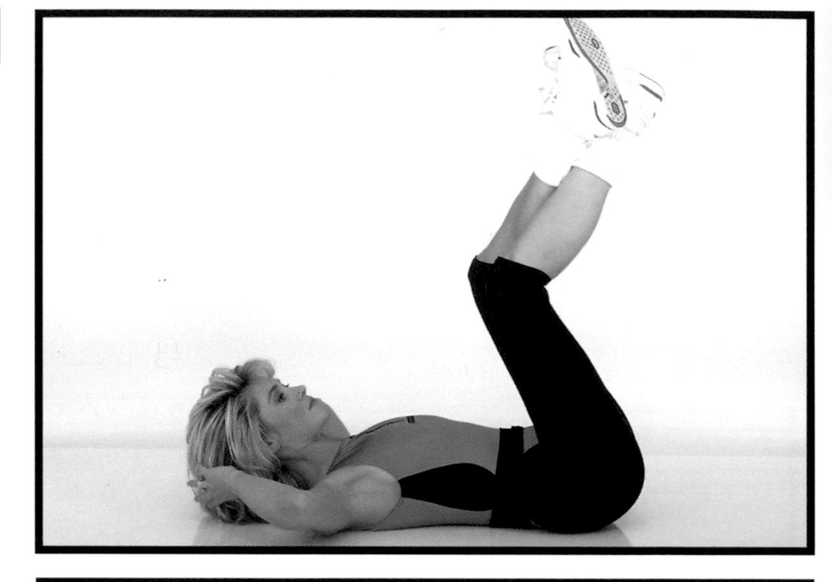

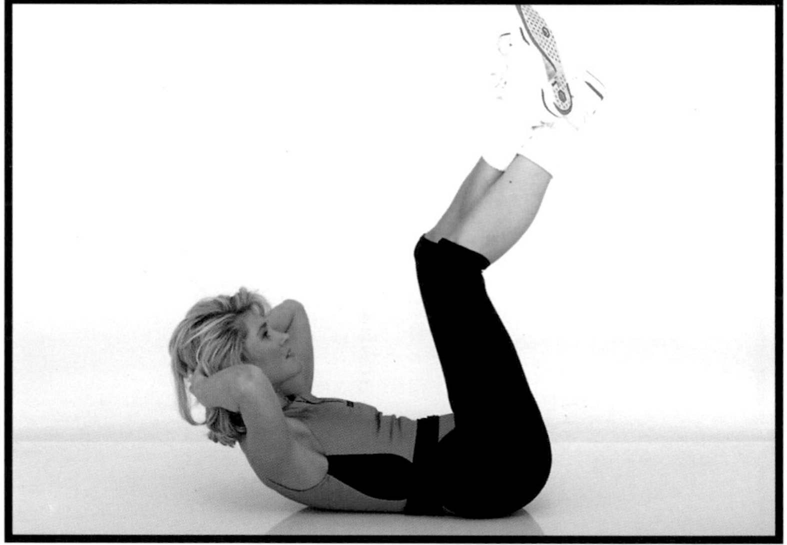

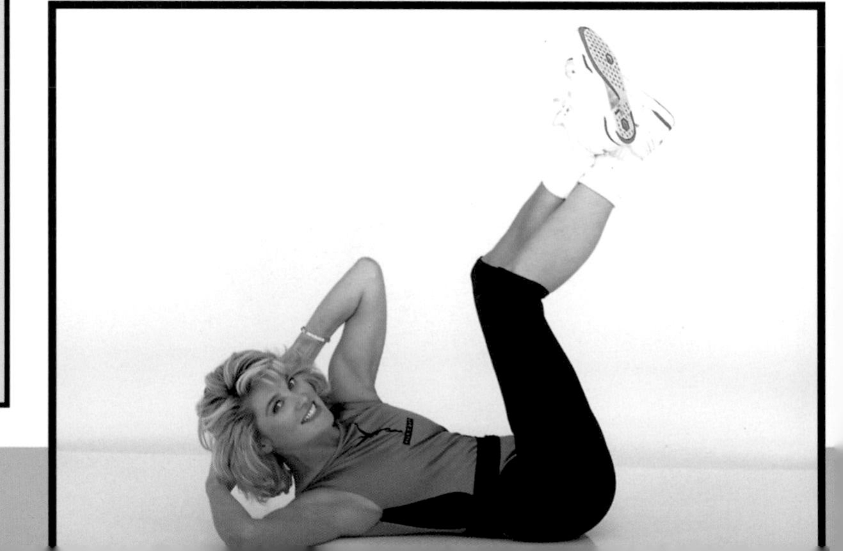

Exercise 7

REPEAT OF CURL-UPS WITH KNEE IN

REPETITIONS
4 Right 4 Left
PURPOSE:
To tone the abdominals (tum)

- Lie on your back with one leg bent and the foot flat on the floor, the other leg extended off the floor so that the thigh is parallel with that of the bent leg. Tilt your pelvis to protect your back and rest your head on your fingertips with your elbows back.

- Holding your tummy in flat and curling your head and shoulders off the floor, bend the extended leg to bring the knee in to meet the face. Recover, ensuring that your lower back stays on the floor as the leg extends.

- Do this 4 times then change legs and repeat 4 more times.

Feel your abdominals working

Breathe out as you curl up and bring the knee in

As your muscles get tired, make the exercise easier by extending the leg higher than the bent knee

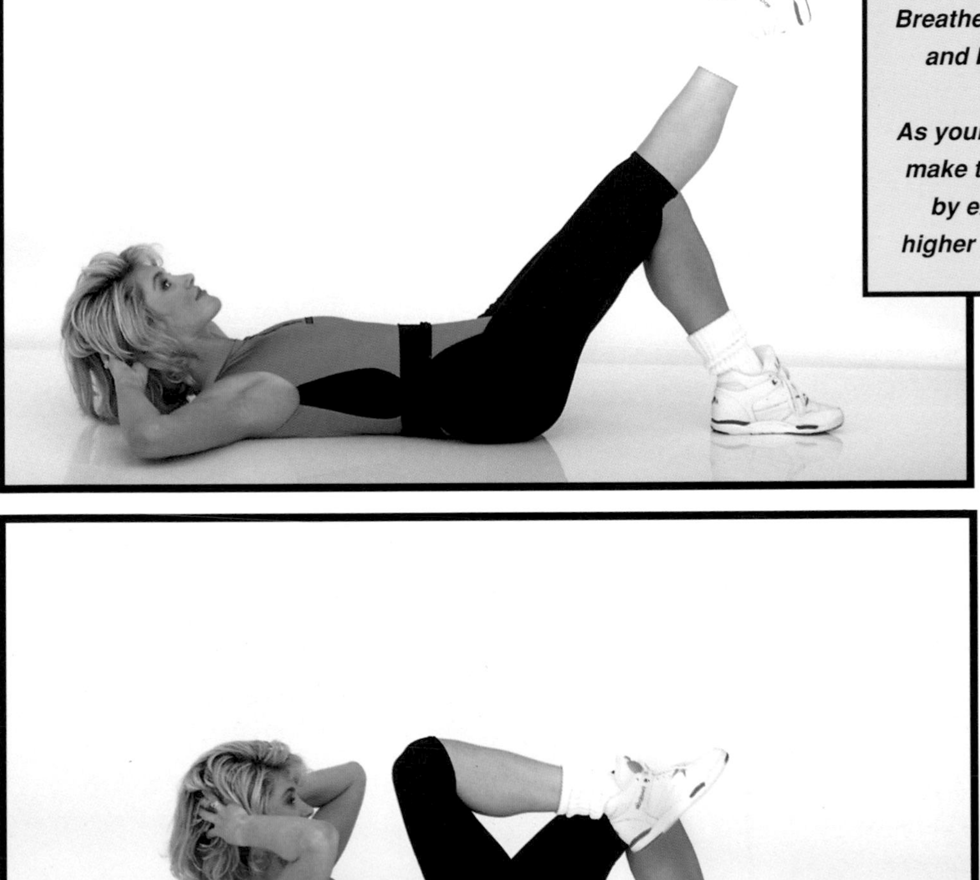

These cool-down stretches cover the major muscle groups worked in Supertone. The three levels of Countdown have covered a variety of stretches for these muscle groups. You could now compile your own set of cool-down stretches if you prefer. Just make sure that you incorporate stretches for all the necessary

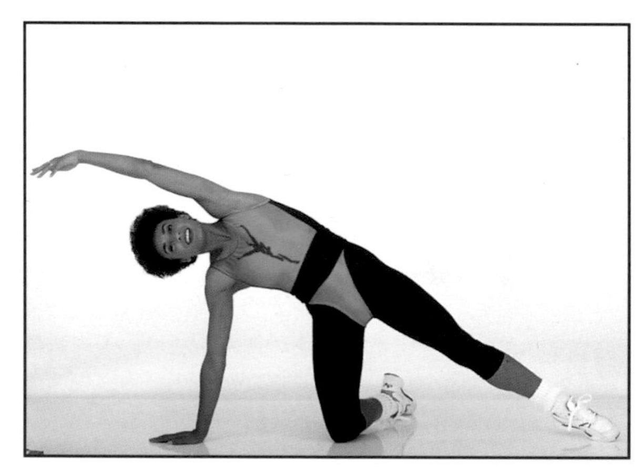

KNEELING SIDE STRETCH
8 counts each side

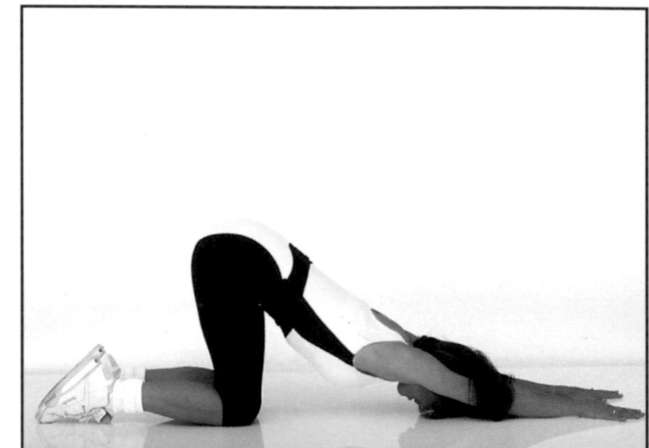

KNEELING SHOULDER STRETCH
8 counts

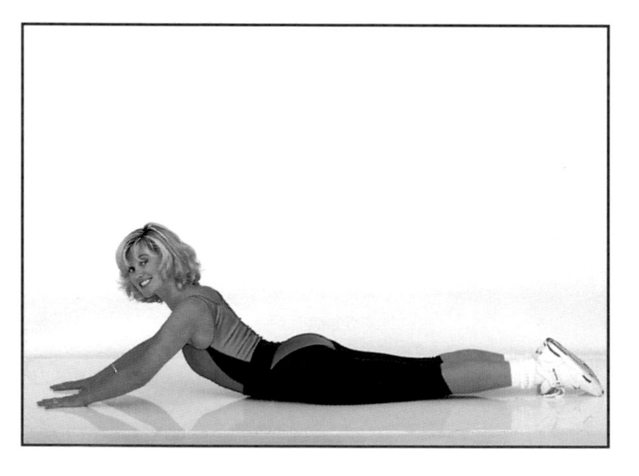

TUM STRETCH
2 x 4 counts

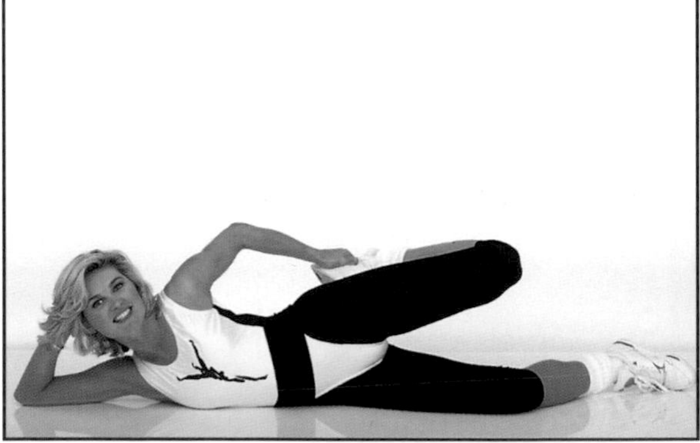

SIDE LYING QUADS STRETCH
16 counts each leg

muscle groups. Remember that stretching at this point in your exercise session is an excellent time to improve your suppleness. To do this you must be comfortable in each stretch and give time for the muscles to relax into the position. The longer you stretch the more you will achieve.

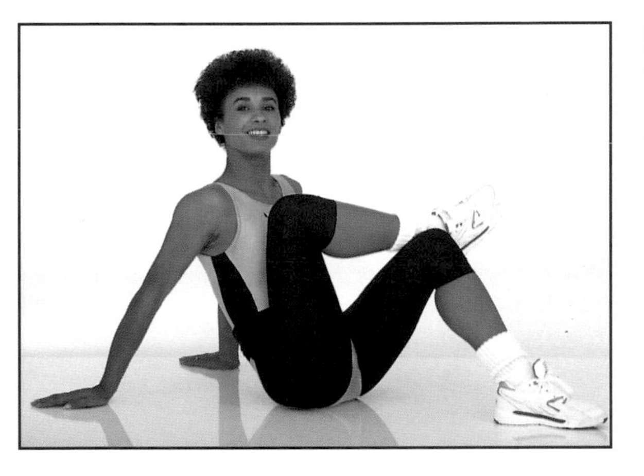

SEATED BUTTOCK STRETCH
16 counts each side

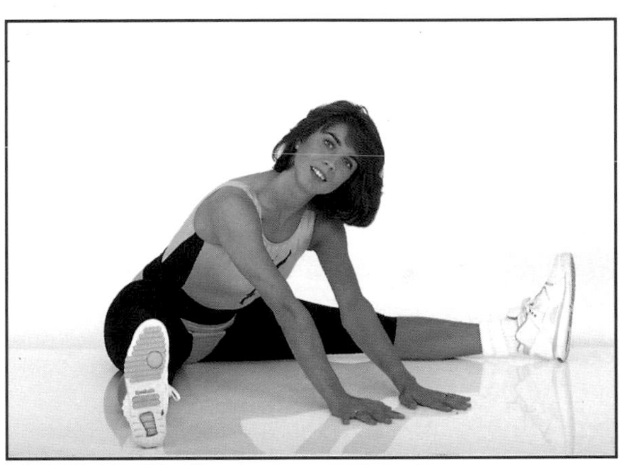

STRADDLE STRETCH
16 counts

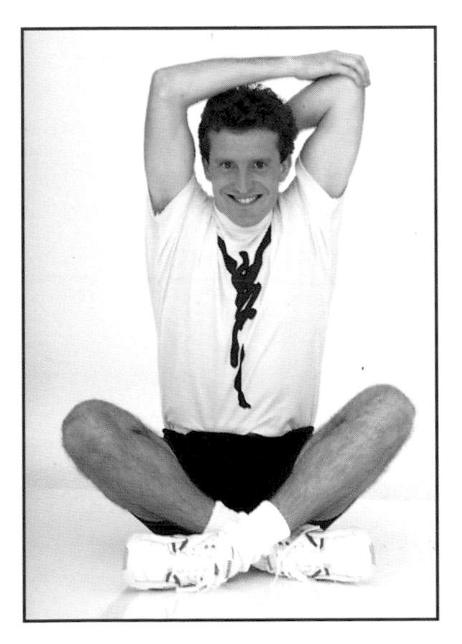

SEATED TRICEPS STRETCH
8 counts each arm

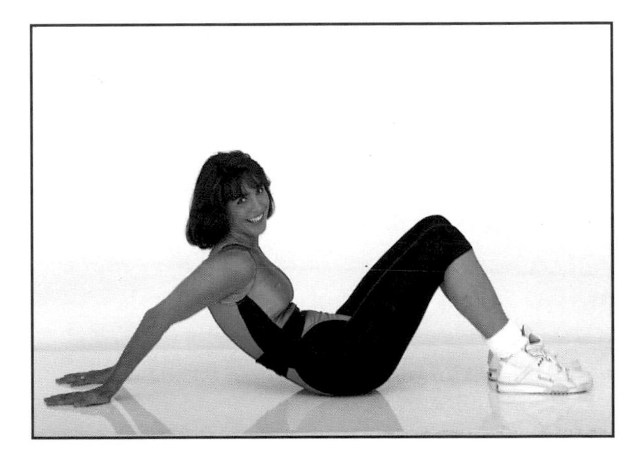

SEATED SHOULDER STRETCH
8 counts

Now you should feel on the way to keeping the firmer, flatter shape that you have developed through the 36-Day Countdown. Keep up the good work.

The Story of Countdown

Myths or Facts?

It is sometimes very difficult to dispel established myths that have grown up around a subject and exercise programmes are still bedevilled by inaccurate information. We, and many others, have been preaching commonsense, proven facts about exercise for 15 years and yet we still have students coming to us to train as fitness teachers who have been given false and out-of-date facts. Some of this information has been around for a while, passed down largely by word of mouth by generations of teachers and coaches. More recently it has been perpetuated in our culture because the media have chosen to promote ill-informed celebrity exercise programmes rather than those offered by expert teachers and exercise physiologists.

The myths associated with fitness programmes are very varied and cover the whole range of exercises. Some cause injury, while others put people off exercising because it sounds too difficult. Some people begin to exercise but soon stop because they are not seeing the results they are led by false claims to expect.

Let's explode those myths particularly relevant to our 36 Day Countdown programme.

Exercise Myths

Myth *Exercise is only doing you good if it hurts.*

Fact Exercise should never be painful. Pain is a sign from the body that you are overdoing it or performing the exercise incorrectly. If any exercise is painful, stop at once, otherwise you may injure a muscle or a joint.

Myth *When doing toning exercises you must 'go for the burn'.*

Fact If the muscle starts to give a burning sensation it is rapidly fatiguing and this is a sign to ease off or stop. Continuing to exercise could result in injury or prevent further exercise for several days.

Myth *If you stop exercising muscle turns to fat.*

Fact A muscle will go flaccid or flabby and waste (atrophy) from a lack of exercise but it cannot turn to fat.

Myth *Weight training and toning exercises make women develop big muscles.*

Fact It is much harder for women to develop big muscles because they possess much less of the muscle building androgen hormone.

Myth *You need to eat lots of protein to build and tone muscles.*

Fact The body needs only a small daily amount of protein for cell production and body maintenance – between 12 and 15 percent of a total day's calories. To keep the body fit and active the muscle needs a food store called glycogen for energy. Glycogen is broken down (or digested) carbohydrate. Carbohydrate should constitute 45 to 55 percent of daily calorie intake.

Myth *A woman shouldn't do press ups.*

Fact If a woman has adequate upper body strength there is no physical reason why she should not do full press ups, provided she does them correctly.

Myth *Exercise makes you gain weight.*

Fact When you exercise you increase muscle mass and muscle weighs more than fat. If you exercise and do not increase your food intake you will gain a little weight but lose fat and inches.

Myth *You can exercise away your cellulite.*

Fact Fat is fat! The journal of the American Medical Association reported: 'There is no medical condition known as cellulite. Cellulite is just plain fat that has accumulated under the surface of the skin.' Special treatments such as massage, creams and rubber pants do not break down fat or cellulite!

Myth *In order to gain any benefits from exercise you have to exercise for long hours every week.*

Fact A little exercise every other day is better than no exercise at all. The fitness required for everyday living is very different to that needed by an athlete or sportsman. Everything you do is relative – the more you put into something, the more you get out of it!

Myth *The more you exercise the better.*

Fact Too much exercise can be harmful. The body needs at least one rest day a week and if the programme is too difficult for people to cope with injuries will occur. People have been known to become addicted and, once addicted, they lose the ability to listen to the body when it is telling them to rest.

Myth *It is dangerous to exercise if you are overweight.*

Fact Exercise is very important for overweight people because it assists weight loss, but the principles of fitness must be carefully followed when embarking on an exercise programme. The programme should begin at a low level and progress gradually.

Myth *If you eat a Mars Bar before exercise it will give you energy straight away.*

Fact A Mars Bar is full of energy but this needs to be broken down and the glycogen stored in your muscles before it can be used as fuel in exercise. This takes several hours.

Myth *In order to get rid of the fat around the stomach you need to do tummy exercises (sit ups) every other day.*

Fact Sit ups every other day will firm up the tummy muscles but will not get rid of excess fat. The body needs regular aerobic exercise and a reduction in food intake to burn up fat. Fat is stored underneath the skin all over the body and excess fat is burnt off from all fat stores gradually. You cannot get a slim tummy by toning exercises alone if you have large amount of excessive fat.

Myth *Women are not as fit as men.*

Fact Women have slightly lower fitness levels than men but this is predominantly to do with cultural rather than biological reasons. Females, because of less muscle bulk than males, are not as strong as men, but in all other areas of fitness they compare favourably and in flexibility they tend to be better.

Myth *You should not exercise during menstruation.*

Fact There is no physical reason why you should not exercise – in fact it may relieve period pains and backache.

Myth *When you exercise vigorously you need to drink lots of water.*

Fact During prolonged exercise you sweat, lose fluids and get a bit dehydrated. It is wise to drink little and often.

The Followers of the Countdown

The Countdown exercise programme is a culmination of 20 years' experience in practical teaching, of which the last 13 years have been specifically related to developing and perfecting exercise 80 programmes to improve all-round physical fitness. During this period we taught num -erous exercise classes, both at London Central

YMCA and around the country. This has given us constant contact with, and feedback from, our class participants, who came in all shapes and sizes, ages and fitness levels and in both sexes. It is this vital practical experience that allowed us to put together the Y Plan exercise series.

As preparation for Y Plan 1 the YMCA Training and Development department set up a mini research project. We devised a draft programme and produced a home video for a group of mixed individuals to follow and periodically tested them to observe improvements. We also had a control group who did not exercise at all to make comparisons. This project helped us enormously with determining the level and sequence of exercise and gave us the indication that the programme was on the right lines.

The feedback from the original Y Plan was invaluable when we came to devise the Countdown. We believe the Y Plan series can only get better as long as we stay close to those for whom it is designed. Therefore, in the Countdown video we included a questionnaire as part of the booklet with the aim of getting much more specific feedback from those who had tried the Countdown exercises.

We feel that these individual comments will be valuable to us when we are designing future programmes and are of interest to you, just starting out on the Y Plan road to exercise and health. Remember that the more help we can get from our followers the better programmes you will receive in the future.

In the opening chapter we identified some key points that our followers had liked about the Countdown. The following examples, which are just two of the many success stories we have received, should motivate you to want to take up and maintain exercise.

The following is an extract from a letter from Karen Steed:

As a 29-year-old who was extremely unfit, I have found it both enjoyable and possible! I am in the process of losing weight at a Slimming Club. I've lost 2½ stone so far, but this tape has really helped to tone my muscles and trim my shape, giving me confidence and encouragement. I found the tape to be easy to understand, with your presentation straightforward, no nonsense and informative.

The following is an extract from a letter from Mrs A. Van De Varle:

Many thanks for making such an enjoyable video. At first I thought I was never going to make it, but after a few weeks I really began to enjoy getting up on a morning and beginning my day with my workout.

The centimetres have really fallen off and both my husband and myself are more than pleased with the result. Especially me going down two sizes means a whole new wardrobe.

If you wish to do more exercise in a safe and social environment, seek out your local trained and qualified teacher. There are many trained specialists in the field of exercise and teaching but it is important that they have recently trained in up-to-date exercise physiology and teaching methods and are practising teachers.

The minimum requirement for teaching exercise such as the Countdown is the YMCA or RSA Basic Certificate in the teaching of Exercise to Music.

Best of luck and happy exercising !